Advances in
Myocardiology
Volume 5

Advances in Myocardiology
Series Editors: N. S. Dhalla and G. Rona

A Continuation Order Plan is available for this series. A continuation order will bring delivery of each new volume immediately upon publication. Volumes are billed only upon actual shipment. For further information please contact the publisher. Volumes 1 and 2 of this series were published by University Park Press, Baltimore.

Advances in Myocardiology
Volume 5

Edited by

Peter Harris
and
Philip A. Poole-Wilson

Cardiothoracic Institute
University of London
London, England

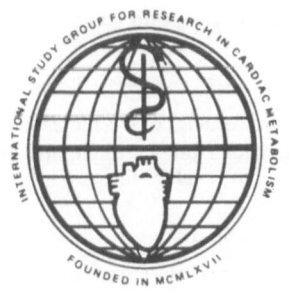

Springer Science+Business Media, LLC

ISBN 978-1-4757-1289-6   ISBN 978-1-4757-1287-2 (eBook)
DOI 10.1007/978-1-4757-1287-2

Library of Congress card number 80-643989

Derived from the proceedings of the Eleventh Congress of the
International Society for Heart Research, held July 11-14, 1983,
in London, England

© Springer Science+Business Media New York

Originally published by Plenum US in 1985.

Softcover reprint of the hardcover 1st edition 1985

Preface

The Eleventh World Congress of the International Society for Heart Research 1983 provided an opportunity to review some of the growing points in our knowledge of the structure and function of the myocardium. Those at the meeting will recall how London suddenly went tropical. Yet a series of scintillating reviews held over six hundred scientists captive in the lecture halls of Imperial College. There were sessions on nuclear magnetic resonance, the molecular basis of electrophysiology, calmodulin, protein synthesis and degradation, oxygen free radicals, the structural components of the myocyte, sarcolemmal sodium exchange, and the influence of lipids on membranes.

Here we have gathered together, as quickly as possible, a number of the presentations of the speakers invited to the symposia. They give, we believe, a striking picture of the diversity of technology and scientific enquiry which underlies this immensely active domain of modern cardiology. If only our clinical colleagues were more aware of it!

Peter Harris
Philip A. Poole-Wilson

London

Contents

STRUCTURAL COMPONENTS OF THE MYOCYTE AND ITS MATRIX

SARCOLEMMAL SODIUM EXCHANGE

INFLUENCE OF LIPIDS ON MEMBRANES

Evolution, Cardiac Failure, and Water Metabolism
Presidential Address

Peter Harris

Cardiothoracic Institute
London W1N 2DX, England

Abstract. In this essay, I take the liberty of doubting the widely held view that congestive cardiac failure is due to an inability of the heart to provide enough oxygen for the needs of the body. Instead, the syndrome is best explained by an inappropriate and prolonged stimulation of the neurohumoral defense reaction that developed during evolution to support exercise and preserve life.

DIFFUSION AND CONVECTION

Theology and science alike are agreed that life had its origins in the sea. In these primeval waters, the first cells floated freely. Special devices were developed to transport molecules across the cell wall, but the movement of substances toward and away from these was by diffusion, aided by the random currents of the outside world. As multicellular organisms developed and increased in size, they needed to impose their own convective streams on the surrounding water in order to ensure an exchange of materials that could no longer be achieved by simple diffusion

Many simple organisms, such as the sponges and coelenterates, use the water in which they live as the sole means of convective transport. This system serves the combined functions of respiration, ingestion, and excretion. In more complex organisms, the transport distances within the body became too great to be maintained without the development of a mechanically propelled internal convective system. In the fishes, the function of the external convective system is still mixed. In addition to being used for the exchange of respiratory gases, it is used for the excretion of ammonia, the chief end-product of nitrogenous metabolism, and, to a variable degree, for ingestion.

The motility of the body as a whole is also a mechanism of external convection. This is so even in a unicellular organism such as paramecium. Does it just stir the water, or is it swimming? And what is the purpose of locomotion except to renew the environment? Many fishes have to swim in order to ventilate the gills. Predators rely on movement to capture food.

1

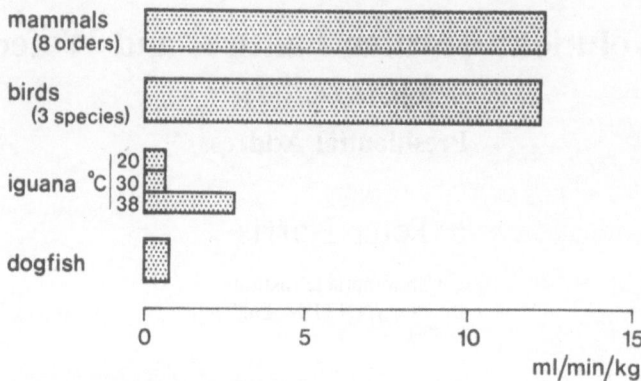

Figure 1.   Basal oxygen uptake of mammals and birds compared with that of the iguana and the dogfish. Data from Altman and Dittmer [1].

And we all walk away from our own excrement. In this way, locomotion takes its place as a form of external convection.

This essay considers three great convective systems of the body: the flow of air, the flow of blood, and the flow of urine. They do not work in isolation, and when the heart is diseased, both the lungs and the kidneys suffer. The combined system is under greatest strain when locomotion, the fourth convector, comes into operation. We shall see how the demands of physical exercise have necessitated the development of a specific neuro-hormonal response and how the inappropriate and prolonged evocation of this response leads to the clinical syndrome of cardiac failure.

EVOLUTION OF THE LUNGS

Life began without oxygen, and the primitive pathways for the anaerobic production of high-energy phosphate groups persist to this day in every cell of our body. The bath of oxygen in which we now find ourselves is the result of the activity of photosynthetic organisms. With the arrival of oxygen, opportunistic forms of life took advantage of the greater efficiency with which biologically useful energy could be derived from the combustion of hydrogen, and this process has been a dominating evolutionary force. It is probable that the mitochondria invaded the primitive eukaryotic cell as parasitic microorganisms in past eons and have stayed there ever since.

A survey of the oxygen consumption of the vertebrates leads us to the first of a group of "evolutionary jumps" that coincide with the development of warm blood (Figure 1). The oxygen consumption of mammals and birds is many times that of the cold-blooded vertebrates and is not due simply to the higher temperatures of the body (Figure 1). It was accompanied by an equally striking jump in the cardiac output (Figure 2).

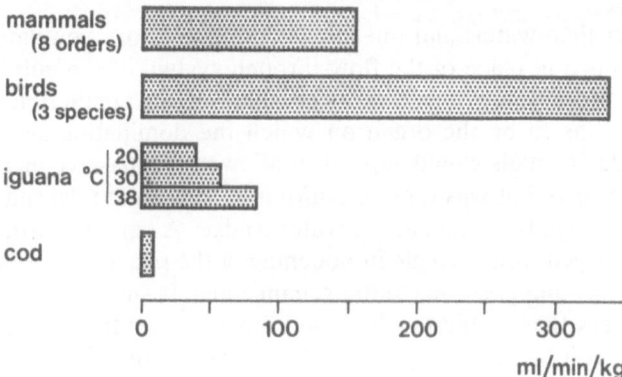

Figure 2. Basal cardiac output of mammals and birds compared with that of the iguana and the cod. Data from Altman and Dittmer [1].

At the same time, radical changes were occurring in the design of the cardiovascular and ventilatory systems. In the fish, a single ventricle pumps blood first to the gills and subsequently to a second capillary network in the body. The mammals and birds developed a two-pump system, one pump being responsible for respiratory exchange with the outside world, the other for supplying the tissues of the body. The amphibian heart is a halfway step between the two.

With the emergence of life onto the land and into the air, the ventilatory system became converted from water to air. The use of air carried two bonuses. Oxygen is poorly soluble in water, so that air allowed an impressive reduction in the volume of ventilation (Figure 3). At the same time, air is

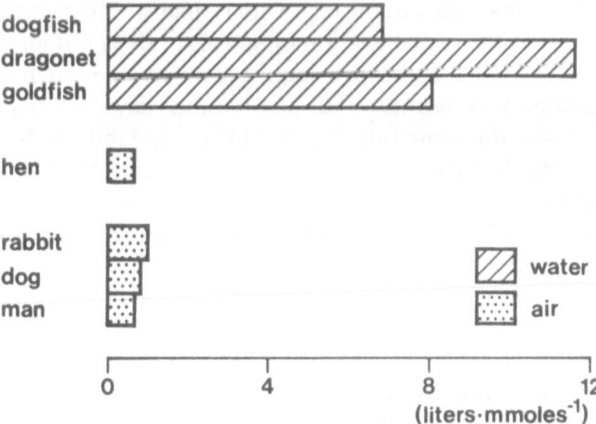

Figure 3. Ratio of ventilation to oxygen uptake in various fishes, in the hen, and in mammals. Data from Dejours [4].

much lighter than water, and this allowed an oscillatory ventilatory system to be developed in place of the flow-through system of the gills.

The two redesigned systems of circulation and ventilation met in the lungs. This was to be the organ on which the dominating success of the warm-blooded animals would depend. It allowed the massive increase in the uptake of oxygen that was required during exercise and released the organism from the need to remain at the water's edge. A complex arborization of air tubes emerged from a single in-pouching of the pharyngeal ectoderm and ended in a vast and gossamer-thin exchange membrane. The alveolar membrane was less than a micron thick and would cover the area of a squash court, and yet it had been organized within the volume of a football.

The design was brilliant, yet it carried with it the seeds of disaster—a susceptibility to flooding. Pulmonary edema could never have occurred in the fish. It is one of the prices of evolution.

ECONOMY OF WATER

The threat of flooding came more from within than from without. The pulmonary extravascular space is as susceptible as the systemic to changes in water balance.

Economy of water affects cells as well as the extracellular liquids. Within each cell, there are some 2000–3000 different enzymes, each with one or two substrates and many with cofactors. If all these molecules were present in simple solution, the cell would be impossibly big.

Very early in evolution, a number of devices were developed that allow the cell to contain within a small space the vast number of molecules necessary to its function. Fuel may be stored in an insoluble form such as glycogen or triglyceride. Enzymes may be embedded in membranes so that only their active sites stick out into the watery phase. Most enzymes operate at a low K_m so that the concentration of substrate does not have to be high, and K_m values tend to be similar in a sequence of enzymes so that the product of one reaction may be fed into the next without large fluctuations in concentration. Finally, the formation of activated compounds such as the thioesters of coenzyme A drastically reduces the concentrations at which a reaction can occur.

The economy of water in the extracellular space is no less important. This has been greatly helped by the development of a closed circulatory system. In the crustaceans and the molluscs, the arteries deliver blood directly into the intercellular spaces, from which it returns to the heart through ostia. The relatively closed circulatory system of the vertebrates has led to a considerable reduction in the volume of extracellular liquid.

Despite all these economies, both inside and outside the cells, the body is still predominantly water.

EVOLUTION OF RENAL FUNCTION

The overall control of body water rests largely with the kidney. It seems likely that the primary function of this organ was to rid the body of excess water. According to Homer Smith [11], the fishes had their origin in fresh water. The problem that faced these progenitors of the vertebrates was the same problem that faces the freshwater fishes of today—a surfeit of water that was continually absorbed by osmosis into the gills. The kidney disposed of water by a process of filtration followed by the reabsorption of salts. This devious system was necessitated by the universal inability of the vertebrates to design a pump through which water could be actively transported across cell membranes. At this stage in evolution, the kidney was not used for the excretion of nitrogenous waste, which was eliminated as ammonia by simple diffusion across the gills.

Migration into salt water brought opposite problems. Now the sea drew water out of the circulation by osmosis through the gills. The kidney was useless; in many marine species, its tubular system is rudimentary, and in some it has lost its glomeruli. To counteract the loss of water, most species drink the seawater, which is reabsorbed in the intestine. The reabsorbed salt is then removed by chloride cells in the gills. Once again, the body uses the active transport of sodium or chloride ions; the movement of water is passive.

With migration onto land, the ingestion of water was intermittent, and the main concern was its conservation. At the same time, it became no longer possible to eliminate nitrogenous waste as ammonia through the gills. Ammonia is toxic above a very low concentration, so that it had to be converted to a more acceptable form. For this purpose, the mammals chose urea, while the birds and reptiles chose uric acid. The kidney now took on the responsibility for both water and salt balance and for the excretion of nitrogenous waste. It was now required not only, on occasion, to produce a highly dilute urine in the way it had originally functioned, but also, on other occasions, to produce a highly concentrated urine in order to conserve water. To provide this latter function, the kidney developed the concentrating mechanism associated with the loop of Henle. The overall control of water and salt balance was the responsibility of a neurohumoral mechanism that comprised the sympathetic nervous system in coordination with renin–angiotensin, aldosterone, and vasopressin.

At this stage, we come across another remarkable evolutionary jump—a great increase in the glomerular filtration rate (Figure 4). Such a high rate could be achieved only by a high flow of blood through the kidney, since the colloidal osmotic pressure of the plasma sets a limit to the filtration fraction. Thus, in man, the kidneys receive as much as one quarter of the output of the heart.

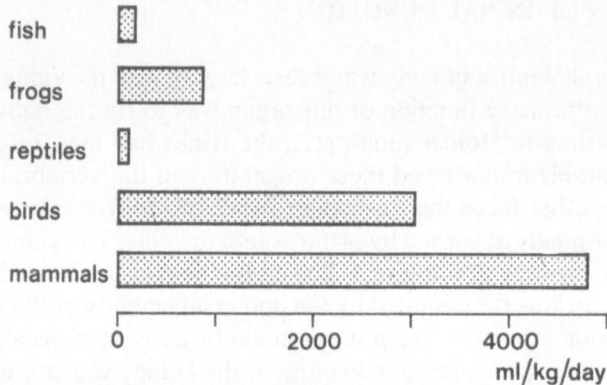

Figure 4.   Average values for the glomerular filtration rates of various classes of vertebrates. Data from Schmidt-Nielsen and Mackay [10].

DISTRIBUTION OF THE CARDIAC OUTPUT

The necessity for such a large flow of blood to the kidney is, as we have seen, the mechanical requirement of filtration and not a metabolic requirement for oxygen. The case is similar for the skin, where a large flow of blood is required for the dissipation of heat. Thus, these organs receive a share of the total cardiac output that is disproportionately high in relation to their requirement for oxygen. It follows that the rest of the body has to be content with less than its share (Figure 5). Such inequalities lead to wide discrep-

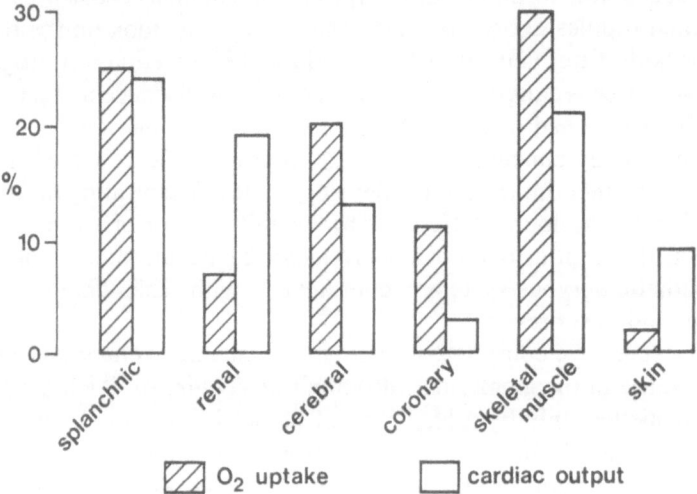

Figure 5.   Percentage of total oxygen consumed and percentage of total cardiac output received by various organs in a normal person at rest. Data from Wade and Bishop [12].

ancies in the arteriovenous differences for oxygen. Of these, the most notable is that for the myocardium, which extracts two thirds of the oxygen brought to it. Skeletal muscle is affected in a similar way.

During physical exercise, the oxygen uptake of skeletal and cardiac muscle may increase many times. To support this increase, they have been endowed with a powerful and overriding local vasodilatory mechanism. At the same time, activation of the sympathetic nervous system constricts the blood supply to those parts of the body that are not immediately necessary for the purposes of exercise [12]. This vasoconstriction particularly affects the kidney.

Thus, during evolution, the mechanical necessity for a high renal blood flow has, in this indirect fashion, caused the myocardium to be utterly dependent on local vasodilatation during physical exercise. The consequences are tragic when the coronary arteries are rendered rigid by atheroma in a population that has outgrown the age during which the forces of natural selection have operated.

THE BLOOD PRESSURE

An important factor underlying the development of atheroma is the level of the blood pressure. We do not need epidemiology to tell us this; we each carry our own control. Atheroma is limited and late in the normal pulmonary circulation, but becomes prominent when, in disease, the pulmonary arterial pressure reaches the level of the systemic. And here we meet our last and most striking evolutionary jump (Figure 6). The systemic blood pressure of fishes, amphibians, and reptiles averages about 30 mm Hg. But all mammals have a blood pressure similar to ours, and birds average somewhat higher. Why this has come to be so has nothing to do with standing upright, although advantage is taken of the mechanism for this purpose [6].

CONGESTIVE CARDIAC FAILURE

We start with a semantic disadvantage. The difficulty is that the term carries its own definition. To take a recent example [3], congestive cardiac failure is:

> The pathophysiological state in which an abnormality of cardiac function is responsible for failure of the heart to pump blood at a rate commensurate with the requirements of the metabolizing tissues.

The heart can fail only in pumping enough blood. But enough blood for what? The metabolic requirements of the tissues. Then what are those requirements? Oxygen, glucose, free fatty acids? Only for oxygen does the entire cardiac output pass through the point of entry into the body. But, if

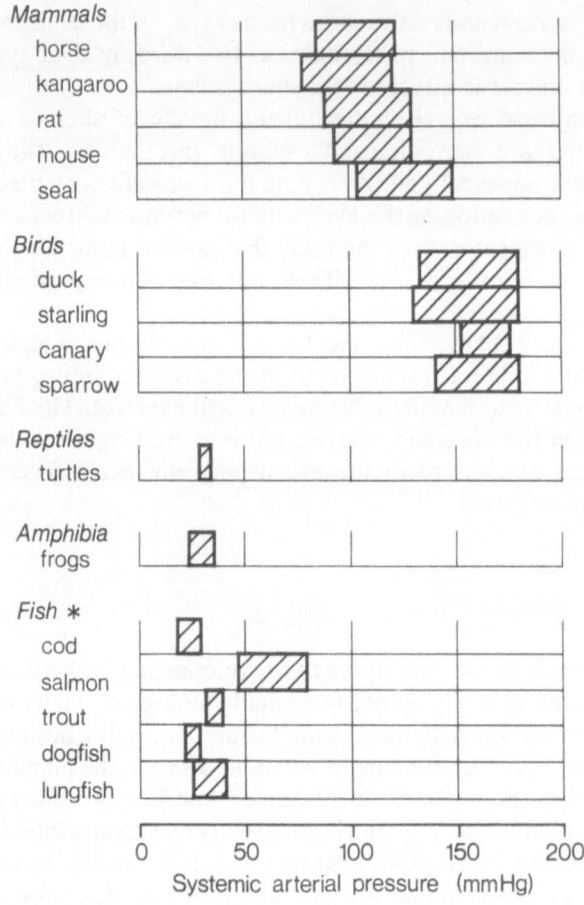

Figure 6. Systolic and diastolic blood pressures in various animals. Data from Altman and Dittmer [1]. *Ventral aorta.

the needs of the body for oxygen are not being met, it follows that the oxygen uptake is reduced. And yet we have known for over three decades that this is not the case [7].

If we were wise, we would discard the term. Call it cardiac edema or cardiac congestion, perhaps. But custom is too strong, and doubtless we are stuck with it.

This "forward-failure" way of looking at the condition has been fashionable for several decades, but the older "backward-failure" view persists. According to this view, cardiac edema is due to blood being held back behind a failing ventricle. The venous pressure rises and squeezes liquid out into the tissue.

There is limited truth in the concept owing to the different volumes of blood contained in the pulmonary and systemic circuits. The pulmonary blood volume is about one tenth of the systemic and is extremely vulnerable to overfilling. Suppose, for instance, that the left ventricle puts out one drop of blood less than the right each beat (a quantity utterly unrecognizable by any modern clinical technique). Then, in two hours, the pulmonary blood volume will have doubled, the pulmonary vascular pressures will have greatly increased, and the patient will be dying from pulmonary edema. That can clearly be called left ventricular failure.

Students are still taught that the systemic edema of cardiac failure is caused by a similar failure of the right ventricle; but it cannot be so. If the right ventricle pumps less blood than the left, the most that can happen is that the entire pulmonary blood volume is transferred to the systemic circuit. It would be roughly equivalent to giving a "unit" of blood to a normal man. Is that what is meant by "right heart failure"?

If systemic edema were caused simply by a mechanical expulsion of liquid into the tissues, the blood volume should decrease. But it increases. Simple studies [13], long since forgotten in a world of differentiated pressures and feedback Chinese puzzles, showed that at the early stages of cardiac failure, the weight of the body increased before there was any perceptible increase in venous pressure.

The syndrome of congestive cardiac failure, then, depends on the retention of water and salt by the kidneys, so that the total body water and exchangeable sodium increase [2]. The reason for this is an activation of the neurohumoral mechanism: sympathetic, renin–angiotensin, aldosterone, and vasopressin. The cardiac output is redistributed in a way that preserves the blood supply to skeletal and cardiac muscle due to vasoconstriction in the kidneys, the skin, and the gut. The diminished flow of blood to the kidneys is partly responsible for the retention of water and salt, but, in addition, aldosterone is active. Thus, in congestive cardiac failure, there is widespread vasoconstriction, increased levels of angiotensin II and aldosterone in the blood, and retention of water and salt by the kidney.

One has come to assume that how the body reacts to disease should be for the best. For instance, vasoconstriction should maintain the blood pressure and preserve flow to vital regions. Yet vasodilators are now widely used to treat cardiac failure. The renal retention of water expands the blood volume and helps to fill a weakened ventricle. Yet the diuretics are the most successful form of treatment that we have. Similarly, the beneficial effects of angiotensin II and aldosterone might be argued; and yet captopril and spirolactone are widely used to treat cardiac failure.

If the reaction of the body in cardiac failure has evolved in order to preserve life, why, at every turn, are we able to help our patients by reversing those processes that nature has set in motion? The probable answer is that these processes evolved for some entirely different purpose. Cardiac failure is, after all, a rare event. So exotic a condition would not have any perceptible effect on the survival of the species. The mechanisms that we find in cardiac failure are more likely to have evolved to deal with circumstances

Table 1. Comparison of the Response of the Body in Cardiac Failure with Its Response in Hypoxia, Salt Lack, Shock and Hemorrhage, Standing and Exercise [6]

	Heart failure	Hypoxia	Salt lack	Shock and hemorrhage	Standing	Exercise
Sympathetic	+	0	+	+	+	+
Renal blood flow	−	0+	−	−	−	−
Urine volume	−	+	−	−	−	−
Na$^+$ excretion	−	+	−	−	−	−
Renin: angiotensin	+	0 +	+	+	+	+
Aldosterone	+	?	+	+	+	+
Vasopressin	+	0	0+	+	+	+

vital to preservation that are far more plebeian. Has it happened, then, rather by accident, that damage to the heart calls up these mechanisms by somehow simulating the circumstances for which they had properly been developed?

To pursue this thesis, we need to consider what such circumstances might be. Perhaps the reduced cardiac output causes a lack of oxygen in the tissues and thus simulates an elemental threat to life. Perhaps it suggests shock. Perhaps the escape of liquid into the tissue spaces simulates a shortage of water or salt. Or the consequent decrease in blood volume might suggest hemorrhage. All these conditions are far more likely to endanger the survival of the species than heart failure. So let us compare how the body responds to them with how it responds in cardiac failure.

Table 1 tells us immediately that the effects of global hypoxia hardly begin to mimic those in cardiac failure. On the other hand, the reactions of the body to salt depletion or shock or hemorrhage closely resemble those in cardiac failure. These last are circumstances that clearly threaten life and are common in a hazardous and predatory world, so that it would have been reasonable for mechanisms to have evolved to protect against them. But notice that during muscular exercise, the body responds in precisely the same way. And here we have a function that is essential to daily survival, as vital to the hunted as to the hunter. Would it not seem most likely that it is to support physical exercise that the mechanisms that we find in cardiac failure were originally evolved?

To appreciate the relevance of the effects of exercise to those that occur in cardiac failure, it is necessary to consider the response of the body to prolonged exertion such as hill-walking [9]. After a few days of such prolonged exercise, there can be a retention of water and salt sufficient to cause pitting edema.

The stereotyped response of the sympathetic system that is found in all these conditions has been identified as the "defense reaction" [8]. It carries with it the relevant endocrine responses, some of them vasoconstrictive and some leading to the retention of saline in the body. The entire sympathetic–endocrine system functions as a coordinated unit, the endocrine element acting as an "effector arm" of the nervous system [5].

In congestive cardiac failure, there is a prolonged and inappropriate stimulation of the defense reaction. When the output of the diseased heart becomes diminished, the body responds in exactly the way it has been programmed to do in exercise or shock. It cannot distinguish the primary cause. But the programming was designed to service the body during a few hours of exercise or a few days of traumatic shock. Now, it is maintained in action over months or years, and an overretention of saline ensues. Why this retention of saline is so harmful is explained by the vulnerability of the lungs to flooding, discussed at the beginning of this address. It is congestion of the lungs that dominates the symptoms of patients in cardiac failure.

A man in cardiac failure is a hero. We meet him every day in the hospital, and we owe it to him to understand him better. A study of our ancestors helps us to do so.

REFERENCES

1. Altman, P. L., and Dittmer, D. S. 1973. *Biological Handbooks: Respiration and Circulation.* *Federation of American Societies for Experimental Biology*, Bethesda, Maryland.
2. Birkenfeld, L. W., Leibman, J., O'Meara, M. P., and Edelman, I. S. 1958. Total exchangeable sodium, total exchangeable potassium, and total body water in edematous patients with cirrhosis of the liver and congestive heart failure. *Invest.* 37:687–698.
3. Braunwald, E. 1983. The definition of heart failure. *Eur. Heart J.* 4:446–447.
4. Dejours, P. 1975. *Principles of Comparative Respiratory Physiology.* North-Holland, Amsterdam.
5. Ganong, W. F. 1981. Neuroendocrine responses to injury and shock. *Adv. Physiol. Sci.* 26:35–44.
6. Harris, P. 1983. Evolution and the cardiac patient. *Cardiovasc. Res.* 17:313–319, 373–378, 437–445.
7. Hickam, J. B., and Cargill, W. H. 1948. Effect of exercise on cardiac output and pulmonary arterial pressure in normal persons and in patients with cardiovascular disease and pulmonary emphysema. *J. Clin. Invest.* 27:10–23.
8. Hilton, S. M., and Spyer, K. M. 1980. Central nervous regulation of vascular resistance. *Annu. Rev. Physiol.* 42:399–411.
9. Milledge, J. S., Bryson, E. I., Catley, D. M., Hesp, R., Luff, N., Minty, B. D., Older, M. W. J., Payne, N. N., Ward, N. P., and Withey, W. R. 1982. Sodium balance, fluid homeostasis and the renin–aldosterone system during the prolonged exercise of hill walking. *Clin. Sci.* 62:595–604.
10. Schmidt-Nielsen, B. M., and Mackay, W. C. 1980. Comparative physiology of electrolyte regulation. In: M. H. Maxwell and C. R. Kleeman (eds.), *Clinical Disorders of Fluid and Electrolyte Metabolism*, pp. 37–88, McGraw-Hill, New York.
11. Smith, H. W. 1951. *The Kidney.* Oxford University Press, New York.
12. Wade, O. L., and Bishop, J. M. 1962. *Cardiac Output and Regional Blood Flow.* Blackwell, Oxford.
13. Warren, J. V., and Stead, E. A., Jr. 1944. Fluid dynamics in chronic congestive heart failure. *Arch. Intern. Med.* 73:138–147.

NUCLEAR MAGNETIC RESONANCE

Phosphorus Two-Dimensional NMR Spectroscopy of Perfused Rat Hearts

Pamela B. Garlick*

Department of Pharmacology
Columbia University College of Physicians and Surgeons
New York, New York 10032

Christopher J. Turner

Department of Chemistry
Columbia University
New York, New York 10027

Abstract. The theory behind the technique of two-dimensional (2-D) NMR is presented with particular reference to 2-D J-spectroscopy and 2-D exchange spectroscopy. Experiments are described in which both these types of 2-D NMR are applied to the isolated perfused rat heart. Possible advantages of 2-D techniques and future applications to physiological systems are discussed.

INTRODUCTION

NMR, in its infancy, was applied to the investigation of molecules in solution, but in the last decade its range has been extended to many different physiological systems [1,2]. One of the differences between the two types of studies lies in the spectral linewidths obtained—narrow, well-resolved lines from solutions and rather broad poorly resolved lines from biological tissues and organs. Typical examples of these are illustrated in Figure 1. The upper panel (A) shows a ^{31}P spectrum of a solution of Mg^{2+}-ATP, while the lower panel (B) shows a spectrum from a perfused heart. [The frequency axis is usually expressed in terms of a "chemical shift" (in ppm) relative to a chosen standard the position of which is taken to be zero.] In the solution spectrum, the three ATP peaks are each split into several lines (multiplets); the γ- and α-peaks are seen as doublets and the β-peak as a triplet. These multiple peaks are due to spin–spin coupling, a phenomenon whereby nuclear spins communicate with each other through covalent bonds, causing changes in the magnetic energy levels available to each of the individual nuclei. If a phosphorus nucleus is bonded to n other phosphorus nuclei, its

* Present address: Heart Research Unit, The Rayne Institute, St. Thomas' Hospital, London S.E.1.

15

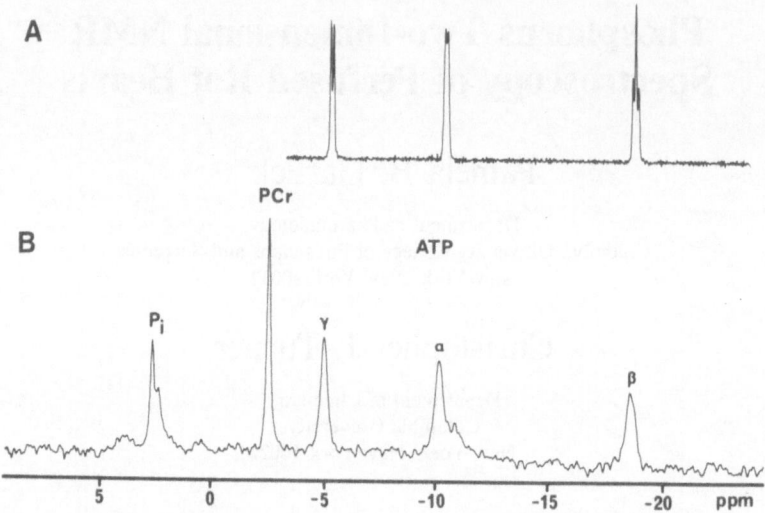

Figure 1.   One-dimensional ^{31}P spectra at 121.5 MHz of a solution of Mg^{2+}-ATP at pH 7 (A) and an isolated perfused rat heart (B). (P_i) Inorganic phosphate; (PCr) phosphocreatine; (γ, α, β) γ-, α-, and β-phosphates of ATP. Frequencies (ppm) are expressed relative to the position of 85% phosphoric acid.

signal will be split into $(n + 1)$ peaks; thus, it is only the central, β-phosphorus of ATP the signal of which appears as a triplet. The separation between the individual peaks of a multiplet, when expressed in Hz, is known as the coupling constant, J. For a particular molecule, J is not in fact constant, but is dependent on a variety of factors such as bond angles and the binding of ions or molecules. In contrast to the ATP peaks in the solution spectrum, those in the heart spectrum (Figure 1B) contain no visible multiplet structure, nor could any be obtained by resolution-enhancement techniques [3]. It would thus seem that the information available from the coupling constants of ATP is lost in the case of heart spectra.

A second aspect of the situation that is not visible in conventional physiological spectra is that of chemical exchange. Thus, for example, although biochemists know that creatine kinase is causing the continuous interconversion of γ-ATP and PCr in the heart, there is no evidence for this in the spectrum in Figure 1B. The question that therefore arises is, "Is there any way in which one can visualize these two 'hidden' aspects of metabolites in spectra of intact hearts?" The answer to this question is yes, and the technique that makes it possible is that of two-dimensional (2-D) NMR [4–7].* A complete understanding of the theoretical basis of this technique requires complex analysis with the aid of density matrices [4,7]. Since such a

---

* Evidence of exchange could also be obtained using 1-D "magnetization transfer" methods [8].

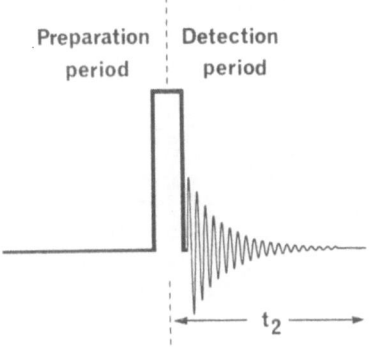

Figure 2. Pulse diagram for a conventional 1-D experiment. The signal is acquired during the detection period (t_2) following the application of the radiofrequency pulse. The preparation period enables the nuclear magnetization to return toward its equilibrium value between successive pulses.

treatment would be inappropriate in this chapter, a more pragmatic and considerably less detailed approach is offered in the following section.

THEORY

Conventional one-dimensional (1-D) NMR utilizes the behavior of the nuclei *following* the detection pulse to obtain frequency information. Experimentally (see Figure 2), a single radiofrequency pulse is applied to the sample nuclei, and the resultant signal (amplitude vs. time) is recorded during the detection period (t_2); the amplitude of this signal decays exponentially due to "relaxation processes." If several pulses in succession are required to obtain a signal of sufficient size, they are each separated by the "preparation period"; without such an interval, the signal would gradually disappear because of "saturation." The process of Fourier transformation (with respect to t_2) is then used to convert the final signal acquired into a spectrum of amplitude vs. frequency. Two-dimensional or double Fourier transform NMR utilizes, in addition, the "memory" of the nuclei for their behavior *prior to* the detection pulse, i.e., during what is called the evolution period (t_1). Changing the length of the evolution period allows information about the phase and/or amplitude of the nuclear magnetization during t_1 to be transferred to the signal that is detected subsequently during t_2. (It has been suggested by Freeman [9] that this information transfer is analogous to a runner in a relay race passing the baton to the next member of the team.) Experimentally, a series of signals (amplitude vs. t_2) is accumulated that corresponds to different but evenly spaced values of the evolution period (t_1) Fourier transformation of these signals with respect to both t_2 (real time) and t_1 (evolution period) produces a 2-D spectrum of amplitude vs. frequencies (F_1 and F_2). The interpretation of the F_1 frequency axis and of its exact relationship with F_2 will depend on the particular pulse sequence chosen and on the conditions prevailing during the interpulse periods. In all types of 2-D spectra, however, visual simplification is achieved because

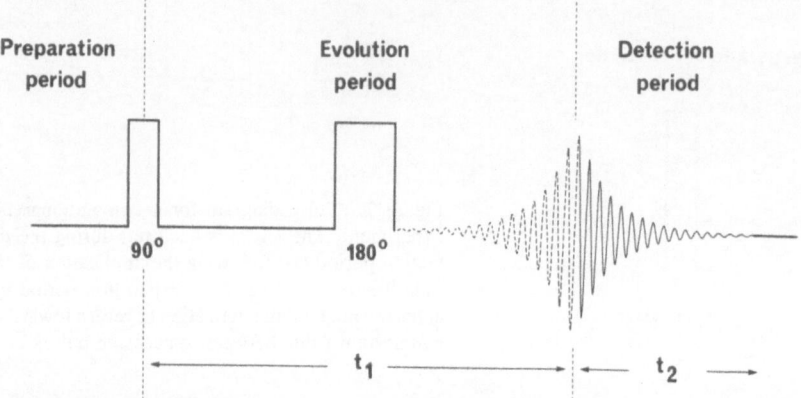

Figure 3.   Basic two-pulse sequence used in the acquisition of 2-D J-spectra. The 180° pulse causes the formation of the "echo envelope," and the second half of this is the signal that is detected during t_2.

some aspect of the "normal" spectrum has been projected into a second dimension. Since the application of both 2-D J-spectroscopy and exchange spectroscopy to perfused hearts will be presented in this chapter, the theory of each will now be discussed briefly.

TWO-DIMENSIONAL J-SPECTROSCOPY

The two-pulse sequence used in this type of experiment and the "echo envelope," the second half of which is the detected signal, are shown in Figure 3. When spin–spin coupling (see the Introduction) occurs between sample nuclei, it induces phase modulation of the echo as a function of t_1 (the evolution period). Thus, if a series of echo signals, with different t_1 values, are detected and Fourier transformed with respect to both t_1 and t_2, the chemical shift information from the "normal" spectrum appears in the F_2 dimension, while any resolvable multiplet structure appears in F_1. The resolution along the F_1 axis is superior to that in a conventional 1-D spectrum because the 180° pulse eliminates the effects of static magnetic field inhomogeneities, which, if present, would broaden the lines. A 2-D J-spectrum of ATP in solution is shown, as an example, in Figure 4 (cf. Figure 1A). In the F_2 dimension, peaks can be seen at -5, -10, and -18 ppm, corresponding to the central frequencies of the γ-, α-, and β-multiplets of ATP; in the F_1 dimension, the γ- and α-peaks are resolved into doublets and the β-peak into a triplet. By plotting cross sections parallel to the F_1 axis at the appropriate chemical shifts, one can measure the coupling constants (J) with some accuracy.

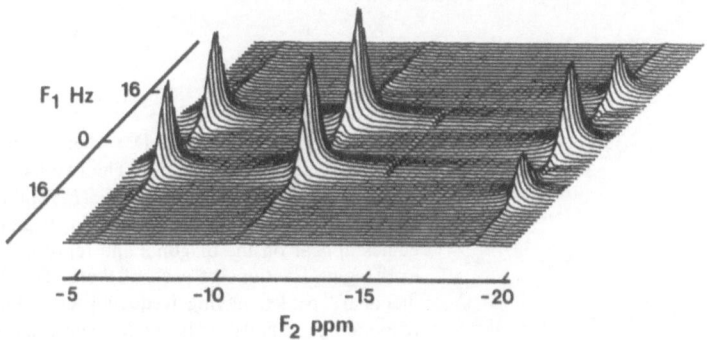

Figure 4. A 2-D J-spectrum (as a stacked plot) of a solution of Mg^{2+}-ATP at pH 7. The multiplets occurring at -5, -10, and -18 ppm (F_2) are the γ-, α-, and β-phosphates of ATP, respectively.

TWO-DIMENSIONAL EXCHANGE SPECTROSCOPY

The three-pulse sequence used in this type of experiment is shown in Figure 5. During the evolution period (t_1), the nuclear magnetization becomes "frequency-labeled," (i.e. the signal amplitudes become a defined function of the signal frequencies) and during the mixing period (τ_m), this labeled magnetization is exchanged between chemically or enzymatically interconverting nuclei. The signal that is finally detected thus has a frequency with respect to real time t_2 and an amplitude that is modulated as a function of t_1. By incrementing t_1, a series of signals is obtained that, on Fourier transformation with respect to both t_1 and t_2, yields a 2-D exchange spectrum with frequency axes F_1 and F_2. F_1 and F_2 correspond to the frequencies of the nucleus before and after the mixing period, respectively. A hypothetical

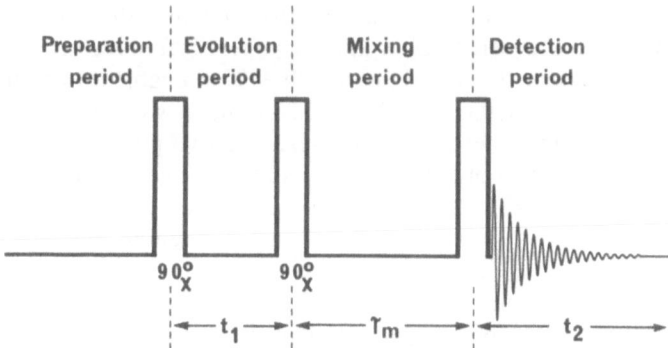

Figure 5. Basic three-pulse sequence used in the 2-D exchange experiment. The nuclear magnetization becomes "frequency-labeled" during the evolution period (t_1), and exchange can occur during the mixing period (τ_m). The third pulse is a conventional detection pulse.

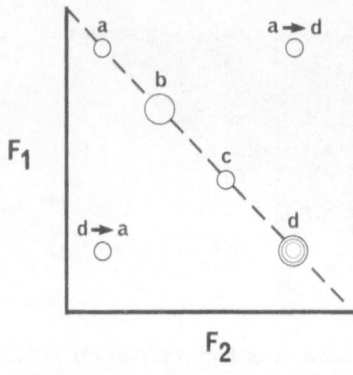

Figure 6. A hypothetical 2-D exchange spectrum of four molecules, a, b, c, and d. The two axes give the frequencies of the molecules before (F_1) and after (F_2) the mixing period. Peaks corresponding to all four molecules appear on the diagonal and represent the non-exchanging fractions of each of them. The two "off-diagonal" peaks, having frequency coordinates corresponding to a and d, indicate the occurrence of chemical exchange between these two molecules.

2-D exchange spectrum of four molecules, a, b, c, and d, is shown in Figure 6 as a contour plot; in this type of plot, contours are drawn around the central frequency of each peak, as in a geographical map. Nonexchanging nuclei (e.g., b and c), having equal frequencies before and after the mixing period and thus equal coordinates in both dimensions, will have peaks that lie on the diagonal (i.e., at 45°); these are referred to as "auto" or "diagonal" peaks. Exchanging nuclei (e.g., a and d) will have peaks both on the diagonal (corresponding to that fraction that has not undergone exchange during τ_m) and off the diagonal (corresponding to that fraction that has exchanged during τ_m). The "off-diagonal" or "cross" peaks will have coordinates that give the frequency of the nucleus before (F_1) and after (F_2) the mixing period. Thus, the 2-D exchange spectrum provides an excellent way of visualizing the exchange processes occurring in a sample; quantification of the rates of these processes can be achieved by variation of the mixing period [10,11].

METHODS

Hearts from male Sprague–Dawley rats weighing 300–350 g were perfused with Krebs–Henseleit buffer in the Langendorff mode in a system that had been modified, as described previously [12] to enable it to be interfaced with an NMR spectrometer. ^{31}P NMR measurements were made on a Bruker WM-300 WB spectrometer, at 121.5 MHz. The two-pulse sequence shown in Figure 3 was used to obtain the 2-D J-spectra. The sweepwidths were 4 kHz (F_2) and 64 Hz (F_1). A 16×1024 data matrix was collected and zero-filled to 128×1024; a 10-Hz Lorentzian line-broadening was applied in the F_2 dimension, while a Lorentzian-to-Gaussian transformation was used in F_1. Artifacts were minimized by using 16-transient phase-cycling [13] and self-compensating 180° pulses [14,15]. The three-pulse sequence shown in Figure 5 was used for the 2-D exchange experiments. Quadrature detection was used in both dimensions, and the sweepwidths were equal at 4000 Hz. Unwanted signals were suppressed by phase-cycling [7]. A 128×1024 data

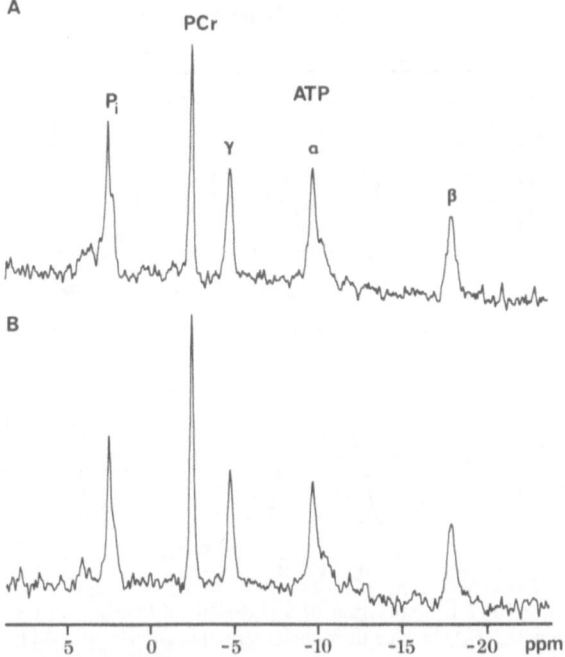

Figure 7. ^{31}P 1-D spectra of a perfused rat heart acquired before the collection of one of the 2-D J-spectra, after 1 hr of perfusion (A), and after the collection of the 2-D data file, following 10 hr of perfusion (B). Each spectrum is the sum of 40 90° pulses applied at 15-sec intervals.

matrix was collected and zero-filled to 1024 × 1024; a 10-Hz Lorentzian line-broadening was applied in each dimension. The collection of each type of 2-D data file took on the order of 10 hr, and because of this extended time period, it was necessary to establish the metabolic stability of each heart preparation. This was achieved by measurement of 1-D spectra.

RESULTS AND DISCUSSION

Figure 7 shows two 1-D spectra that were acquired before (A) and after (B) the collection of a typical 2-D data file. The constancy of the peak heights testifies to the long-term metabolic stability of the heart preparation. By the use of 2-D J-spectroscopy, it was possible to resolve the γ- and α-ATP peaks of the heart spectra into doublets, although the β-peak always remained as a single broad resonance.* The two doublets can be seen in Figure 8 both in a contour plot and in cross sections through that plot at the appropriate chemical shifts. From the cross sections, one can measure the coupling

---

* The inability to resolve the multiplet structure of the β-peak was subsequently explained by 1-D echo experiments [16].

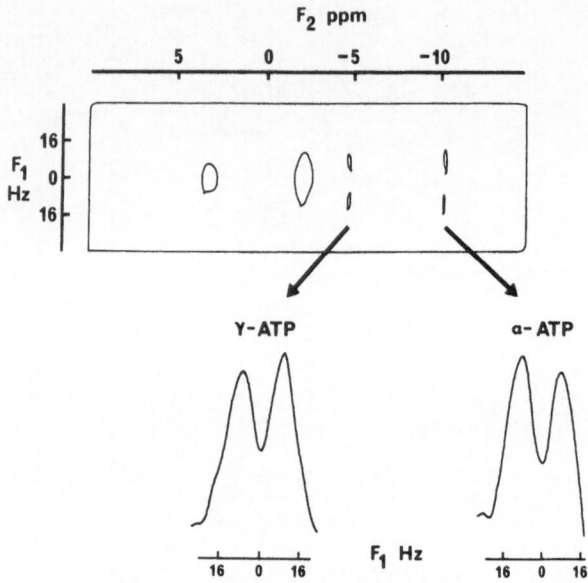

Figure 8.   Part of a ^{31}P 2-D J-spectrum of a perfused rat heart, with cross sections at the appropriate frequencies (F_2) showing the doublet structures of γ- and α-ATP. The singlet peaks at 3.0 and −2.5 ppm (F_2) are from inorganic phosphate and phosphocreatine, respectively.

constants $J_{\alpha\beta}$ and $J_{\beta\gamma}$, and they are found to be the same as the values published for ATP when complexed to magnesium [17,18]. Our results thus confirm those obtained from chemical shift data, namely, that within experimental error, all the ATP in the myocardial cell is in the form of Mg^{2+}-ATP. This has important consequences when calculating the free magnesium content of the cell.

A 2-D exchange spectrum of a rat heart, both as a contour plot (a) and as a stacked plot (b), is shown in Figure 9; the mixing period was 0.4 sec. As explained in the Theory section, the "normal" spectrum, with peaks from P_i, PCr, γ-, α-, and β-ATP, is seen along the diagonal. The appearance of the two "cross" peaks x and y indicates the occurrence of chemical exchange. Since these peaks have coordinates corresponding to γ-ATP and PCr, the exchange that is visualized is obviously that catalyzed by creatine kinase:

$$PCr + ADP + H^+ \rightleftharpoons ATP + creatine$$

Experiments are now in progress with different mixing times to enable the rate constants of the reaction to be quantified. Preparations with increased work loads will be used to measure the ATPase rates.

The results thus show that the technique of 2-D NMR can be applied to the study of intracellular metabolites in the perfused heart. Because of

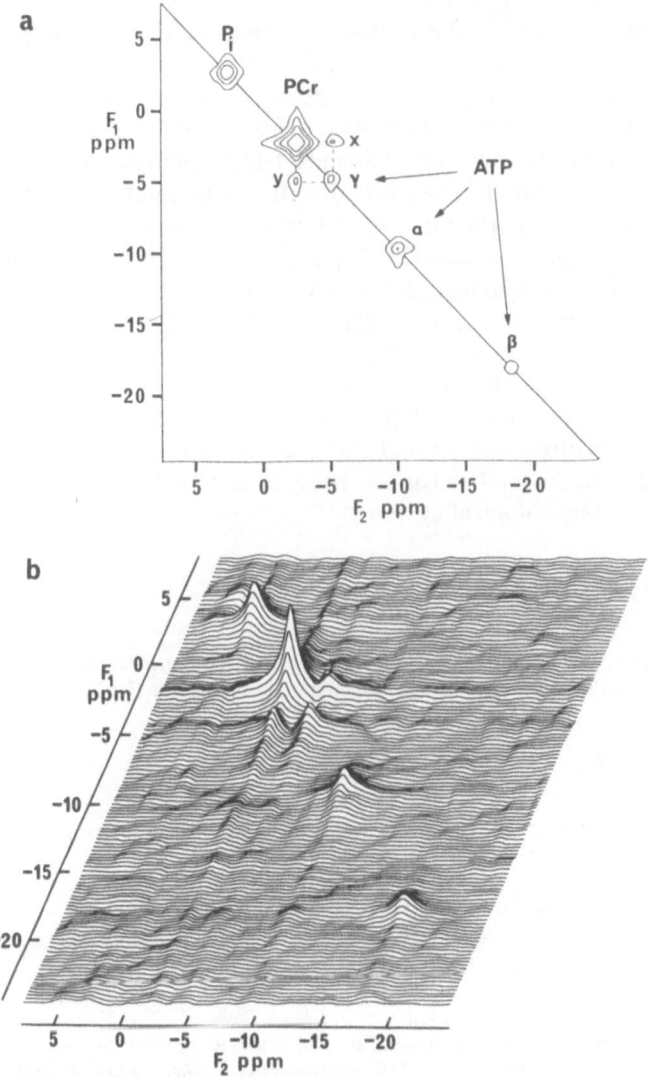

Figure 9. A ^{31}P 2-D exchange spectrum of a perfused rat heart, shown as a contour plot (a) and a stacked plot (b). The mixing time was 0.4 sec, the preparation time was 5 sec, and the total time for the accumulation of the data file was 10.5 hr. The "diagonal" peaks are identified as labeled; the "off-diagonal" peaks x and y correlate the phosphocreatine (-2.52 ppm) and the γ-phosphate of ATP (-4.94 ppm).

the length of time required for the acquisition of the 2-D data files, long-term metabolic stability of the heart preparation is essential and should be carefully checked in each experiment. Two-dimensional J-spectroscopy may prove to be a useful technique for the study of physiological systems, particularly when applied to the observation of ^{13}C or ^{1}H nuclei. In the case of carbon, for example, if the proton–carbon coupling were removed during the period t_2 but not during t_1, the resultant projection of the multiplets and chemical shifts into two different dimensions would considerably aid in the difficult process of peak assignment. Two-dimensional exchange spectroscopy may provide a useful alternative to 1-D magnetization transfer methods for the investigation of in situ kinetics. It will be interesting to see whether the "discrepancy" in the flux rates of creatine kinase observed in 1-D NMR studies of heart preparations [19–21] is still detected by 2-D techniques. Two-dimensional NMR also has certain advantages over 1-D methods for kinetic studies in that it minimizes problems associated with overcrowded spectra and it has no requirements for extra hardware, such as frequency synthesizers or amplifiers; the extra software that is necessary for the 2-D experiments is now uniformly available on most commercial spectrometers. Thus, 2-D NMR spectroscopy should now be added to the ever-growing list of biophysical methods that can be used to obtain biochemical information about intact physiological systems.

ACKNOWLEDGMENTS

The authors thank the National Science Foundation for generous support of this research, and Pamela Garlick also acknowledges funding from NIH Grant HL-27318.

REFERENCES

1. Ingwall, J. S. 1982. Phosphorus nuclear magnetic resonance spectroscopy of cardiac and skeletal muscles. *Am. J. Physiol.* 242:H729–H744.
2. Iles, R. A., Stevens, A. N., and Griffiths, J. 1982. NMR studies of metabolites in living tissue. *Prog. NMR Spectrosc.* 15:49–200.
3. Lindon, J. C., and Ferrige, A. G. 1980. Digitization and data processing in Fourier transform NMR. *Prog. NMR Spectrosc.* 14:27–66.
4. Aue, W. P., Bartholdi, E., and Ernst, R. R. 1976. Two-dimensional spectroscopy: Application to nuclear magnetic resonance. *J. Chem. Phys.* 64:2229–2246.
5. Jeener, J., Meier, B. H., Bachmann, P., and Ernst, R. R. 1979. Investigation of exchange processes by two dimensional NMR spectroscopy. *J. Chem. Phys.* 71:4546–4553.
6. Nagayama, K. 1981. Two-dimensional NMR spectroscopy: An application to the study of flexibility of protein molecules. *Adv. Biophys.* 14:139–204.
7. Bax, A. 1982. *Two Dimensional Nuclear Magnetic Resonance in Liquids.* Delft University Press, Delft, Holland.
8. Forsén, S. H., and Hoffman, R. A. 1963. Study of moderately rapid chemical exchange reactions by means of nuclear magnetic double resonance. *J. Chem. Phys.* 39:2892–2901.
9. Freeman, R. 1980. Nuclear magnetic resonance spectroscopy in two frequency dimensions. *Proc. R. Soc. Lond. Ser. A* 373:149–178.
10. Bodenhausen, G., and Ernst, R. R. 1982. Direct determination of rate constants of slow dynamic processes by two-dimensional "accordion" spectroscopy in nuclear magnetic resonance. *J. Am. Chem. Soc.* 104:1304–1309.
11. Balaban, R. S. and Ferretti, J. A. 1983. Rates of enzyme-catalyzed exchange determined by two dimensional NMR: A study of glucose 6-phosphate anomerization and isomerization. *Proc. Natl. Acad. Sci. U.S.A.* 80:1241–1245.

12. Garlick, P. B., Radda, G. K., and Seeley, P. J. 1979. Studies of acidosis in the ischemic heart by phosphorus nuclear magnetic resonance. *Biochem. J.* 184:547–554.
13. Bodenhausen, G., and Turner, D. L. 1980. Artifacts in two-dimensional J-spectra. *J. Magn. Reson.* 41:200–206.
14. Levitt, M. H. 1982. Symmetric composite pulse sequences for NMR population inversion. I. Compensation of radiofrequency field inhomogeneity. *J. Magn. Reson.* 48:234–264.
15. Levitt, M. H. 1982. Symmetric composite pulse sequences for NMR population inversion. II. Compensation of resonance offset. *J. Magn. Reson.* 50:95–110.
16. Turner, C. J., and Garlick, P. B. 1984. One- and two-dimensional ^{31}P spin echo studies of myocardial ATP and phosphocreatine. *J. Magn. Reson.* 57:221–227.
17. Son, T. D., Roux, M., and Ellenberger, M. 1975. Interaction of Mg^{2+} ions with nucleoside triphosphates by phosphorus magnetic resonance spectroscopy. *Nucleic Acids. Res.* 2:1101–1110.
18. Jaffe, E. K., and Cohn, M. 1978. ^{31}P Nuclear magnetic resonance spectra of the thiophosphate analogues of adenine nucleotides; effects of pH and Mg^{2+} binding. *Biochemistry* 17:652–657.
19. Brown, T. R., Gadian, D. G., Garlick, P. B., Radda, G. K., Seeley, P. J., and Styles, P. 1978. Creatine kinase activities in skeletal and cardiac muscle measured by saturation transfer NMR. In: L. Dutton, J. Leigh, and A. Scarpa (eds.), *Frontiers of Biological Energetics: Electrons to Tissues.* pp. 1341–1349. Academic Press, New York.
20. Nunnally, R. L,, and Hollis, D. P. 1979. ATP compartmentation in living hearts—a phosphorus nuclear magnetic resonance saturation transfer study. *Biochemistry* 18:3642–3646.
21. Matthews, P. M., Bland, J. L., Gadian, D. G., and Radda, G. K. 1982. A ^{31}P NMR saturation transfer study of the regulation of creatine kinase in the rat heart. *Biochim. Biophys. Acta* 721:312–320.

High-Time-Resolution ^{31}P NMR Studies of the Perfused Ferret Heart

Peter Gordon Morris

MRC Biomedical NMR Centre
National Institute for Medical Research
London NW7 1AA, England

David G. Allen and Clive H. Orchard

Department of Physiology
University College London
London WC1E 6BT, England

Abstract. A cell is described that has enabled isolated Langendorff-perfused ferret hearts to be studied in a Bruker WM200 widebore superconducting nuclear magnetic resonance (NMR) spectrometer. Left ventricular pressure was monitored with a latex balloon catheter, and the hearts were paced with a stimulator triggered from the spectrometer's central computer, enabling gated studies to be performed. Suitable radiofrequency filtering for the pacing leads is described. Phosphorus (^{31}P) NMR was used to determine internal pH and the concentration of phosphorylated metabolites under resting conditions. The perfusion rate is shown to affect the phosphocreatine/ATP ratio at low flow rates, but the removal of phosphate from the perfusate is shown not to affect metabolite levels or the internal pH. The time resolution of the method is assessed and its potential for monitoring transient effects illustrated by studies of the effects of acetylcholine and cyanide-induced anoxia. The cardiac gated ^{31}P NMR experiment is discussed and four spectra, corresponding to mid- and end systole and mid- and end diastole are presented. No effects of cycling of high-energy phosphates are evident in these results.

INTRODUCTION

Since the first demonstration in 1974 that nuclear magnetic resonance (NMR) could be applied to living tissues [1], the perfused heart has been widely studied both by ^{31}P [2–6] and by ^{13}C [7] NMR. Our aim was to develop a system with sufficiently good time resolution to enable us to use ^{31}P NMR to correlate observed transient changes in developed tension with pH (as determined from the chemical shift of the inorganic phosphate resonance [8]) and the status of the NMR-visible high-energy phosphorylated metabolites: free (unbound) sugar phosphates, phosphocreatine (PCr), and ATP. Taken together with parallel aequorin determinations of intracellular free calcium in ferret papillary muscle [9], these measurements allow us to investigate in considerable depth the processes that regulate cardiac performance.

27

The effects we wish to follow are transient in nature, occurring over time scales of 0.5–10 min. Unfortunately, NMR is in general a rather insensitive analytical technique, and the ^{31}P nucleus, although it is the only naturally occurring isotope of phosphorus, has a rather low magnetic moment, giving it a sensitivity (at constant field) only 0.08 times that of the proton. To maximize the NMR signal, and hence the time resolution, it is therefore important to use the largest amount of tissue consistent with magnetic-field homogeneity. Such considerations led us to use a perfused ferret heart, which fits comfortably within a 25-mm ^{31}P probe, the largest commercially available for the MRC Biomedical NMR Centre's widebore WM200 spectrometer used in these experiments.

We were also interested in monitoring changes that occur over the time scale of the cardiac cycle. This required the interfacing of the pacing stimulator with the central computer of the WM200 to gain precise control over the position of the NMR sampling interval within the cardiac cycle.

METHODS

We used a Langendorff retrograde perfusion method under constant flow conditions. Hearts were removed from anesthetized animals and placed in Tyrodes solution (see the chapter by Orchard, Allen, and Morris for details) at room temperature. Perfusion was started at 1–2 min following excision. All remaining pericardium and lung were trimmed away at this stage to prevent reception of signal from these unwanted sources.

Temperature regulation (at 30 or 37°C) was effected in three stages by: (1) preheating the perfusate reservoir in a temperature-controlled water bath, (2) surrounding the downlead with an outer jacket through which water from the same bath was cirulcated at a high flow rate, and (3) using a variable-temperature gas-flow system in the sample chamber itself. In this matter, the temperature was maintained to an accuracy of better than 1°C.

Butyl XX rubber was used for the perfusion leads, since it has a very low gas permeability, an important consideration since we require a considerable length of tubing to gain access to the center of the magnet bore. It is also important to insert a good filter (we used a sintered glass filter porosity No. 3) into the downlead to avoid blockage of the coronary capillaries. If the perfusate is recirculated, a filter is particularly valuable, and a good protocol is to discard the first few hundred milliliters of perfusate following commencement of perfusion, since it is at this stage that the bulk of "debris" is released. Inadequate filtering, resulting in decreased efficiency of coronary perfusion, is evidenced by a monotonic rise in perfusion pressure over the course of the experiment. For similar reasons, the use of one or more bubble traps is mandatory. The heart itself is located in a 25-mm o.d. glass NMR tube and is bathed in Tyrodes solution, which is removed by a return line located above the NMR coil. It has been the experience of other researchers [4] that a tissue–water interface disturbs the magnetic-field homogeneity rather less than a tissue–air one, hence our decision to opt for this arrangement.

Both perfusion pressure and left ventricular pressure are continuously monitored, the latter with the aid of an isovolumic balloon catheter, and recorded on a Gould 2200S high-speed chart recorder.

Following destruction of the sinoatrial node, hearts are paced at a rate of 1–2 Hz using a Digitimer DS9A stimulator. This is either operated in "free-run" mode or triggered via the Aspect 2000 computer that oversees the operation of the whole spectrometer. In this way, the NMR acquisition can be synchronized with the cardiac cycle. The electrodes consist of two fine-gauge platinum wires that are inserted into the left ventricle. It is important to take steps to prevent introduction of noise and stray radiofrequency (r.f.) into the receiver system via this source: we used r.f. traps (a 15-pF variable capacitor and a parallel inductor, adjusted for resonance at 81 MHz, our 31P operating frequency). These are located immediately outside the receiver coil. In addition, low-pass π filters are inserted in the screened leads as they enter the bore of the superconducting magnet. Such an arrangement introduces negligible additional noise and is more convenient than the use of high-impedance electrodes.

The Bruker WM200 widebore spectrometer used in these experiments is equipped with an Oxford Instruments 4.7 T magnet having a room-temperature bore of 98 mm. Radiofrequency irradiation is used to excite transitions between the Zeeman energy levels that correspond to different orientations of the nuclear magnetic moment in the applied magnetic field. In the case of a spin $\frac{1}{2}$ nucleus such as 31P, only two orientations are possible: parallel or antiparallel. The resonance frequency is proportional to the energy splitting and hence to the strength of the magnetic field. Perturbations in field at the nuclear site that arise from the electronic environment enable chemically distinct 31P atoms to be distinguished by virtue of their different resonance frequencies. These so-called chemical shifts are normally quoted in ppm relative to a fixed standard—in our case PCr, taken to have a shift of 0 ppm. The WM200 operates in Fourier transform mode using a short ($\approx$30 μsec) intense ($\approx$100 W) r.f. pulse to simultaneously excite all 31P resonances. The NMR signal or free induction decay (fid) is detected as the voltage induced in a coil forming part of a tuned circuit. After amplification, detection, digitization, and signal-averaging, the spectrum is obtained from the fid by fast Fourier transformation.

EFFECTS OF PERFUSION RATE AND EXTRACELLULAR PHOSPHATE ON CONTROL CONDITIONS

We perfused our hearts with Tyrodes solution equilibrated with 95% O_2–5% CO_2. The flow rate was established by observing the [PCr]/[ATP]

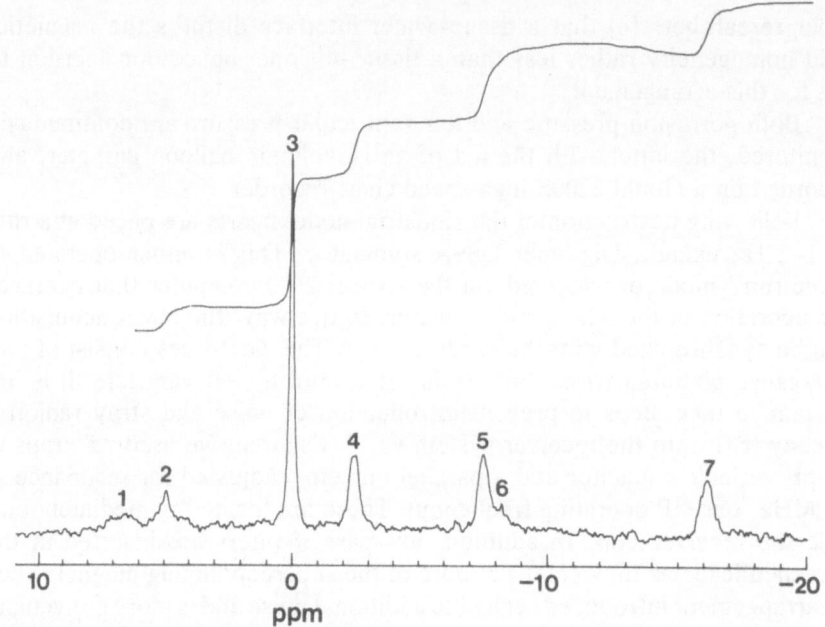

Figure 1. ^{31}P NMR spectrum of a ferret heart perfused in phosphate-free Tyrodes solution at 30°C. Acquisition details: sweepwidth 7.5 kHz, spectral size 8 K, interpulse interval 8 sec, pulse length 45 μsec (90° pulse), number of scans 300, exponential line-broadening 5 Hz. Peak assignments: (1) sugar phosphate; (2) internal P_i, (3) PCr, (4) γ-NTP and β-NDP, essentially γ-ATP; (5) α-NTP and NDP, essentially α-ATP; (6) NAD/NADH; (7) β-NTP, essentially β-ATP. The integral shown above the spectrum is for illustration only; actual areas were determined by cutting and weighing.

ratio. This increased steadily from a value of 1.5–2.0 at a flow rate of 4 ml · g^{-1} · min^{-1}, reaching a plateau value of typically 2.6 at a rate of 10 ml · g^{-1} · min^{-1}. This observation of a sustained improvement in [PCr]/[ATP] ratio at high flow rates suggests that some of the lower values reported in other species may be (at least partially) the result of inadequate perfusion.

The control spectrum of Figure 1 is shown with an exponential line-broadening of 5 Hz, but without application of any convolution difference or other resolution-enhancing procedure. It was obtained with an interpulse delay of 8 sec, sufficient to allow virtually complete relaxation of the spins. It enables one to compare concentrations of the metabolites from the relative integrals of the resonance lines (assignments are indicated in the figure caption). These are shown relative to [ATP] = 1 in the first column of Table 1. Absolute concentrations were also assigned (second column) on the basis of standard biochemical determinations of [ATP] using identically perfused ferret hearts that were freeze-clamped. Note that no resonance is observed in the so-called phosphodiester region of the spectrum (1–4 ppm relative to PCr). This is in contrast to the situation with guinea pig and rabbit hearts,

Table 1. Concentrations of Phosphorylated Metabolites in Perfused Ferret Heart as Determined by ^{31}P NMR

| Metabolite | Concentration | | Saturation factor (1-sec 40° scans) | Uncertainty for 1-min block (N = 5) |
	Relative [ATP] = 1	Absolute (mM)[a]		
Sugar phosphate	0.43	3.8	2.7	—
P_i	0.65	5.7	1.2	10%
PCr	2.65	23.3	1.35	5%
ATP	1	8.8	1.0	7%
NAD/NADH	0.32	2.8	1.0	31%

[a] Based on a value of [ATP] = 4.4 $\mu M \cdot g^{-1}$ wet weight determined by standard biochemical assay.

in which glycerophosphorylcholine is normally observed in substantial amounts. Notice, too, the broad nature of the P_i peak ($\approx$40 Hz), probably to be interpreted in terms of a heterogeneity of pH environment ($\approx$0.4 unit); it is certainly not an artifact caused by magnetic-field inhomogeneity, since the PCr resonance is narrow, usually less than 10 Hz. As is generally the case in perfused tissue, free ADP is below the detection threshold ($\approx$0.2 mM), and the ATP would appear to be completely Mg^{2+}-bound [12].

There has been some controversy regarding the requirement for external phosphate [5,6]. Although under favorable circumstances this can be resolved in the ^{31}P spectrum by virtue of its higher pH [see Figure 2A, wherein external and internal phosphate resonances are seen at shifts (relative to PCr) of 5.177 and 4.94 ppm, corresponding respectively to an external pH of 7.34 and an internal resting one of 7.11], it nevertheless adds uncertainty to the measurement of internal [P_i] and pH and is clearly undesirable in situations in which alkalosis can occur. For these reasons, we normally switch from 1 mM P_i to a P_i-free Tyrodes solution some minutes prior to data acquisition. It has been suggested that internal phosphate is lost to the perfusate during P_i-free perfusion [10]. This has not been the experience of groups working on rat heart preparations perfused with pyruvate, although they do observe an initial fall in [PCr] of about 20% followed by reestablishment of a steady state [11]. We have not observed any fall in [PCr], nor have we seen any evidence of leaking of P_i over a time scale of some hours. This is clearly demonstrated in Figure 2, which compares a control ^{31}P spectrum in the presence of 1 mM P_i (A) with spectra obtained after 4 min (B) and 28 min (C) of P_i-free perfusion. The internal pH remains at 7.11 within 0.01 pH unit, and the PCr concentrations stay within 2% of the P_i-perfused value as determined from the integrals of the PCr resonances. Similarly, no change in any of the other metabolite levels is evident.

In general, the signal available from a single scan (see Figure 3A) will be insufficient for all but the crudest estimate of [PCr], and some tens or perhaps hundreds of scans will be necessary for accurate quantifications. It

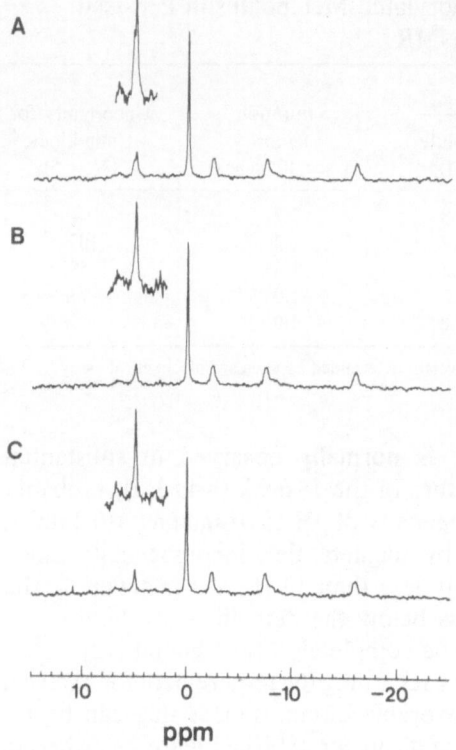

Figure 2.   Effect of removal of phosphate from perfusion medium. (A) Block of 240 1-sec scans with 1 mM external P_i present; (B, C) blocks of 240 1-sec scans 4 min (B) and 28 min (C) following removal of P_i from perfusate. Section plots are ×4. Sweep width 6 kHz, size 8 K, pulse width 20 μsec (40° pulse), line-broadening 8 Hz.

is therefore inconvenient or impossible to wait for 8 sec between r.f. pulses, and the usual solution is to decrease the interpulse interval to about 1 sec while at the same time reducing the r.f. pulse from a 90° to a 45° or 30° one to optimize the signal-to-noise obtained per unit time. Unless the relaxation times of the different metabolites are all equal, this procedure will affect the peak intensities in a differential fashion. However, provided the magnitude of this effect is determined, one can scale each peak by the appropriate "saturation factor" to revert to a true intensity measure. Saturation factors, determined as the ratio of peak areas in 8-sec and 1-sec spectra, are shown in Table 1.

TIME RESOLUTION

The time resolution of the method will of course depend on what quantity we wish to measure and on the accuracy with which the measurement is made. As regards concentrations, the percentage accuracy (of the control values) available from a 1-min block of 1-sec scans is shown for the different metabolites in Table 1. Signal-to-noise and hence accuracy increase as the square root of the number of pulses or equivalently of the elapsed time.

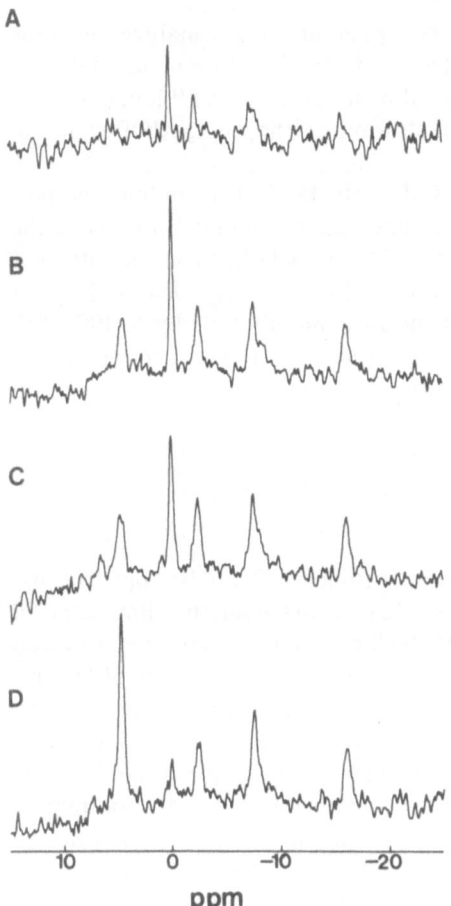

Figure 3. (A) ³¹P NMR spectrum of perfused ferret heart obtained from a single scan. Line-broadening 12 Hz; other acquisition parameters as for Figure 1. (B–D) Blocks of 60 1-sec scans, as control (B) and after 2-min (C) and 10-min (D) exposure to 2 mM NaCN. Sweep width 6 kHz, size 4 K, pulse width 20 μsec (40° pulse), line-broadening 12 Hz.

When it comes to determining the pH, one is interested solely in the position of the P_i resonance, rather than its integral. Unfortunately, as discussed above, the P_i peak is not particularly intense and is relatively broad. This makes the job of pH measurement difficult, particularly under control conditions. We estimate the pH uncertainty in a 1-min data block to be 0.03 unit (1 standard deviation, $N = 5$). Note that this refers to changes in pH and should not be taken as the absolute accuracy of the method, which depends on the particular choice of pH calibration curve.

We have been interested in monitoring the pH following cyanide-induced hypoxia with a view to explaining the transient increase in tension that has previously been shown not to be mirrored in any change in Ca^{2+} level (see the chapter by Orchard, Allen, and Morris). Figure 3 shows the spectra obtained in 1-min blocks as control (B); after 2–min exposure to NaCN, where a slight but definite alkalosis is apparent (C); and after 10-min exposure to NaCN, when the PCr level has dropped virtually to zero and the lactic acidosis is manifest (3). This phenomenon is analyzed in some depth in the chapter by Orchard, Allen, and Morris. Note incidentally (in spectrum D) that even though [PCr] is almost zero, the ATP levels remain undiminished—an unequivocal demonstration of the energy-buffering capacity of PCr.

It has also been possible to follow the effects of drugs on cardiac performance in the guinea pig heart with a time resolution of 0.5 min using the same perfusion system. For example, 10^{-6}M acetylcholine causes a 30–40% reduction in ventricular pressure followed by slow recovery. The ATP levels are sustained during this process, but the PCr initially falls by 5–10%, followed by a recovery. Subsequent treatments show a slower recovery of left ventricular pressure and larger (20–30%), though still reversible, changes in [PCr] [13].

GATED STUDIES

From the foregoing discussion of signal-to-noise, it will be apparent that one cannot in general follow a process that occurs over the time scale of the cardiac cycle unless the process is itself a periodic event synchronized to the cycle. In this case, it is possible to signal-average a series of spectra each collected over the same relative time interval in different heart cycles. Our system lends itself to this type of investigation, since the timing pulses for stimulation and for acquisition are derived from the same source. Suitable software-controlled delays then enable the acquisition period to be moved to any interval within the cardiac cycle. The timing scheme is illustrated in Figure 4. Note that it is not essential to collect data during every cycle; in the studies to be described, the heart was stimulated at a rate of 1.5 Hz and data were collected every fourth cycle, giving 2.64 sec for relaxation recovery between r.f. pulses.

Although it is possible to position the NMR acquisition interval with great precision (1 μsec in our case), this is not the true time resolution of the method as has sometimes been implied [14]—a measurement at a single point in time would clearly give no spectral information! One has to sample for a time that is the inverse of the frequency resolution required and, to fulfill the Nyquist condition, at a rate corresponding to twice the maximum frequency present. In practice, one samples for a relatively long period, perhaps 50–100 msec, and supplements the data set with an equivalent number of zeros prior to Fourier transformation. This process of "zero filling" gives a (genuine) increase in spectral resolution. The true time resolution then is related to the spin–spin relaxation time of the resonance (or alternatively to the inverse of their linewidths), i.e., between 20 and 100 msec depending on the particular metabolite.

We used this method to take essentially 50-msec averages over different parts of the cardiac cycle. Figure 5 shows a series of such spectra obtained

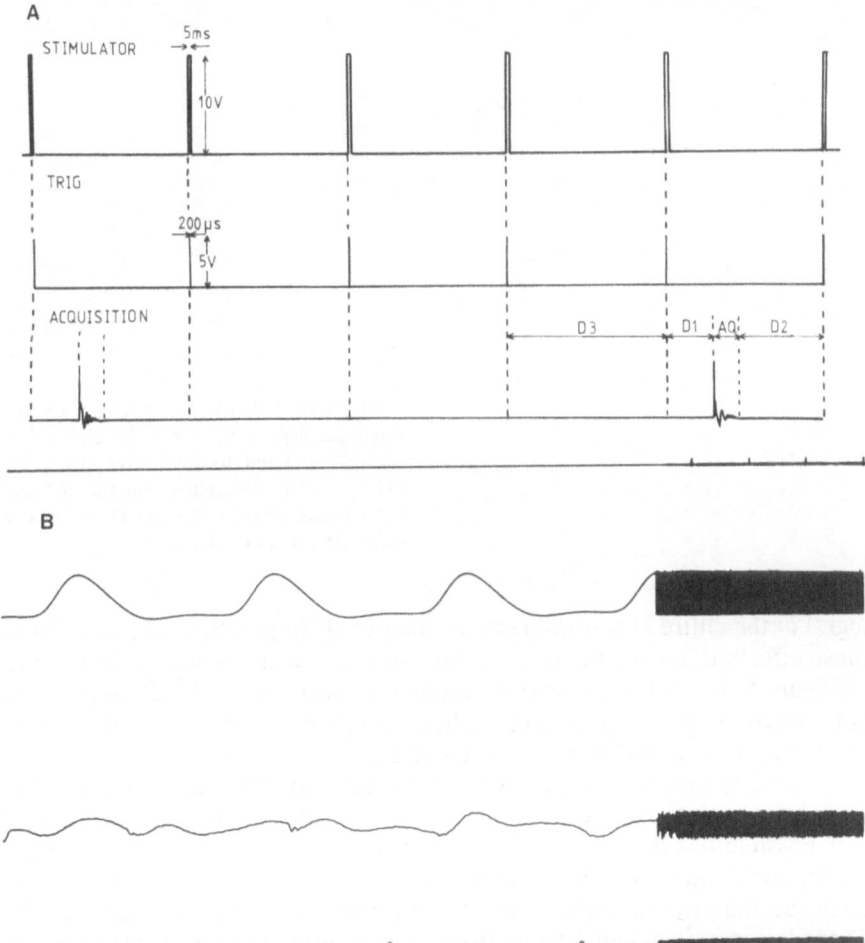

Figure 4. (A) Pulse scheme for gated heart studies. Narrow TTL pulses (TRIG) from the WM200 are used to trigger the stimulator. Location of the acquisition interval (AQ) is achieved by varying D1,D2. For results of Figure 5, D3 = 0.66 sec, AQ = 0.1352 sec, and D1,D2 are chosen such that D1 + D2 + AQ = D3. (B) Gould 2200S chart recording showing left ventricular pressure (upper trace), perfusion pressure (lower trace), and TRIG pulses (lower marker). The left-hand sections of the plots were recorded at higher chart speeds than the right.

at midsystole (A), end systole (B), middiastole (C), and end diastole (D). Great care was taken to ensure that the heart remained entirely within the confines of the receiver coil. Any excursion beyond this limit would have led to the recording of artifactual changes. Similarly, since the receiver-coil response is nonuniform at radial distances greater than 0.7 times the coil radius [15], a change in either the volume or the location of the region occupied by the heart is a potential source of error. It is therefore essential to check that the concentration of total phosphate (as measured from the in-

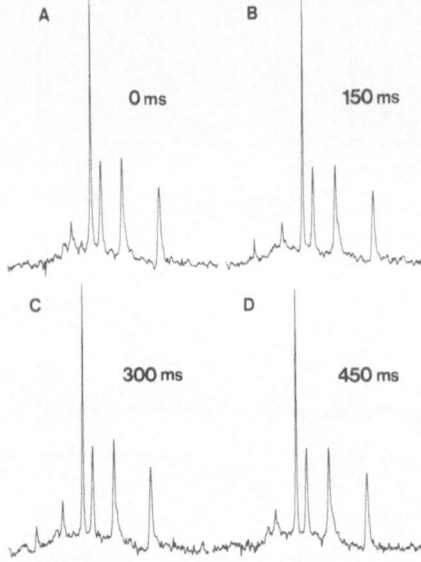

Figure 5.   Set of four gated ^{31}P ferret heart spectra recorded with D1 values (see Figure 4) of 0 (A), 150 (B), 300 (C), and 450 (D) msec, corresponding to mid- and end systole and mid- and end diastole. Sweep width 7.5 kHz, size 2 K, interpulse interval 2.64 sec, pulse length 45 μsec (90° pulse), number of scans 200, line-broadening 12 Hz.

tegral of the entire spectrum) remains unaltered. In practice, we have found these effects to be small, and no correction has been applied to the spectra of Figure 5. In contrast to earlier results on a working rat heart preparation [14], we found no suggestion of cyclical variation in high-energy phosphate concentrations to within an accuracy of 2%.

There is considerable evidence that the performance of the heart is strongly substrate-related [16], and in particular it has been suggested that it is possible to observe phosphate cycling with glucose as sole substrate. Under such conditions, it is possible that the malate aspartate shuttle [17] could become rate-limiting, leading to cyclical variations of NAD/NADH. There is some evidence for this from lactate/pyruvate ratio measurements. Any cycling of NAD/NADH would in turn drive corresponding variations in ADP, ATP, and PCr. Although we have not examined this possibility in the perfused ferret heart, similar studies on Langendorff-perfused guinea pig hearts have failed to demonstrate a positive effect.

ACKNOWLEDGMENTS

We would like to thank Dr. Paul Matthews both for helpful discussion and for his determination of the [ATP] on which the absolute concentrations of Table 1 are based. D.G.A. and C.H.O. would like to acknowledge support from the British Heart Foundation and a grant from the MRC.

REFERENCES

1. Hoult, D. I., Busby, S. J. W., Gadian, D. G., Radda, G. K., Richards, R. E., and Seeley, P. J. 1974. Observation of tissue metabolites using P-31 nuclear magnetic resonance. *Nature* (*London*) 252:285–287.

2. Jacobus, W. E., Taylor, G. J., IV, Hollis, D. P., and Nunnally, R. L. 1977. Phosphorus nuclear magnetic resonance of perfused working rat hearts. *Nature (London)* 265:756–758.
3. Garlick, P. B., Radda, G. K., Seeley, P. J., and Chance, B. 1977. Phosphorus NMR studies on perfused heart. *Biochem. Biophys. Res. Commun.* 74:1256–1262.
4. Ingwall, J. S. 1982. Phosphorus nuclear magnetic resonance spectroscopy of cardiac and skeletal muscles. *Am. J. Physiol.* 242:H729–H744.
5. Dawson, M. J. 1983. Nuclear magnetic resonance. In: A. J. Drake-Holland and M. I. M. Noble (eds.), *Cardiac Metabolism.* pp. 309–337. Wiley and Sons, Chichester.
6. Dawson, M. J., and Wilkie, D. R. 1983. Muscle and brain metabolism studied by ^{31}P nuclear magnetic resonance. In: P. Baker (ed.), *Recent Advances in Physiology.* pp. 247–276. Churchill Livingstone, Edinburgh.
7. Neurohr, K. J., Barrett, E. J., and Shulman, R. G. 1983. In vivo carbon-13 nuclear magnetic resonance studies of heart metabolism. *Proc. Natl. Acad. Sci. U.S.A.* 80:1603–1607.
8. Moon, R. B., and Richards, J. H. 1973. Determination of intracellular pH as observed by 31-P magnetic resonance. *J. Biol. Chem.* 248:7276–7278.
9. Allen, D. G., and Orchard, C. H. 1983. Intracellular calcium concentration during hypoxia and metabolic inhibition in mammalian ventricular muscle. *J. Physiol.* 339:107–122.
10. Salhany, J. M., Pieper, G. M. Wu, S., Todd, G. L., Clayton, F. C., and Eli, R. S. 1979. P-31 nuclear magnetic resonance measurement of cardiac pH in perfused guinea-pig hearts. *J. Mol. Cell Cardiol.* 11:601–610.
11. Matthews, P. M. 1982. Applications of NMR to the study of cardiac metabolism. Ph.D. thesis, Oxford.
12. Gupta, R. K., Benovic, J. L., and Rose, Z. B. 1978. The determination of the free magnesium level in the human red blood cell by P-31 NMR. *J. Biol. Chem.* 253:6172–6176.
13. Morris, P. G., Burgen, A. S. V., Harbird, C. J., and Callingham, B. W. 1982. Unpublished results.
14. Fossel, E. T., Morgan, H. E., and Ingwall, J. S. 1980. Measurement of changes in high-energy phosphates in the cardiac cycle using gated P-31 NMR. *Proc. Natl. Acad. Sci. U.S.A.* 77:3654–3658.
15. Mansfield, P., and Morris, P. G. 1982. NMR Imaging in Biomedicine. *Advances in Magnetic Resonance*, Supplement 2. Academic Press, New York.
16. Matthews, P. M., Williams, S. R., Seymour, A. M., Schwartz, A., Dube, G., Gadian, D. G., and Radda, G. K. 1982. A phosphorus-31 NMR study of some metabolic and functional effects of the inotropic agents epinephrine and ouabain, and the ionophore Ro2-2985 (X537A) in the isolated perfused rat heart. *Biochim. Biophys. Acta* 720:163–171.
17. La Noue, K. F., and Schoolwerth, A. C. 1979. Metabolic transport in mitochondria. *Annu. Rev. Biochem.* 48:871–922.

MOLECULAR BASIS OF ELECTROPHYSIOLOGY

Molecular Approach to the Calcium Channel

H. Glossmann, D. R. Ferry, A. Goll, and T. Linn

Rudolf Buchheim-Institut für Pharmakologie
Justus Liebig Universität, Giessen
D-63 Giessen, Federal Republic of Germany

Abstract. Tritiated 1,4-dihydropyridines (nimodipine, nitrendipine, nifedipine, PN 200-110) and [^{3}H]D-*cis*-diltiazem as well as [^{3}H]verapamil were employed to directly identify calcium channels in membranes from excitable tissues. The channels, when probed with 1,4-dihydropyridines, exhibit the following properties:

1. 1,4-Dihydropyridine calcium channel blockers bind in a temperature-dependent, reversible manner and with high affinity (dissociation constants 0.2–2 nM at 37°C) to a finite number of sites. For chiral 1,4-dihydropyridines, the binding is stereoselective. Hill slopes of approximately 1.0 are observed.
2. In brain, heart, and solubilized skeletal-muscle membranes, an absolute requirement for certain divalent cations exists in order to bind the ligands with high affinity. Cooperativity (negative and positive) between Me^{2+} and 1,4-dihydropyridine binding sites is observed.
3. 1,4-Dihydropyridine binding sites are down-regulated in a complex manner by the optically pure enantiomers of D-600 and verapamil. These channel blockers induce, to a different extent, a low-affinity state of the 1,4-dihydropyridine binding site. It is postulated that this allosteric site, at which these blockers act, is closely coupled to the 1,4-dihydropyridine binding site and that a spectrum of compounds exists that differ in their affinity as well as their intrinsic activity to induce the down-regulation.
4. The 1,4-dihydropyridine binding sites are up-regulated by D-*cis*-diltiazem and KB-944. The up-regulation is temperature-dependent and induces a high-affinity state for 1,4-dihydropyridine channel blockers, accompanied by distinct alterations of the kinetics as well as the pharmacological profile of the 1,4-dihydropyridine binding sites. Complex interactions exist between the channel blockers that induce up-regulation and those that induce down-regulation of the binding.
5. For a given radiolabeled 1,4-dihydropyridine, a tissue-specific (but not species-specific) equilibrium binding dissociation constant is observed. Thus, all hearts (human, rat, guinea pig, frog, bovine) have the same K_D (0.25 nM at 37°C) for, [^{3}H]nimodipine. The same is observed for brain (K_D = 0.5 nM) and for skeletal muscle (K_D = 1–2 nM). Three subtypes of channels can be distinguished on the basis of the K_D and the tissue-specific up-regulation by D-*cis*-diltiazem. Subtype-selective drugs exist; e.g., AQA 39 is an inhibitor of [^{3}H]nimodipine binding at skeletal-muscle calcium channels, but not at brain channels.
6. Despite their different pharmacological and kinetic profiles, calcium channels in skeletal muscle and brain have the same molecular size (M_r) when probed by radiation inactivation. The apparent M_r of the brain channel (probed with [^{3}H]nimodipine) is 185,000; the M_r of the skeletal-muscle channel is 178,000.
7. The M_r of the channel, as evaluated by radiation inactivation, is decreased by 60,000–75,000 when channels are up-regulated by D-*cis*-diltiazem. The action of D-*cis*-diltiazem is stereospecific, since L-*cis*-diltiazem is inactive. In addition, neither benzodiazepine receptor M_r (in brain) nor acetylcholinesterase M_r (in skeletal muscle) is decreased by D-*cis*-diltiazem.

8. Different 1,4-dihydropyridines do not label the same density of binding sites, e.g., in skeletal-muscle membranes, in the absence or presence of D-*cis*-diltiazem. The concept of intrinsic activity for a given 1,4-dihydropyridine is introduced, based on its ability to induce or stabilize a high-affinity state. Most notable is that [^{3}H]-PN 200-110 labels more sites in skeletal muscle than nifedipine, nimodipine, or nitrendipine.

9. [^{3}H]-PN 200-110 binding to skeletal-muscle microsomes is stimulated by the allosteric regulator D-*cis*-diltiazem. However, although the kinetic constants are changed by D-*cis*-diltiazem, there is, in contrast to [^{3}H]nimodipine or [^{3}H]nitrendipine, only a small increase with respect to the density of sites labeled by [^{3}H]-PN 200-110.

10. The M_r of the skeletal-muscle calcium channel, determined by radiation inactivation and with [^{3}H]-PN-200-110 as ligand, is 138,000, this being 40,000 mass units smaller than that determined with [^{3}H]nimodipine. These findings, taken together with the stereospecific effects of D-*cis*-diltiazem on the M_r of [^{3}H]nimodipine-labeled channels in brain and skeletal muscle, are indicative of an oligomeric nature of the channel and support the concept of a continuum of 1,4-dihydropyridines ranging from agonists to antagonists.

11. The allosteric regulatory sites that interact with the 1,4-dihydropyridine site have been directly labeled with [^{3}H]D-*cis*-diltiazem in skeletal muscle. Binding of [^{3}H]D-*cis*-diltiazem is temperature-dependent, and maximal labeling of 11 pmole binding sites with a K_D of 39 nM occurs at 2°C. The ratio of allosteric sites to 1,4-dihydropyridine binding sites appears to be 1:1 or 1:2, depending on the radioligand. Binding of D-*cis*-diltiazem is regulated in a complex manner by calcium-channel agonists and antagonists. At temperatures greater than 20°C, 1,4-dihydropyridine-channel antagonists stimulate; at 2°C, they are inhibitors. The rank order of efficacies (as well as the respective IC_{50} or EC_{50} values) differs for stimulation and inhibition and is typical for a given 1,4-dihydropyridine. On the basis of these findings, agonists and antagonists (which keep channels in unshut and shut states) are discriminated.

12. Skeletal-muscle calcium channels can be purified in t-tubular membranes. The density of channels is extremely high ($\approx$60,000 fmoles/mg protein). The channel has been solubilized in good yield with detergents and is stable at 4°C with a half-life of 60 hr or more. The $S_{20,w}$ value is 12.9 S, and sucrose-gradient-purified channels are still up-regulated by D-*cis*-diltiazem. The channel is a glycoprotein, since it is selectively adsorbed by lectin-affinity columns and desorbed (17- to 40-fold purified) by corresponding sugars.

INTRODUCTION

Inward transmembrane currents dependent on the presence of extracellular calcium have been measured for nearly two decades. These currents have been recorded in dendrites, presynaptic terminals, smooth-muscle cells, mammalian myocardium, and molluscan neurons.

The study of calcium currents has proved more difficult than that of sodium currents. This is due in part to the lack of an electrical preparation equivalent to the squid giant-axon preparation for sodium-current dissection. Although the electrical study of the calcium channel may be regarded as somewhat behind the level of sophistication already applied to the sodium channel, the biochemical study of the membrane structure(s) associated with calcium currents (calcium channels) in contrast to sodium channels has hardly started. In part, this may be related to the fact that no toxins, with the exception of maitotoxin, equivalent in potency to tetrodotoxin, the scorpion toxins, sea anemone toxins, or lipid-soluble polycyclic alkaloids such as veratridine and batrachotoxin have been described that modulate calcium-channel function at low concentrations (<100 nM). However, numerous man-made drugs have been synthesized that regulate calcium channels by block-ade. In contrast to many sodium-channel toxins, these calcium-channel drugs are not highly toxic to mammals. Calcium-channel blockers are ef-fective therapeutic agents in man for arrhythmias, angina, vasospastic dis-orders, and hypertension. Perhaps this low toxicity of the man-made cal-cium-channel blockers explains why nature has found no advantage in preserving genes for the synthesis of calcium-channel-blocking toxins. When relatively selective calcium-channel-blocking drugs became available, it was found experimentally that their action was equivalent to removal of extra-cellular calcium. The electric current due to Ca^{2+} conductance disappears and there is a simultaneous loss of the contractile responses of, for example, the myocardium [1]. For these reasons, the calcium-channel blockers have become known as "calcium antagonists." Calcium antagonists are chemi-cally a highly diverse set of substances. Of all the known calcium antagonists, 1,4-dihydropyridines are the most potent. In electrophysiological and classic pharmacological experiments, nifedipine has ED_{50} values in the range 10–100 nM for cellular responses dependent on the presence of extracellular Ca^{2+} [2,3]. Although nifedipine is a powerful calcium antagonist, certain chiral 1,4-dihydropyridines are significantly more potent, at least in vascular smooth muscle [4]. The chiral 1,4-dihydropyridine nitrendipine lowers the blood pressure of renal hypertensive dogs, and of rats with either renal hypertension or deoxycorticosterone acetate hypertension, in doses as low as 1 mg·kg^{-1}. The high potency, apparent channel selectivity, and stereo-specificity of the action of the 1,4-dihydropyridines suggested that they could be employed in radiolabeled form as ligands to directly identify the site of action (assumed to be the putative calcium channel) in membranes of ex-citable tissues.

The sections that follow cover the main findings of the Giessen group in this field. The basic properties of the binding sites (or drug receptors) for 1,4-dihydropyridines are presented, the cooperative interactions of divalent cations with the binding sites are exemplified for the brain calcium channel, the concept of multiple drug-receptor sites within the channel is developed, and evidence for the existence of subtypes of calcium channels (which occur in a tissue- but not species-specific manner) is given. Data on the molecular size of the calcium channel in situ, as probed by radiation-inactivation with high-energy electrons, are presented. The fascinating finding that up-regu-lation of 1,4-dihydropyridine binding by the allosteric regulator D-cis-dilti-azem is accompanied by a reduction in the apparent M_r of the channel is discussed in light of the differential labeling of the channels by different 1,4-dihydropyridines. Further support for the multiple-receptor-site concept comes from direct labeling of the other receptor sites (e.g., with [^{3}H]D-cis-diltiazem and [^{3}H]verapamil), and finally, the solubilization and partial pu-rification of the calcium channel are reported. We realize that at the time of writing, most of our work (as well as that of others) has concentrated on brain, heart, and skeletal muscle. For adult brain and skeletal muscle, no obvious pharmacological actions of the potent 1,4-dihydropyridine calcium-channel blockers have been reported, and large discrepancies exist between the measured binding constants for calcium-channel blockers in vitro and the constants derived from pharmacological experiments with isolated heart cells.

However, the three tissues are quite rich with respect to 1,4-dihydro-pyridine binding sites, and skeletal muscle can be truly termed the electric eel for the biochemist who is trying to purify the channel. So far, no obvious differences are apparent (with the exception of the existence of subtypes) between the properties of the channels in tissues in which a good correlation to the pharmacological data exists (smooth muscle) and those tissues in which either such a correlation is not yet possible (brain, skeletal muscle) or discrepancies are evident (heart). The discrepancies may result from (1) the partial agonism of the drugs, which may be a function of the chemical structure as well as of the tissue; (2) the existence of intracellular, tissue-specific factors that antagonize or modulate the action of calcium-channel blockers; (3) failure to ask the appropriate question with respect to channel function in a given tissue; (4) a biased selection of drugs; or a combination of any of these points.

BASIC PROPERTIES OF 1,4-DIHYDROPYRIDINE-LABELED CALCIUM CHANNELS

Figure 1 shows the radioligands that were employed to label calcium channels. Findings with [^{3}H]verapamil and [^{3}H]D-*cis*-diltiazem are summarized in the section entitled "Labeling of the drug receptors that allo-sterically regulate the binding of 1,4-dihydropyridines to calcium channels."

Table 1 shows the tissue distribution of 1,4-dihydropyridine binding sites, labeled by [^{3}H]nimodipine at 37°C. Clearly, skeletal muscle, heart, and brain offer excellent signals, whereas other tissues are somewhat problematic to work with. It was decided to investigate the properties of the calcium channels in heart (a partially purified sarcolemma preparation from bovine heart was employed), guinea pig brain, and guinea pig hindlimb skeletal muscle.

Bovine Heart Calcium Channel

[^{3}H]Nimodipine binds to a single class of binding sites in bovine sar-colemma with a K_D of 0.25 nM and a B_{max} of 350–900 fmoles/mg; the Hill slope is 1.0. Equilibrium binding parameters in comparison with hearts from other species are shown in Table 2. In competition experiments against [^{3}H]nimodipine in this tissue, Bay e (−)6927 had an IC$_{50}$ of 300 pM and Bay e (+)6927 an IC$_{50}$ of 20 nM; Bay e (−)6927 was 66 times more potent than

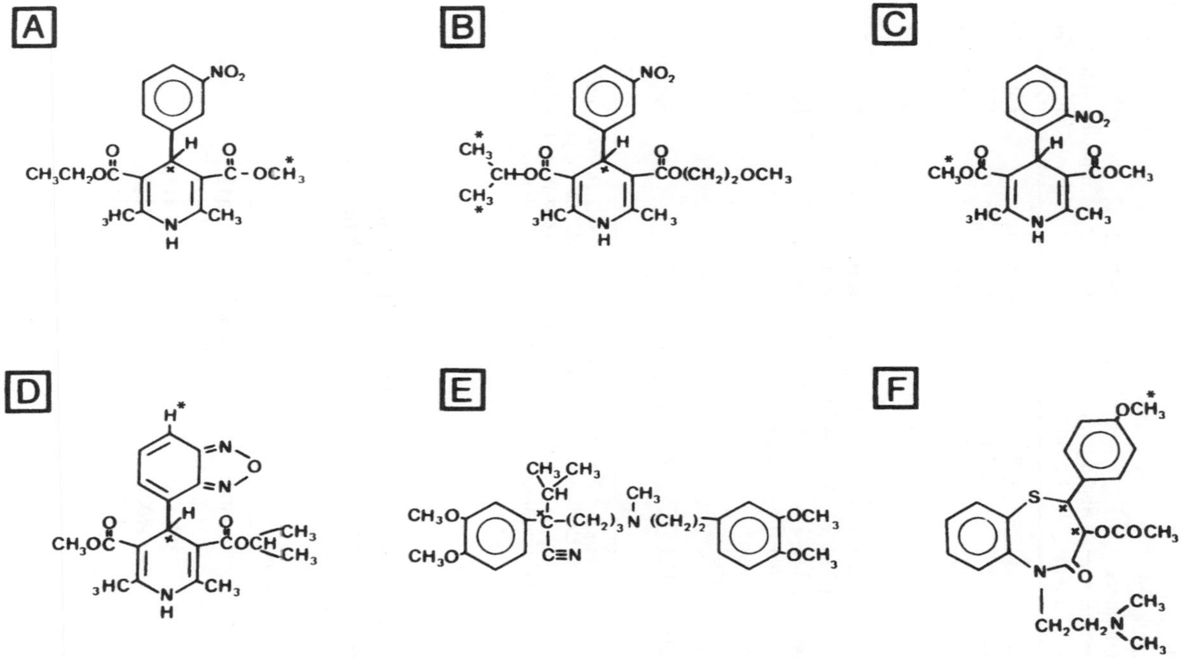

Figure 1. Structures of radiolabeled 1,4-dihydropyridines, verapamil, and diltiazem. (*) position of T; (×) an asymmetrical carbon atom. (A) (±) [³H]nitrendipine [1,4-dihydro-2,6-dimethyl (3-nitrophenyl)-3,5-pyridine carboxylic acid, 3 ethyl-5-methyl ester]; (B) (±) [³H]nimodipine [isopropyl (2-methoxymethyl)-1,4-dihydro-2,6-dimethyl-4-(3-nitrophenyl)-3,5-pyridinedicarboxylate]; (C) [³H]nifedipine [dimethyl,1,1,4-dihydro-2,6-dimethyl 1,4-(2-nitrophenyl)-3,5-pyridine dicarboxylate]; (D) (±) [³H]-PN 200-110 [isopropyl 4-(2,1,3-benzoxadiazol-4-yl)-1,4-dihydro-2,6-dimethyl-5-methoxy carbonyl-pyridine-3-carboxylate]; (E) (±) verapamil [5-N-(3,4-dimethoxyphenethyl)-N-methylamino-2-(3,4-dimethoxy phenyl)-2-isopropylvaleronitrile; (F) D,L-cis,trans-diltiazem [3-acetoxy-2,3-dihydro-5-2-(diethylamino)ethyl-2-(p-methoxy phenyl)-1,5-benzothiazepine-4-(5H)-one hydrochloride]. The labeled compound is D-cis-diltiazem.

Table 1.   Distribution of [^{3}H]Nimodipine Binding[a]

Tissue	Bound radioligand (dpm/filter)		Signal-to-noise ratio	Protein/assay tube (μg)	Specific binding (fmoles/mg protein)
	Total	Blank			
Skeletal muscle	33,062	2,710	11.2	48.2	1770
Heart	15,291	3,287	3.65	91.2	371
Adrenal gland	2,890	1,303	1.22	21.1	212
Hippocampus	9,716	3,224	2.01	91.3	200
Olfactory tubercle	4,666	1,200	2.89	60.0	163
Cerebral cortex	13,518	2,582	4.24	200.0	153
Uterus	3,241	1,276	1.54	36.4	152
Duodenum	5,006	2,331	1.15	60.5	124
Kidney	19,179	15,880	0.21	300.5	31
Liver	39,698	30,926	0.28	530.0	48
Fat-cell membranes	434	585	0	3.6	—
Blood-platelet membranes	1,082	1,023	0	35.2	—

[a] Tissues were prepared from the guinea pig. [^{3}H]Nimodipine was 0.98 nM. Values are from duplicate incubations that varied less than 10%. Skeletal muscle, heart, and cerebral cortex have excellent signal-to-noise ratios. Fat-cell membranes (which were from hamsters) and human blood platelets did not bind [^{3}H]nimodipine specifically under the conditions employed. Signal-to-noise ratio is defined as (total dpm − blank dpm)/(blank dpm).

Table 2. B_{max} and K_D Values for [^{3}H]Nimodipine Binding to Heart Membranes from Various Species[a]

Species	B_{max} (fmoles/mg protein)	K_D (nM)	Reference
Guinea pig	350	0.26	[12]
Rat	400	0.24	[13]
Bovine	350–980	0.25	[14]
Frog	1700	0.29	[15]
Human	100	0.28	[16]

[a] Saturation isotherms were constructed with 0.05–2 nM [^{3}H]nimodipine (without taking account of its racemic nature) and for the rat heart with 0.026–0.7 nM [^{3}H]nimodipine. Guinea pig, bovine, and human heart (intraventricular wall from patients with hypertrophic cardiac myopathy) equilibrium binding experiments were performed at 37°C; the frog and rat heart experiments were performed at 22°C.

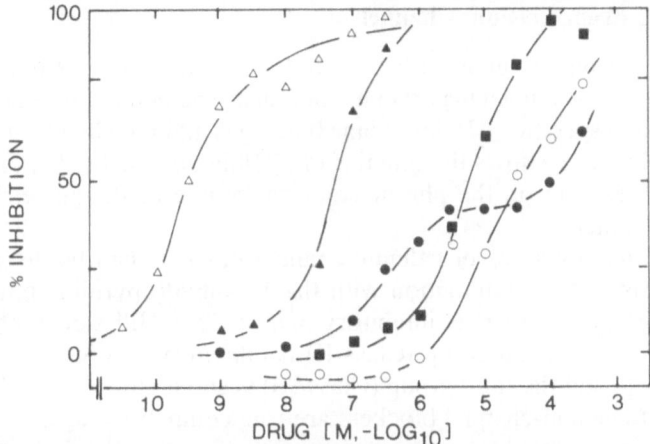

Figure 2.   Pharmacological profile of [³H]nimodipine binding in bovine heart sarcolemma. Purified bovine sarcolemma (11–15 μg/0.25 ml) and [³H]nimodipine (0.3–0.7 nM) were incubated for 30 min at 37°C in the presence of increasing concentration of unlabeled calcium antagonists. The figure illustrates the stereospecific nature of [³H]nimodipine binding for the Class I 1,4-dihydropyridine calcium antagonists (−)6927 (△) and (+)6927 (▲), and (+)fendiline (■), with slope factors close to unity. In contrast, the Class II calcium antagonist (−)D-600 (●) displays a markedly biphasic inhibition profile; (+)D-600 (○) shows a rather flat inhibition profile, but lacks the high-affinity component seen with (−)D-600.

the Bay e (+)6927 (Figure 2). Fendiline is a calcium antagonist structurally unrelated to 1,4-dihydropyridines and competed with [³H]nimodipine binding with Hill slopes close to unity. The optically pure enantiomers of D-600 inhibited specific [³H]nimodipine binding in a stereoselective manner in bovine sarcolemma. A typical example of this competition behavior is shown in Figure 2. (−)D-600 displays a high-affinity component with an IC_{50} value of 500 nM and a low-affinity component with an IC_{50} value of 300 μM. The (+)D-600 competition profile is not as markedly biphasic as that of the (−)D 600. In addition, (+)D-600 has no component of as high affinity as the (−)D-600 high-affinity site. D-*cis*-Diltiazem stimulated specific [³H]nimodipine binding in bovine sarcolemma. These observations in bovine sarcolemma indicated that the calcium antagonists were a subdividable set on the basis of their interaction with [³H]nimodipine binding sites. Three main classes (I–III) of antagonists appeared to exist: Class I (e.g., the 1,4-dihydropyridines), which competed in a monophasic manner; Class II (e.g., the enantiomers of D-600), which displayed complex inhibition behavior; and Class III (e.g., D-*cis*-diltiazem), which did not inhibit [³H]nimodipine binding, but stimulated it. To generalize our findings, we have performed a detailed study of the structure–function relationship of various calcium antagonists to the calcium channel in membranes from guinea pig brain.

Guinea Pig Brain Calcium Channel

[^{3}H]Nimodipine binds with a K_D of 0.62 nM at 37°C to 350–600 fmoles of binding sites in guinea pig brain membranes. The binding sites are trypsin-sensitive, and specific [^{3}H]nimodipine binding is inhibited by phospholipases A and C. Figure 3 shows the kinetics of [^{3}H]nimodipine binding, and Table 3 summarizes data on the pharmacological profile of the guinea pig brain calcium channel.

Three main classes of calcium-channel blockers can be discriminated on the basis of their interaction with the 1,4-dihydropyridine binding site. The first group (Class I) is inhibitory and exhibits Hill slopes of approximately 1.0, the second group (Class II) is inhibitory and has Hill slopes of less than 1.0, and the third group (Class III) is stimulatory (at 37°C). Among the Class I calcium-channel blockers are true competitive agents, allosteric regulators, and mixed-type compounds. They can be discriminated by kinetic and saturation experiments and also by the effects of D-*cis*-diltiazem on the binding-inhibition profile. The latter calcium-channel blocker is the prototype of a novel class of agents that allosterically up-regulate the 1,4-dihydropyridine binding in a temperature-dependent manner. KB-944 is another representative of this group.

The interaction of the Class II channel blockers with the 1,4-dihydropyridine binding site is complicated. In general, these agents are negative allosteric regulators of 1,4-dihydropyridine channel blocker binding. The complications arise from the fact that the optical enantiomers of D-600 and verapamil, which are prototypes, behave quite differently. For example, in some tissues, e.g., the human heart, (–)verapamil has less intrinsic activity but apparent higher affinity compared with (+)verapamil to induce a low-affinity state for 1,4-dihydropyridine channel blocker binding. In skeletal muscle, (–)D-600 is not inhibitory at all; in contrast, when the channel is up-regulated by D-*cis*-diltiazem at 37°C, it is inhibitory.

Figure 4 demonstrates that the optically pure enantiomers of the racemic Class II channel blockers are needed to evaluate their interaction with the 1,4-dihydropyridine binding site. The Class III calcium-channel blockers not only regulate the binding of the 1,4-dihydropyridines (mainly by decreasing the half-life of the channel–ligand complex) but also change, in a rather dramatic way, the regulation by the Class II channel blockers. For example, in guinea pig brain membranes, both (+) and (–)verapamil exhibited complex competition profiles (Figure 4). The binding-inhibition data could be adequately described under the assumption of two (high- and low-affinity) binding sites. The (–)verapamil high-affinity site had a K_D (K_D high) of 61 nM, which was of 3.1-fold higher affinity than the (+)verapamil high-affinity site (K_D high 191 nM). The (–) verapamil high-affinity component represented 30% of the total (–)verapamil binding, but the high-affinity (+)verapamil site represented 67% of the total (+)verapamil binding (Table 3). The (+)verapamil low-affinity site was of higher affinity than the (–)verapamil low-affinity site by a factor of 4.

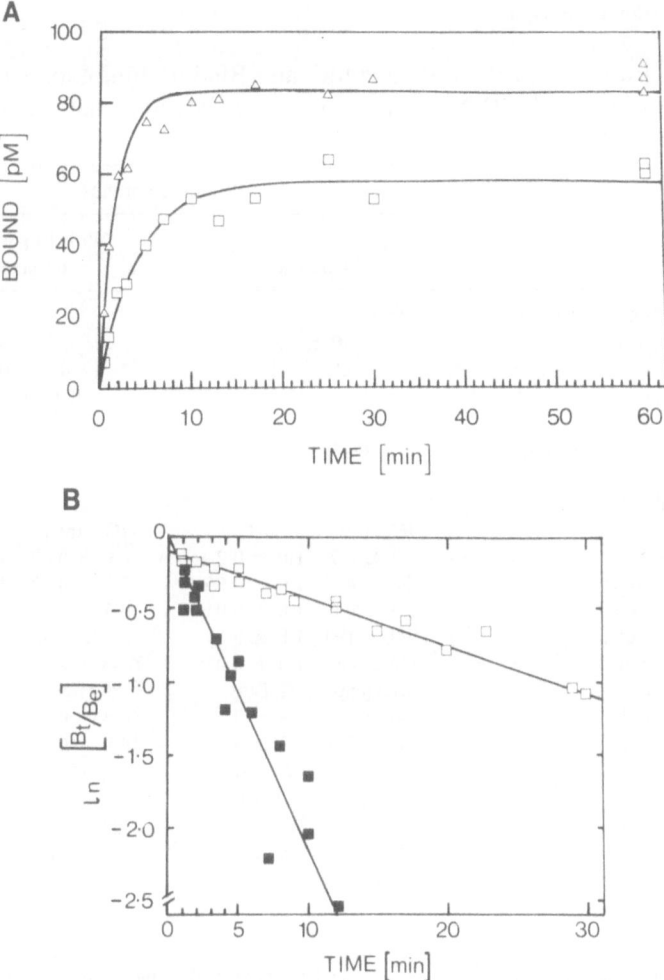

Figure 3. (A) Association kinetics of [^{3}H]nimodipine with guinea pig brain membranes. Guinea pig brain membranes were preincubated in buffer A for 30 min at 30°C in a volume of 0.2 ml at a protein concentration of 460 µg/ml. Association reactions were initiated by adding 50 µl [^{3}H]nimodipine that was prewarmed to 30°C. The association reactions were performed at [^{3}H]-ligand concentrations (bindable enantiomers) of 0.28 nM ($\square$) and 1.11 nM ($\triangle$). Calculating the bound/free ratios at the radioligand concentrations allows the B_{max} to be estimated (300 fmoles/mg, which corresponds to a receptor concentration of 138 pM). Data points are fitted directly to the differential form of the second-order rate equation by the error-sum-of-squares principle. At a [^{3}H]nimodipine concentration of 0.28 nM, the best parameter estimates (± asymptotic standard deviation) were k_{+1} (association rate constant) = 0.135 ± 0.34 nM^{-1}·min^{-1} and k_{-1} (dissociation rate constant) = 0.12 ± 0.02·min^{-1}, and at a [^{3}H]nimodipine concentration of 1.11 nM, k_{+1} = 0.279 ± 0.026 nM^{-1}·min^{-1} and k_{-1} = 0.22 ± 0.03 min^{-1}. (B) Temperature dependence of [^{3}H]nimodipine dissociation from calcium channels. [^{3}H]Nimodipine was allowed to associate for 30 min at 37 or 25°C with guinea pig brain membranes. Nimodipine (25 µM, 10 µl) was added for up to 30 min prior to the separation of bound and free radioactivity. The plot of the natural logarithm of the ratio of specific binding after a given time of addition of unlabeled drug (B_t) to specific binding at equilibrium (B_e) is linear. At 37°C ($\blacksquare$), the dissociation rate constant (k_{-1}), calculated from the slope of the plot, is 0.19 min^{-1}. At 25°C ($\square$), k_{-1} is 0.032 min^{-1}; thus, the mean half-life of channel–[^{3}H]nimodipine complexes is 5.9 times longer at 25°C.

Table 3. Equilibrium Binding, Kinetic, and Binding-Inhibition Constants for Various Drugs of [^{3}H]Nimodipine-Labeled Calcium Channels in Brain[a]

	Brain membranes			
	Control		With 10 μM D-*cis*-diltiazem	
Equilibrium binding and kinetic parameters				
B_{max} (fmoles/mg protein)	570 ± 99		452 ± 35	
Dissociation constant (nM)	0.6 ± 0.1		0.2 ± 0.01	
Association rate constant [nM^{-1} · min^{-1}]	0.32 ± 0.05		0.37 ± 0.10	
Dissociation rate constant [min^{-1}]	0.18 ± 0.01		0.05 ± 0.005	
Binding-inhibition data				
Drug	IC$_{50}$ [nM]	nH	IC$_{50}$ [nM]	nH
Niludipine	5.7 ± 2.7	1.0 ± 0.2	0.6 ± 0.07	1.0 ± 0.07
(−)Nicardipine	28 ± 4	1.0 ± 0.06	3.2 ± 0.07	1.0 ± 0.01
(+)Nicardipine	2.3 ± 0.6	1.0 ± 0.04	0.7 ± 0.07	1.0 ± 0.01
(−)Prenylamine	590 ± 190	1.0 ± 0.05	1200 ± 300	1.1 ± 0.2
(+)Prenylamine	420 ± 45	1.0 ± 0.05	1200 ± 230	1.4 ± 0.11
	% High	% Low	% High	% Low
(−)Verapamil	30 ± 7	69 ± 7	46.3 ± 0.8	54 ± 0.8
(+)Verapamil	67 ± 5	33 ± 5	14.0 ± 6	86 ± 6
	K_D high (nM)	K_D low (nM)	K_D high (nM)	K_D low (nM)
(−)Verapamil	61 ± 30	280 ± 80	2200 ± 330	246 ± 75
(+)Verapamil	191 ± 20	70 ± 30	450 ± 210	23 ± 0.6
Diltiazem diastereoisomers	IC$_{50}$ (μM)		EC$_{50}$ (μM)	
D-*cis*-Diltiazem	—		0.38 ± 0.07	
L-*cis*-Diltiazem	221 ± 60		—	

[a] Equilibrium binding and kinetic parameters were calculated without taking into account the racemic nature of [^{3}H]nimodipine. The biphasic verapamil inhibition curves for brain membranes were analyzed with the LIGAND computer package. (nH) Hill slope. Data are from 37°C experiments. For D-*cis*-diltiazem, the EC$_{50}$ value for stimulation is given.

The inclusion of diltiazem (10 μM) led to characteristic and highly reproducible changes in the binding-inhibition profiles of the verapamil enantiomers. Diltiazem reduced the affinity of the (−)verapamil high-affinity site by a factor of 36, whereas the K_D of the low-affinity site of verapamil was unchanged. The effect of diltiazem on (+)verapamil was to reduce the proportion of high-affinity sites from 66.7 to 14.5%. However, the affinity of [^{3}H]nimodipine for the low-affinity (+)verapamil site increased by a factor of 3 (Table 3).

Metalloprotein Nature of the Calcium Channels as Revealed by 1,4-Dihydropyridine Channel Blocker Binding

The binding of tritiated 1,4-dihydropyridines to brain and heart membranes as well as solubilized skeletal-muscle membranes is inhibited by che-

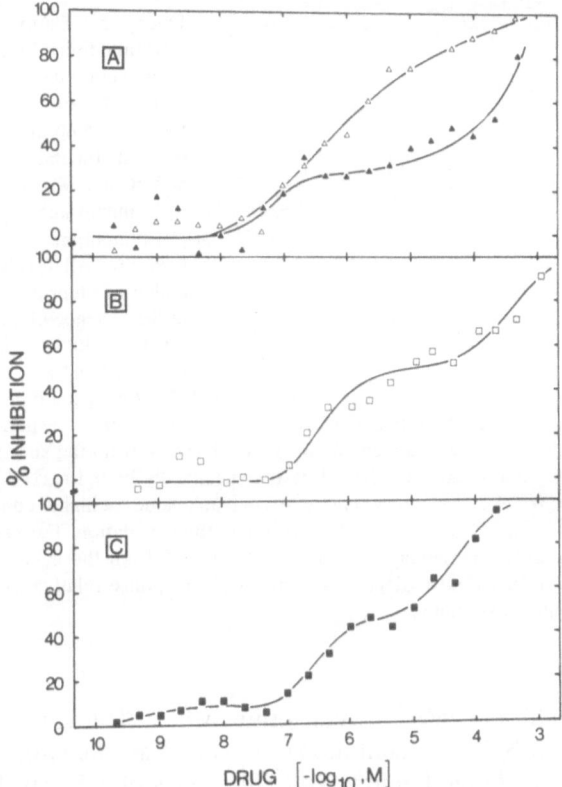

Figure 4.   Inhibition of [^{3}H]nimodipine binding by ($-$)verapamil, ($+$)verapamil, and ($\pm$)verapamil in guinea pig brain membranes. (A) ($-$)Verapamil (▲) and ($+$)verapamil (△) exhibit complex biphasic inhibition profiles, indicative of the heterogeneity of the receptor sites for these Class II calcium antagonists. The experiment was performed with 0.069 mg guinea pig brain membrane protein and 0.88 nM [^{3}H]nimodipine. (B) Algebraic addition of the ($-$) and ($+$)verapamil inhibition curves shown in (A). (C) Inhibition profile of ($\pm$)verapamil. The experiment was performed as in (A). The [^{3}H]nimodipine concentration was 0.78 nM.

lators. Addition of EDTA or CDTA to guinea pig brain membranes inhibits specific [^{3}H]nimodipine binding in a dose-dependent manner. The ED_{50} for EDTA is in the range of 10–20 μM. The inhibition by EDTA is due to chelation of divalent cations and is reversible. Saturation experiments revealed that the chelation of endogenous cations reduces the B_{max} for [^{3}H]nimodipine without changing the K_D (not shown). When guinea pig brain membranes are incubated with 5 mM EDTA for 30 min at 37°C and subsequently washed thoroughly in buffer to remove the chelator, the specific [^{3}H]nimodipine binding is lost to a large extent (95–100%).

High-affinity binding can be restored by addition of Me^{2+}, this reconstitution by Me^{2+} occurring in a dose-dependent manner. The ED_{50} of Mn^{2+} is 11 μM, for Ca^{2+} 14 μM, and for Mg^{2+} 43 μM. Sr^{2+} is less potent, with an ED_{50} of 99 μM. The slope factors of the divalent cation reconstitution is-

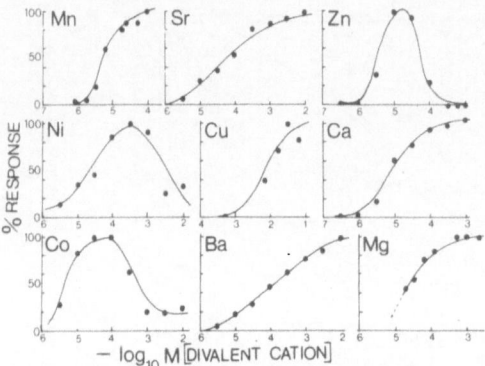

Figure 5. Cation dependence of [^{3}H]nimodipine binding in guinea pig brain membranes. Representative example of cation refilling of EDTA-treated membranes as described in the text. Incubation time was 30 min at 37°C in a volume of 1.0 ml with 80 μg membrane protein/ml. The [^{3}H]nimodipine concentration was 0.78 nM. All divalent cations were added as chloride salts. The binding in the absence of exogenously added divalent cations was 3.57% (0.3 pM) of that when Ca^{2+} at 1 mM was added (8.4 pM) (96.43 ± 0.2% reduction). Blank values were defined by 1 μM unlabeled nimodipine and were measured for every salt concentration. To calculate the "response," the specific binding (cpm) in the absence of added cations was subtracted from the specific binding in the presence of added cation and was divided by the specifically bound maximum observed and multiplied by 100. When cations caused increases in blank values at higher concentrations (e.g., Ni^{2+}, Co^{2+}, Zn^{2+}, Cu^{2+}), this was accounted for in the calculation. For cations giving bell-shaped refilling profiles, percentage response is calculated from the maximum of the filling curve. See Table 4 for average ED$_{50}$ values, maximum response relative to Ca^{2+}, and slope factors of the refilling experiments.

otherms are different. Mn^{2+} reconstitutes with a Hill slope of 2–3, while the Hill slope for Sr^{2+} reconstitution is 0.4–0.5; Ca^{2+} and Mg^{2+} reconstitute specific [^{3}H]nimodipine binding with Hill slopes of 1.5–2.0. Examples are shown in Figure 5. Average data for the reconstitution experiments are given in Table 4.

Monovalent cations up to 150 mM have little effect on [^{3}H]nimodipine binding, but trivalent cations such as La^{3+} inhibit specific [^{3}H]nimodipine binding in a dose-dependent manner. In guinea pig brain membranes, La^{3+}

Table 4. Summary of Data from Cation Refilling Experiments in Guinea Pig Brain Membranes.

Cation	ED$_{50}$ (μM)	Efficacy[a]	Slope factor
Ca^{2+}	14	100	1.7–2.5
Mn^{2+}	11	94	2.0–3.0
Mg^{2+}	43	86	1.5–2.0
Co^{2+}	8	82	1.5–2.0
Ni^{2+}	12	55	1.0–1.5
Zn^{2+}	4	36	1.8–2.0
Cu^{2+}	5000	57	1.8–2.0
Ba^{2+}	306	64	0.3–0.5
Sr^{2+}	99	105	0.4–0.5

[a] Efficacy is expressed as the percentage of maximum filling relative to Ca^{2+}.

has an ID_{50} value of 90 μM. When 100 μM La^{2+} was included in an assay to measure Ca^{2+}-reconstitution of EDTA-pretreated membranes, the reconstitution was completely blocked.

Kinetic experiments at different temperatures with EDTA show that the dissociation of the 1,4-dihydropyridine induced by the chelator is different from that induced by blockade of the forward reaction. The results are in accord with the simplified scheme below, in which Me^{2+}, 1,4-dihydropyridine, and channel form a ternary, high-affinity complex. If we represent the 1,4-dihydropyridine binding site by R, radioactive nimodipine as L, and the divalent cation as Me^{2+}, the following coupled equilibria describe the interactions among R, L, and Me^{2+}:

$$[Me^{2+}] + [R] \underset{k_{-1}}{\overset{k_{+1}}{\rightleftarrows}} [Me^{2+} \cdot R] \tag{1}$$

$$[Me^{2+} \cdot R] + L \underset{k_{-2}}{\overset{k_{+2}}{\rightleftarrows}} [Me^{2+} \cdot L \cdot R] \tag{2}$$

$$[Me^{2+} \cdot R \cdot L] \underset{k_{-3}}{\overset{k_{+3}}{\rightleftarrows}} [Me^{2+}] + [R \cdot L] \tag{3}$$

$$[R \cdot L] \underset{k_{-4}}{\overset{k_{+4}}{\rightleftarrows}} [R] + [L] \tag{4}$$

R requires Me^{2+} to possess high affinity for L. Once the trimolecular complex $[Me^{2+}L \cdot R]$ is formed, L can dissociate via two pathways. The first is via k_{-2} and involves debinding of L while Me^{2+} is still bound to R. The second is via k_{-3} and k_{-4}, where Me^{2+} first dissociates, followed by the rapid dissociation of the thermodynamically unstable complex $[R \cdot L]$. It is therefore obvious, because of additional rate-limiting steps, that the dissociation can be slower when induced by removal of Me^{2+} from the system (by addition of an excess of EDTA) than the blockade of the forward reaction by addition of unlabeled nimodipine.

These kinetic considerations may be helpful in understanding the mechanism by which the 1,4-dihydropyridines alter the conductivity of the calcium channels because there is good electrophysiological evidence that saturable binding sites for divalent cations exist within calcium channels.

Tissue-Specific Dissociation Constants for 1,4-Dihydropyridine Calcium Channel Blockers and D-*cis*-Diltiazem Effects on 1,4-Dihydropyridine Binding

Figures 6 and 7 demonstrate that each tissue has a characteristic equilibrium dissociation constant at 37°C for, for example, [³H]nimodipine and that the Class III channel blocker D-*cis*-diltiazem has a tissue-specific action. It should be noted that the effects of D-*cis*-diltiazem are dependent not only on temperature but also on the structure of the 1,4-dihydropyridine that is

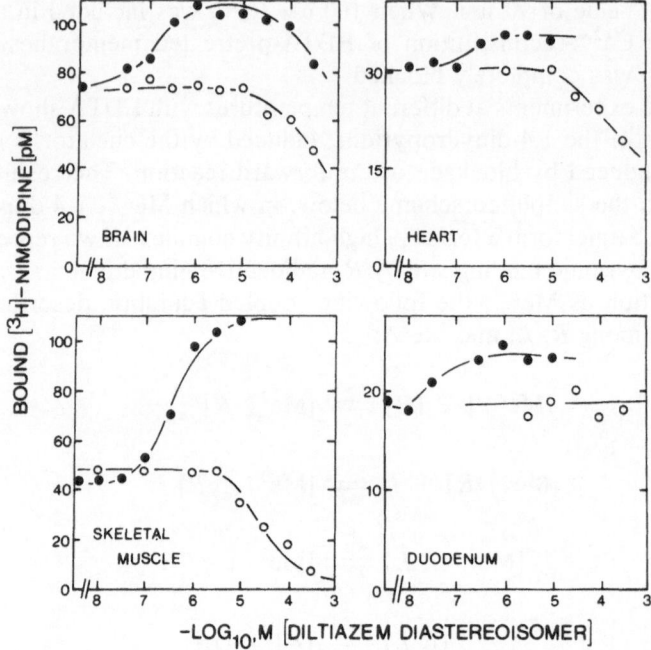

Figure 6. Tissue-specific regulation of [^{3}H]nimodipine binding to guinea pig tissues by the diltiazem diastereoisomers. The effects of d-*cis*-diltiazem (●) and L-*cis*-diltiazem (○) on [^{3}H]nimodipine binding to guinea pig tissues at 37°C are illustrated. The experiments were performed with 0.7–1.5 nM [^{3}H]nimodipine. The following protein concentrations were employed: brain, 0.3–0.4 mg/ml; skeletal muscle, 0.02–0.04 mg/ml; heart, 0.08–0.1 mg/ml; duodenum, 0.3–0.4 mg/ml.

employed to label the channels. Not shown in the figure (but outlined in Table 2 for the heart) is that we find, with minor variations, the same K_D value for a given 1,4-dihydropyridine in a given tissue from different species. Apparently the channel has highly conserved domains that are, for reasons not understood, preserved in each tissue. The channel subtypes can also be discriminated with subtype-selective drugs.

Skeletal-Muscle Calcium Channel

Calcium channels in skeletal-muscle preparations have been studied with voltage-clamp techniques. The skeletal-muscle channels have many characteristics in common with those of the well-studied calcium channel of the myocardium. Thus, they are permeable to Ba^{2+}, Sr^{2+}, Ca^{2+}, Mn^{2+}, and Mg^{2+}, but are blocked by Ni^{2+} and Co^{2+} [5]. The 1,4-dihydropyridine calcium channel blocker nifedipine inhibits the slow inward current in skeletal muscle [6], as do methoxyverapamil (D-600) [7] and diltiazem [8].

High-affinity ($K_D \approx 2.0$ nM) binding sites for the potent 1,4-dihydropyridine calcium channel blocker [^{3}H]nimodipine have been found in guinea

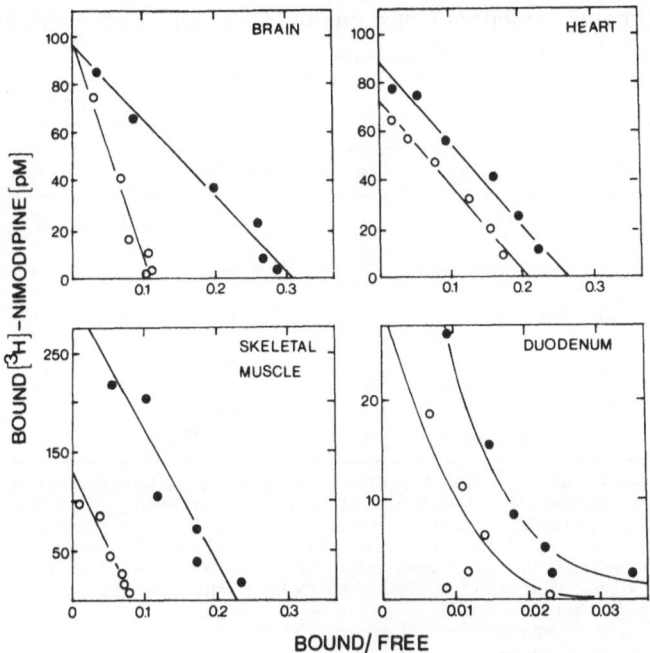

Figure 7.   Tissue-specific regulation of [³H]nimodipine saturation isotherms by D-*cis*-diltiazem. Saturation isotherms in the presence of 10 μM D-*cis*-diltiazem (●) and in the absence of D-*cis*-diltiazem (○) were performed as described. The data are shown as Hofstee plots without taking into account the racemic nature of the radioligand. Mean B_{max} and K_D values for brain membranes are given in Table 3. For guinea pig heart membranes in the absence of D-*cis*-diltiazem, the B_{max} is 333 ± 13 fmoles/mg protein and the K_D of [³H]nimodipine 0.26 ± 0.003 nM. D-*cis*-Diltiazem 10 μM increases the B_{max} to 423 ± 22 fmoles/mg protein without altering the K_D. [³H]Nimodipine high-affinity binding to duodenum membranes has a K_D of 0.2–0.5 nM and a B_{max} of 50–80 fmoles/mg protein; the low-affinity site has a K_D of 2–5 nM and a B_{max} of 170–230 fmoles/mg protein.

pig skeletal-muscle homogenates. These sites could be enriched by differential centrifugation in a crude microsomal fraction. In the microsomal fraction, the density of binding sites was 2–8 pmoles/mg protein. It is shown below that the density of sites labeled is a function of the radioligand. The pharmacological profile of the [³H]nimodipine binding sites suggests that they are part of the putative calcium channel and that [³H]nimodipine binding can be used as a marker for these ionic pores (see Table 5).

In guinea pig brain membranes, [³H]nimodipine labels a single class of sites with a K_D of 0.6 nM, and D-*cis*-diltiazem decreases the K_D by a factor of 3 without a change in the maximum number of receptors. In contrast, D-*cis*-diltiazem (at the optimal concentration of 10 μM) increases the density of the sites in guinea pig skeletal muscle available for [³H]nimodipine with high affinity, and the K_D decreases marginally to 1.0 nM. These effects of D-*cis*-diltiazem are stereospecific, since the pharmacologically inactive dias-

Table 5.   Binding-Inhibition Constants for Drugs of [^{3}H]Nimodipine Binding to Skeletal-Muscle Microsomes[a]

	Control			With 10 μM D-*cis*-diltiazem present			
Drug	IC$_{50}$ (nM)	nH	N	IC$_{50}$ (nM)	nH	N	Shift factor
(+)PN 205-033	2.2 ± 0.55	1.04 ± 0.08	3	3.5 ± 1.6	1.09 ± 0.05	3	1.6
(−)PN 205-034	206 ± 42[b]	0.89 ± 0.07	3	333 ± 88++	1.18 ± 0.06	3	1.6
(±)Fendiline	540 ± 125	0.98 ± 0.10	3	1,209 ± 205[c]	1.23 ± 0.12	3	2.2
Tiapamil	292 ± 74	1.08 ± 0.15	3	12,230 ± 4,260[d]	0.89 ± 0.09	3	42.0
(+)D-600	1,002 ± 267	0.78 ± 0.04	4	5,745 ± 764[e]	0.95 ± 0.14	3	5.7
(−)D-600	—	—	3	1,410 ± 309[f]	0.90 ± 0.14	3	—
La^{3+}	200,000	1.3	2	450,000	1.2	2	1.2
Tetrodotoxin	N.E.		2	N.E.		2	

[a] Average data with standard errors from N separate experiments, each performed in duplicate with 5–10 concentrations of unlabeled drugs. (nH) Hill slope; (IC$_{50}$) concentration of drug causing 50% inhibition of specific [^{3}H]nimodipine binding, as calculated from linear-regression analysis of data transformed into the Hill equation. The shift factor is the ratio of IC$_{50}$ in the presence of 10 μM D-*cis*-diltiazem to IC$_{50}$ in the control experiment. The microsomal protein concentration was between 10 and 25 μg/ml and the concentration of (±) [^{3}H]nimodipine between 0.8 and 1.5 nM. (N.E.) No effect up to 1 μM.
[b] $p < 0.01$ with respect to (+)PN 205-033.
[c] $p < 0.10$ with respect to control.
[d] $p < 0.025$ with respect to control.
[e] $p < 0.001$ with respect to control.
[f] $p < 0.01$ with respect to (+)D-600.

tereoisomer L-*cis*-diltiazem does not stimulate [^{3}H]nimodipine binding, but is inhibitory, albeit at much higher concentrations. It is concluded that a significant fraction of the putative calcium channels has a K_D of 50 nM for [^{3}H]nimodipine and that D-*cis*-diltiazem can increase the affinity of this subpopulation for [^{3}H]nimodipine so that they are detectable in ligand-binding experiments. This will be further outlined in the section on [^{3}H]D-*cis*-diltiazem labeling of the allosteric site that interacts with the 1,4-dihydropyridine drug receptor.

The binding sites for [^{3}H]nimodipine were purified from the crude microsomal pellet by means of sucrose-gradient centrifugation. [^{3}H]Nimodipine binding copurifies with Na$^+$,K$^+$-ATPase and [^{3}H]ouabain binding and is enriched in a vesicular fraction (by a factor of 30- to 60-fold) of low bouyant density [<25% (wt./wt.) sucrose], with a ratio of Na$^+$,K$^+$-ATPase to K$^+$,Ca^{2+}-ATPase activity of 0.77.

Biochemical and electron-microscopic examination suggests that a specialized structure of the sarcolemma, possibly the transverse tubule, is the subcellular locus for the [^{3}H]nimodipine binding site. Since the density of the drug receptors in this purified preparation is extremely high (60 pmoles/mg protein) and exceeds that reported for [^{3}H]saxitoxin binding sites (a specific sodium-channel label) by a factor of 4–10 (with respect to the most highly purified skeletal-muscle membrane isolated), the isolation and puri-

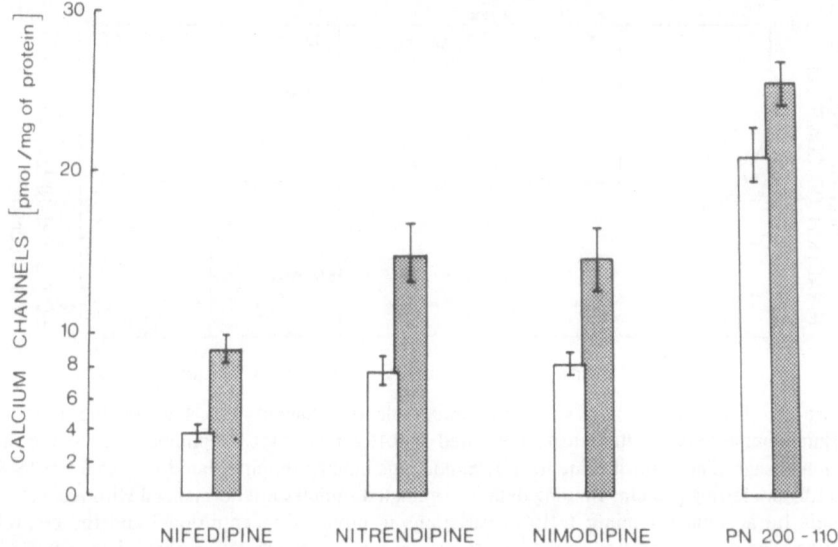

Figure 8. B_{max} values (at 37°C) for the four different radioligands and skeletal-muscle micro-somes. (▨) B_{max} values in the presence of 10 μM D-*cis*-diltiazem.

fication of the putative calcium channel from skeletal muscle is feasible, as will be shown below.

Differential Labeling of Skeletal-Muscle Calcium Channels by Four Different 1,4-Dihydropyridine Calcium Antagonists

When the four 1,4-dihydropyridine calcium-channel blockers [³H]nifedipine, [³H]nitrendipine, [³H]nimodipine, and [³H]-PN 200-110 were employed to label putative calcium channels in guinea pig hindlimb skeletal-muscle membranes, the results described below were obtained at 37°C.

The four radioligands differed with respect to the number of sites (B_{max}) that were labeled. The following rank order of B_{max} values was found: PN 200-110 > nimodipine = nitrendipine > nifedipine. D-*cis*-Diltiazem caused an increase in the density of high-affinity binding sites for all four calcium-channel blockers. The relative stimulation was smallest for PN 200-110 (Figure 8). This rank order of B_{max} values suggests that the different 1,4-dihydropyridines do not interact in an identical manner with the calcium channels in skeletal-muscle membranes, but rather apparently induce or stabilize a channel state with high affinity for these drugs with different efficacy. In analogy to these and related findings shown below, we had put forward the idea that there is a continuum (ranging from agonists to antagonists) for drugs that alter the conductivity of the calcium channel. In this context, it is worth mentioning that with the different radioligands, we measure different molecular sizes of the calcium channel.

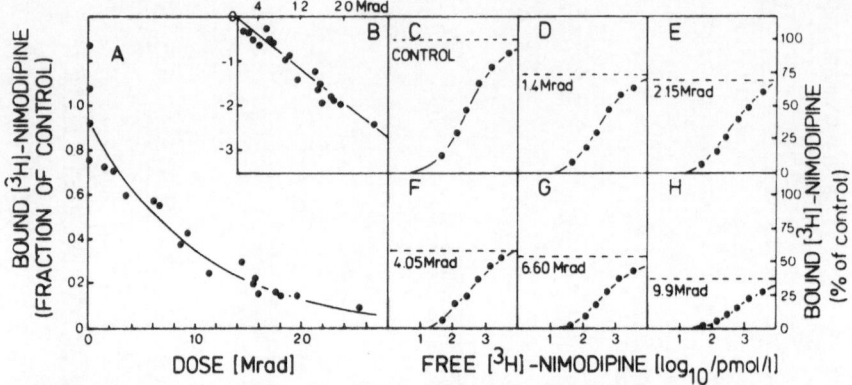

Figure 9. Target-size analysis of the brain calcium channel. (A) Plot of the relative [³H]nimodipine binding-site density measured at 0.16 nmoles/liter [³H]nimodipine vs. the radiation dosage. The control value for [³H]nimodipine binding (nonirradiated samples) was 99.9 ± 11.03 fmoles/mg protein. Binding data for irradiated samples are normalized with respect to protein [to account for minor (<10%) variations in protein concentrations] and the control binding. The data were fitted to the equation: $y = a \cdot e^b$. The correlation coefficient is 0.98, a = 0.94% and b = −0.106 (D_{37} = 9.4 Mrad). (B) Plot of the data in (A) transformed and fitted to the equation [7]: $y = a + b \cdot x$. The correlation coefficient is 0.98, a = −0.09, b = -0.110 (D_{37} = 9.1 Mrad). (C–H) Saturation isotherms of specific [³H]nimodipine binding at various does of irradiation. The data are normalized with respect to control binding (B_{max} value = 100%) and illustrate the B_{max} decrease (−−−) as a function of radiation dose. Each point is the mean value of a duplicate measurement for both total and nonspecific binding. The B_{max} of the control binding amounts to 345 ± 57 fmoles/mg protein (N = 4) in this experiment.

TARGET-SIZE ANALYSIS OF CALCIUM CHANNELS

Brain Calcium Channel

The molecular size of the calcium channel in guinea pig brain membranes labeled with [³H]nimodipine was determined with the radiation-inactivation method. The molecular size of the channel in membranes preincubated and assayed in the presence of 10 μM D-*cis*-diltiazem was also determined.

Saturation experiments with [³H]nimodipine over a concentration range of 0.05–2.5 nM revealed that the irradiation reduced the maximum density of high-affinity [³H]nimodipine binding sites without changing the dissociation constant of [³H]nimodipine for the remaining binding sites. As internal control, the decay of [³H]flunitrazepam-labeled benzodiazepine receptors was monitored. As for the [³H]nimodipine-labeled putative calcium channel, irradiation did not alter the K_D of [³H]flunitrazepam for the residual benzodiazepine receptors, but the density of these receptors was reduced.

When the decay of [³H]nimodipine binding sites is plotted against irradiation dose, a monoexponential relationship is apparent. A semilogarithmic transformation of the data from Figure 9 shows a linear relationship with a correlation coefficient $r = 0.98$, $p < 0.001$, indicating again homogeneity of the [^{3}H]nimodipine binding site population with respect to the target size. Figure 9 also exemplifies the relative decrease in B_{max} (density of [^{3}H]nimodipine binding sites) with respect to nonirradiated samples as a function of radiation dose and the respective occupancies as a function of free [^{3}H]ligand concentration.

Benzodiazepine receptor decay curves were analyzed as described for the [^{3}H] nimodipine binding site (not shown). As reported by other authors [9–11], monophasic plots were obtained. The D_{37} for the [^{3}H]flunitrazepam-labeled benzodiazepine receptor (determined in three different radiation-inactivation experiments) was 24.2 ± 2.32 Mrad. The D_{37} ($\pm$ S.E.M.) of the [^{3}H]nimodipine binding site (from three different experiments) was 10.3 ± 1.3 Mrad. With the temperature-correction factor of 2.8, we calculate the following molecular weights: for the [^{3}H]nimodipine binding site $185,000 \pm 26,800$ ($N = 3$) and for the benzodiazepine receptor $76,500 \pm 7800$ ($N = 3$). Similar experiments were performed with membranes that were preincubated with D-cis-diltiazem and assayed in the presence of 10 μM D-cis-diltiazem. It was found that the D_{37} for the nimodipine-labeled channel was increased to 16.3 ± 1.4 Mrad ($p < 0.01$), which corresponds to an M_r of $110,000 \pm 9800$. In contrast, the benzodiazepine receptor had a D_{37} of 26.4 ± 4.6 Mrad, corresponding to an M_r of $78,000 \pm 9900$. In conclusion, D-cis-diltiazem decreases the M_r of the brain calcium channel by approximately 75,000 mass units.

Target-Size Analysis of the Skeletal-Muscle Calcium Channel

The results shown above demonstrated that the M_r of the calcium channel in guinea pig brain, when labeled with nimodipine, is 185,000 and is decreased, by a large decrement, when D-cis-diltiazem as a positive heterotropic regulator is bound to the channel. The question was whether this finding is a general phenomenon. We therefore determined the M_r of the skeletal-muscle calcium channel.

Guinea pig hindlimb skeletal-muscle membranes were pretreated for 30 min at 37°C in buffer or in buffer supplemented with 10 μM D-cis-diltiazem or 10 μM L-cis-diltiazem. The pretreated membranes were flash-frozen in volumes of 2 ml in polypropylene vials by immersion in liquid nitrogen. The frozen membranes were then irradiated with high-energy electrons (10 MeV).

Control and irradiated membranes were rapidly thawed and diluted 20-fold with ice-cold buffer. The assays for calcium channels were performed in a volume of 0.25 ml (5–25 μg membrane protein) or for diltiazem-pretreated membranes in buffer with the corresponding diastereoisomer at a concentration of 10 μM at 37°C with [^{3}H]nimodipine under equilibrium binding conditions (30 min incubation) prior to collection of membrane-bound [^{3}H]ligand on Whatman GF/C filters after rapid dilution and filtration with ice-cold buffer. Figure 10a shows the decay of calcium-channel binding of

a

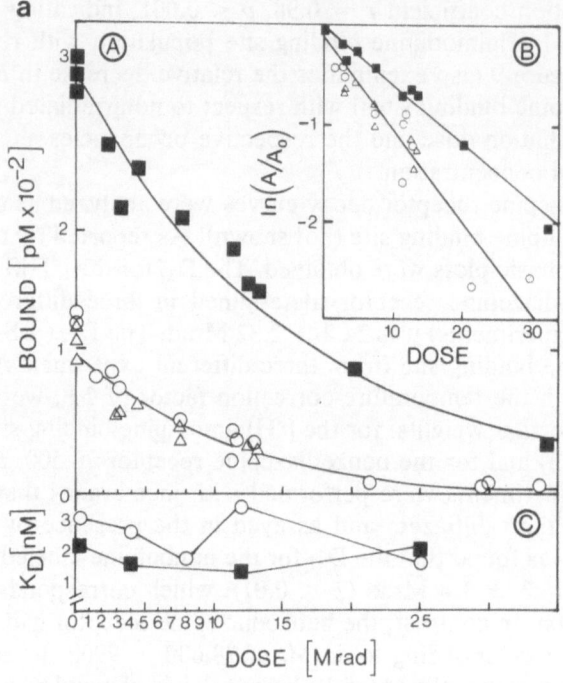

b

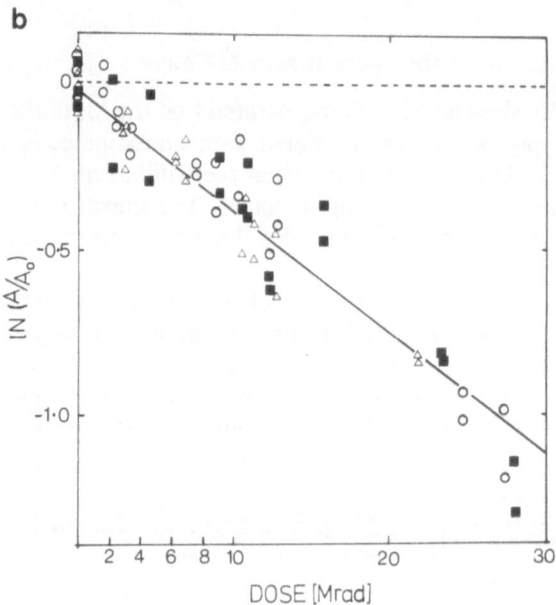

Figure 10.   (a) Radiation inactivation of the [³H]nimodipine-labeled calcium channel in skeletal muscle. (A) Radiation inactivation of the [³H]nimodipine-labeled calcium channel preincubated and assayed in 10 μM D-*cis*-diltiazem (■), preincubated and assayed in 10 μM L-*cis*-diltiazem

[^{3}H]nimodipine for three preincubation conditions of the membranes as a function of radiation dosage; the linear transformations are also shown in the figure. Under all three preincubation conditions, the decay of the [^{3}H]nimodipine-labeled calcium channel is monoexponential, demonstrating the homogeneity of target size. When membranes were preincubated in buffer, the D_{37} of the [^{3}H]nimodipine-labeled calcium channels was 10.1 Mrad, corresponding to a molecular size of 178,000. L-*cis*-Diltiazem preincubation did not significantly alter the D_{37} of the [^{3}H]nimodipine-labeled calcium channel, but D-*cis*-diltiazem preincubation increased the D_{37} by 6 Mrad, corresponding to a loss in M_r of 67,000 mass units. Irradiation of membranes at doses of radiation of up to 25 Mrad did not alter the K_D of [^{3}H]nimodipine for the residual saturable binding sites.

In contrast to the M_r regulation of the [^{3}H]nimodipine-labeled calcium channel by D-*cis*-diltiazem, the M_r of the endogenous acetylcholine esterase was identical for the three different preincubation conditions (see Figure 10b and Table 6).

Similar radiation-inactivation experiments were performed with [^{3}H]PN-200-110 as calcium-channel label. The results are summarized in Table 7.

How can we explain the difference in M_r measured with [^{3}H]-PN 200-110 as opposed to nimodipine and the decrement in functional size induced by D-*cis*-diltiazem? In the absence of more biochemical information on the structural composition of the Ca^{2+} channel, we would like to propose the following model, which uses the assumption that a single hit destroys the total structure of a given "target" whether that target is composed of a single protomer or assembled from heterologous or homologous protomers: Assume that the Ca^{2+} channel consists of four elements (a, b, c, d) that may or may not correspond to the true protomers of the oligomeric channel.

($\triangle$), and preincubated and assayed in buffer A ($\bigcirc$). The membrane samples that received the doses of radiation as indicated were assayed with 1.2 nM [^{3}H]nimodipine at a protein concentration of 20–35 µg/ml. The data points are fitted to the equation $y = ae^b$, where y is bound ligand at the given dose x of radiation, a is the y-axis intercept, and b is the constant of decay (Mrad^{-1}). For all three sets of data, the correlation coefficient is 0.94 or greater. Lines are best fits by the least-squares principle. (B) As in (A), but plotted as the ln [binding at a given dose of irradiation (A)]/[binding in nonirradiated controls (A)] against the dose of irradiation. The D_{37}'s of the [^{3}H]nimodipine-labeled calcium channel are for preincubation with buffer, 10.9 Mrad; for preincubation with 10 µM L-*cis*-diltiazem, 10.8 Mrad; and for preincubation with 10 µM D-*cis*-diltiazem, 16.8 Mrad. (C) Plot of dissociation constants of [^{3}H]nimodipine (nM) for residual calcium channels (vs.) dose of radiation. (■) In the presence of 10 µM D-*cis*-diltiazem; ($\bigcirc$) in the absence of D-*cis*-diltiazem. (b) Radiation inactivation of acetylcholinesterase activity. An example of a single, typical experiment is shown. Membranes were preincubated in buffer A ($\bigcirc$), in 10 µM D-*cis*-diltiazem (■), or in 10 µM L-*cis*-diltiazem ($\triangle$). The ln (activity at a given dose of irradiation/activity in nonirradiated controls) is plotted against radiation dose. In this experiment, the D_{37} of acetylcholinesterase in membranes preincubated in buffer was 25.60 Mrad; preincubated with 10 µM D-*cis*-diltiazem, 25.25 Mrad; and preincubated with L-*cis*-diltiazem, 25.99 Mrad. The line is the best fit to the pooled data points for the three preincubation conditions.

Table 6.   Molecular Sizes of the Skeletal-Muscle Calcium Channel and of Acetylcholinesterase[a]

		Preincubation condition		
		Buffer	D-cis-Diltiazem	L-cis-Diltiazem
[^{3}H]Nimodipine-	D_{37}[Mrad]	10.1 ± 0.4	16.1 ± 0.06	11.3 ± 0.6
labeled calcium	M_r	178,000 ± 7200	111,500 ± 7200[b]	158,000 ± 7100
channel				
Acetylcholine	D_{37}[Mrad]	27.4 ± 1.9	30.9 ± 2.8	26.0 ± 1.2
esterase	M_r	65,500 ± 4500	58,000 ± 5400	68,900 ± 3200

[a] D_{37} and corresponding molecular weights of the [^{3}H]nimodipine-labeled calcium channels and acetyl-cholineesterase. All numbers are arithmetic means ± S.E.M. for three independent irradiations.
[b] $p < 0.003$ with respect to control (buffer-preincubated).

These elements are defined as the largest components required for the measured biological activity, e.g., [^{3}H]-PN 200-110 or [^{3}H]nimodipine labeling after irradiation. Table 8 lists the elements of the model and their measured or deduced M_r's under the different experimental conditions. Element a (carrying the 1,4-dihydropyridine Ca^{2+} antagonist binding site) has to associate with (the facilitatory) element b when PN 200-110 labels the channel, but with (the facilitatory) element c when [^{3}H]nimodipine labels.

The M_r difference (c − b) is 40,000, because under all preincubation conditions (Table 7), the channel assayed by [^{3}H]nimodipine is larger by this increment than when assayed with PN 200-110. The conclusion is that we have not determined the M_r of a, but instead that of the facilitatory

Table 7. M_r Values of the Calcium Channel in Skeletal Muscle as a Function of Radioligand[a]

	Preincubation condition		
	Buffer	D-cis-diltiazem (10μM)	L-cis-diltiazem (10μM)
Skeletal-muscle Ca^{2+} channels labeled with [^{3}H]-PN 200-110	136,000 ± 12,000[b]	75,000 ± 4800[c,d]	123,000 ± 6700[e]
Skeletal-muscle Ca^{2+} channels labeled with [^{3}H]nimodipine	178,000 ± 7,200[b]	111,000 ± 7000[d]	158,000 ± 7100[e]

[a] M_r values are calculated from monophasic decay curves. Means ± S.E.M. for three experiments are shown.
[b] $p < 0.04$ for [^{3}H]-PN-200-110-labeled (vs.) [^{3}H]nimodipine-labeled calcium channels, both preincubated in buffer.
[c] $p < 0.01$ for [^{3}H]-PN-200-110-labeled calcium channels preincubated in 10μM D-cis-diltiazem (vs.) preincubation in buffer.
[d] $p < 0.013$ for [^{3}H]-PN-200-110-labeled calcium channels (vs.) [^{3}H]nimodipine-labeled calcium channels, both preincubated with 10μM D-cis-diltiazem.
[e] $p < 0.06$ for both preincubated in L-cis-diltiazem.

Table 8. Average Target Sizes of Putative Elements of the Calcium Channel in Situ[a]

Element	M_r	Preincubation condition	Ca^{2+} channel label	Proposed function
a	75,000	Derived		Binds 1,4-dihydropyridines
b	75,000	D-*cis*-Diltiazem	[³H]-PN 200-110	Facilitates PN 200-110 binding
c	111,000	D-*cis*-Diltiazem	[³H]Nimodipine	Facilitates nimodipine binding
d	60,000–75,000	Derived		Dissociated by D-*cis*-diltiazem
(b,d)	136,000	Buffer	[³H]-PN 200-110	—
(c,d)	178,000	Buffer	[³H]Nimodipine	—

[a] Elements of the model are the limiting largest structures that allow the data of the target-size analysis to be unambiguously interpreted. In frozen membranes, a always behaves as an independent target, and (b,d) and (c,d) are assembled targets that are dissociated on pretreatment with D-*cis*-diltiazem. The M_r of d is derived by subtracting the M_r of either [³H]nimodipine- or [³H]-PN-200-110-labeled Ca^{2+} channels preincubated with D-*cis*-diltiazem from the M_r of buffer-preincubated channels. The M_r of a, as a condition of the model, must be smaller than any measured M_r. The model is not complete, since the radiation-inactivation data with PN 200-110 labeling of calcium channels in guinea pig brain are not included.

elements (b or c). The following rank order of M_r's must then apply: a < b < c. Because preincubation with D-*cis*-diltiazem decreases the M_r by about 60,000–75,000 in brain or skeletal muscle, we have to postulate that b and c are functionally coupled to element d. Element d is the element that D-*cis*-diltiazem uncouples from either b or c. Therefore, according to the model, in buffer-preincubated membranes frozen at −110°C, the elements exist as a, (b · c), (c · d), where (b · d) and (c · d) are assembled (coupled) elements. In D-*cis*-diltiazem-preincubated membranes, the elements exist uncoupled as a, b, c, d.

Admittedly, this model is speculative, but it can explain the experimental results and gives an estimate of the functional size of the 1,4-dihydropyridine binding site. In any event, our data demonstrate that 1,4-dihydropyridines interact differently with the Ca^{2+} channels as shown by target-size analysis in this study and by comparative ligand-binding experiments. Our experiments have yielded the important result that the allosteric regulator D-*cis*-diltiazem decreases the in situ M_r of the Ca^{2+} channel as labeled by 1,4-dihydropyridines and that slow channel-blocker–channel interactions are of a complex nature at the molecular level.

LABELING OF THE DRUG-RECEPTOR SITES THAT ALLOSTERICALLY REGULATE THE BINDING OF 1,4-DIHYDROPYRIDINES TO CALCIUM CHANNELS

We have employed [³H]verapamil and [³H]D-*cis*-diltiazem to label calcium channels in skeletal-muscle microsomes. Figure 11 shows that the op-

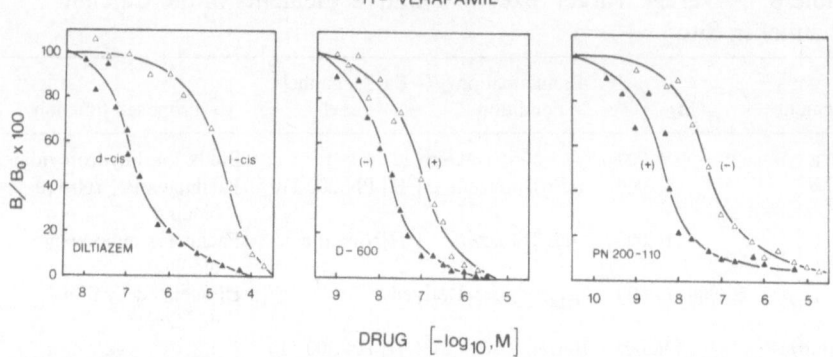

Figure 11.   Inhibition of [³H]verapamil binding by the diastereoisomers D- and L-*cis*-diltiazem, the optically pure enantiomers (−)D-600 and (+)D-600 (gallopamil), and the (+)enantiomer of PN 200-110 (= PN 205-033) and the (−)enantiomer (= PN 205-034) (also see Table 5). The experiment was performed at 2°C with 5.7 nM [³H]verapamil and 0.3 mg/ml of skeletal-muscle microsomal protein. Neither D-*cis*-diltiazem nor the enantiomers of PN 200-110 are competitive inhibitors.

tically pure enantiomers D- and L-*cis*-diltiazem and (−) and (+)D-600 as well as (+)PN 200-110 and (−)PN 200-110 interact in a stereoselective manner with the verapamil binding site. It should be pointed out that, for example, D-*cis*-diltiazem and PN 200-110 are not plain competitive inhibitors of verapamil binding.

Figure 12 shows an experiment in which two tritiated chiral 1,4-dihydropyridines (nitrendipine and nimodipine) were employed to label the Ca²⁺ channel in guinea pig skeletal-muscle microsomal membranes. The experiment was performed in the absence and presence of 10 μM D-*cis*-diltiazem. It can be seen that the stimulatory D-*cis*-diltiazem effect is highly temperature-dependent.

The specific binding of [³H]D-*cis*-diltiazem was measured in parallel. In analogy to the experiment with the labeled 1,4-dihydropyridines, in which D-*cis*-diltiazem was present, several unlabeled 1,4-dihydropyridines were added at the indicated concentrations. The binding-temperature profile shows that an increase in temperature from 2° to 37°C leads to a 5-fold decrease in specific binding of [³H]D-*cis*-diltiazem. However, this binding-temperature profile was characteristically changed by the simultaneous presence of 1,4-dihydropyridines. At 0° and 10°C, all 1,4-dihydropyridines including nimodipine (not shown), nitrendipine, PN 200-110 (not shown) and Bay K 8644 were inhibitory, whereas at temperatures of 20°C or more they were stimulatory to a different extent. As will be shown below, these stimulatory effects are stereospecific for chiral 1,4-dihydropyridines. The most interesting finding is the differential behavior of the various 1,4-dihydropyridines. Included in this series is the novel 1,4-dihydropyridine Bay K 8644, which activates instead of blocks Ca²⁺ channels in guinea pig hearts

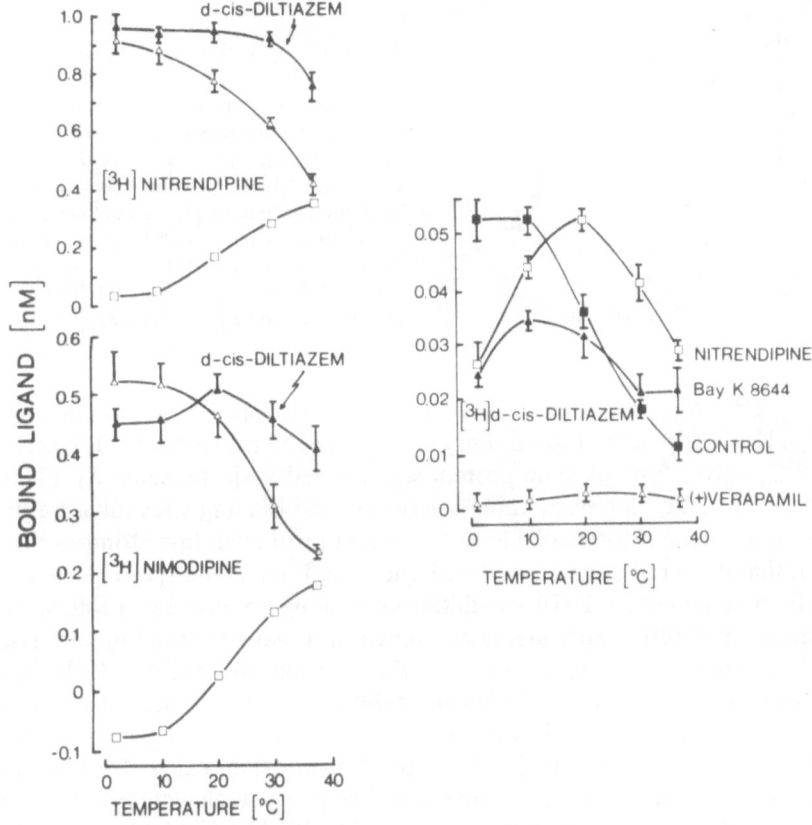

Figure 12. Temperature-dependent binding of [³H]nitrendipine (4.43 nM), [³H]nimodipine (1.56 nM), and [³H]D-*cis*-diltiazem (3.12 nM) to guinea pig skeletal-muscle microsomes (0.16 mg protein/ml). Each point is the mean of three experiments ± S.E.M. In the case where [³H]nitrendipine and [³H]nimodipine labeled the Ca²⁺ channel, D-*cis*-diltiazem (10 μM) (closed symbols) was also present during the incubation; in the case where [³H]D-*cis*-diltiazem labeled the channel, nitrendipine (0.1 μM), Bay K 8644 (1 μM), and (+)verapamil (1 μM) were present during the incubation as indicated. The incubation times for the various temperatures were as follows: 2°C (4 hr), 10°C (3 hr), 20°C (2 hr), 30°C (1 hr), 37°C (30 min). For the 1,4-dihydropyridine labeling experiments of Ca²⁺ channels, the calculated difference between the concentrations of ligand specifically bound in the absence and presence of D-*cis*-diltiazem is plotted (□——□).

and rabbit aortic strips, apparently by binding to the same drug-receptor site as the 1,4-dihydropyridine channel blockers. Bay K 8644 had a K_D value of 50 ± 15 nM for the [³H]nimodipine binding site in skeletal-muscle microsomal membranes.

This agonistic 1,4-dihydropyridine was of high efficacy in inhibiting [³H]D-*cis*-diltiazem binding at low temperatures, but of low efficacy in stimulating binding at higher temperatures. In contrast to these 1,4 dihydropyridines, (+) and (−)verapamil were inhibitory at all temperatures.

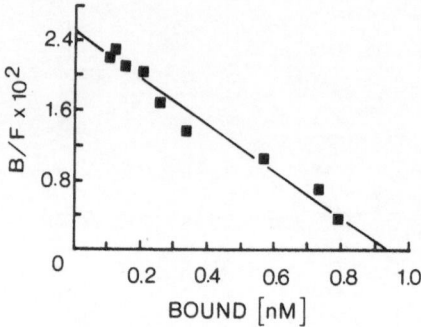

Figure 13. Equilibrium saturation isotherm of [³H]D-*cis*-diltiazem binding to Ca²⁺ channels at 2°C. Each point is the mean from duplicate determinations for both total and nonspecific binding; the data for specific binding are presented as a Scatchard plot. The concentration of guinea pig skeletal-muscle microsomal protein was 0.082 mg/ml. The correlation coefficient for the linear regression was 0.98, B_{max} = 0.94 nM (= 11.465 fmoles/mg protein), and K_D = 37.5 nM.

At 2°C, D-*cis*-diltiazem labeled 11 pmoles/mg protein of binding sites, with a Hill coefficient close to unity and a K_D of 39 nM (Figure 13), whereas at 30°C, only 2.9 pmoles/mg protein was labeled with the same K_D (Table 8). Thus, at 30°C, a considerable fraction of the binding sites must be in a state that is either not available to the ligand or of such low affinity ($K_D \gg$ 5 μM) that it cannot be measured with the filtration technology. The average kinetic parameters for [³H]D-*cis*-diltiazem binding are given in Table 9, and examples of kinetic experiments are shown in Figure 14. Binding of [³H]D-*cis*-diltiazem was fully reversible. The dissociation, induced by blockade of the forward reaction by unlabeled D-*cis*-diltiazem, was monophasic, with a half-life of 35 min at 2°C. The K_D derived from the rate constants (37.7 nM) is in excellent agreement with the dissociation constant calculated from the equilibrium binding saturation isotherms. The pharmacological profile of the D-*cis*-diltiazem binding sites is given in Table 10. Most notable is that the binding sites discriminate between L- and D-*cis*-diltiazem and recognize the structurally different Ca²⁺ channel blockers verapamil, gallopamil, tiapamil, and KB-944, which is an allosteric regulator of 1,4-dihydropyridine binding, as is D-*cis*-diltiazem. The inorganic Ca²⁺ channel blocker La³⁺ also inhibited [³H]D-*cis*-diltiazem binding, whereas several Na⁺ channel drugs were completely inactive.

Figure 15 shows the dose dependency of the stimulatory effect of different 1,4-dihydropyridines at 30°C. It was found that the stimulation was stereospecific, since the enantiomers of PN 200-110 display a eudismic ratio of 150 or greater, which is close to their eudismic ratio for the 1,4 dihydropyridine binding site labeled with [³H]nimodipine. The individual 1,4-dihydropyridines differed with respect to the maximal stimulation and their EC_{50} values. The respective parameters are given in Table 11. Of the 1,4-dihydropyridines investigated, nitrendipine and the (+)enantiomer of PN 200-110 has the highest efficacy for stimulation. Most interesting is that the agonistic 1,4-dihydropyridine Bay K 8644 was extremely weak with respect to stimulation. The benzoxadiazol 1,4-dihydropyridine Vo 2605, which is a 7-bromo-substituted PN 200-110, and about 3 orders of magnitude weaker in affinity for the 1,4-dihydropyridine binding site compared to PN 200 110,

Table 9. Equilibrium Binding Parameters and Kinetic Constants for [^{3}H]D-*cis*-Diltiazem-Labeled Ca^{2+} Channels in Guinea Pig Skeletal-Muscle Microsomes[a]

	Temperature			
	2°C		30°C	
	Nitrendipine		Nitrendipine	
Parameter	Absent	Present	Absent	Present
B_{max} (fmoles/mg protein)	11,020 ± 1380[b] (6)	6170 ± 1250[c] (3)	2911 ± 608[d] (3)	8400 ± 1400 (3)
Dissociation constant (nM)	39.0 ± 5.0 (6)	45 ± 7.6 (3)	37 ± 9 (3)	50 ± 7 (3)
Dissociation rate constant (min^{-1})	0.02 ± 0.01 (3)	N.D.	N.D.	N.D.
Association rate constant (nM · min^{-1})	0.00053 ± 0.0001 (3)	N.D.	N.D.	N.D.

[a] Mean data ± S.E.M. are given. The numbers of experiments are given in parentheses. Equilibrium binding parameters at 2 and 30°C were also determined in the presence of 0.5 μM nitrendipine. (N.D.) Not determined.
[b] $p < 0.05$ for 2°C vs. 30°C.
[c] $p < 0.05$ for nitrendipine present vs. nitrendipine absent at 2°C.
[d] $p < 0.05$ for nitrendipine absent vs. nitrendipine present (Student's two-tailed t test).

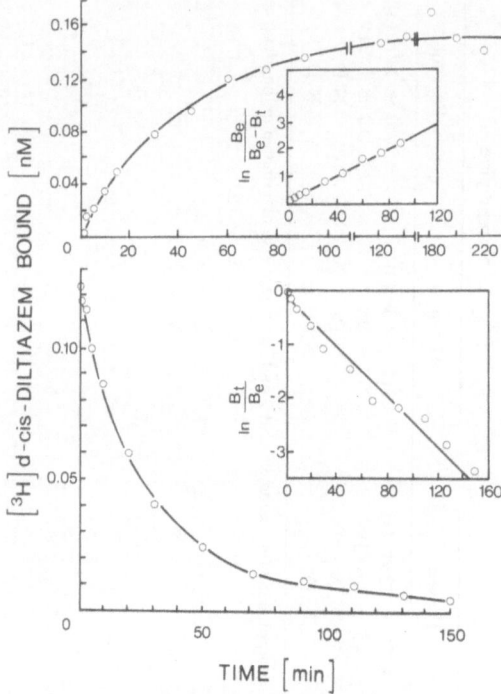

Figure 14. Association and disso-ciation kinetics of [^{3}H]D-*cis*-dilti-azem. *Top:* Guinea pig microsomal membranes (0.16 mg protein/ml) were incubated at 2°C with 7.35 nM [^{3}H]D-*cis*-diltiazem for the indicated times and the concentration of spe-cifically bound ligand determined. Each point is the mean from two ob-servations for both total and non-specific binding (which did not in-crease with time). *Insert:* The kinetic data between 0 and 90 min are plotted according to the K_{obs} method. K_{obs} was 0.024 min^{-1} and k_{-1} (association rate constant) de-rived from K_{obs} and k_{-1} *was 0.0059 nM^{-1}·min^{-1}*. Direct nonlinear curve-fitting of the data to the dif-ferential form of the second-order rate equation yielded (± asymptotic standard deviation) 0.003 ± 0.0002 nM^{-1}·min^{-1} for K_{-1} and 0.019 ± 0.0014 min^{-1} for the k_{-1} and a re-ceptor concentration of 1.6 nM. *Bot-tom:* After 4 hr of incubation of guinea pig skeletal-muscle microsomal protein (0.072 mg/ml) at 2°C with 6.6 nM [^{3}H]D-*cis*-diltiazem (zero time point), the blockade of the forward reaction was initiated by addition of 10 µM D-*cis*-diltiazem. Each point is the mean of duplicate experiments for the given times. *Insert:* Transformation of the dissociation data by plotting ln (B_t/B_e) yielded a slope of −0.022 min^{-1} (correlation coefficient: 0.97), k_{-1} = 0.022 min^{-1}.

was inactive, as was M 5579, which is an inactive nitrendipine derivative with a free carboxyl group. To determine the nature of the [^{3}H]D-*cis*-dilti-azem stimulation, we investigated the effects of nitrendipine (at 0.5 µM) on the equilibrium binding parameters at 30°C (Table 9). The 1,4-dihydropyr-idine channel blocker increased the density of sites labeled by [^{3}H]D-*cis*-diltiazem at 30°C.

Figure 15 demonstrates that the 1,4-dihydropyridines inhibited [^{3}H]D-*cis*-diltiazem binding at 2°C in a concentration-dependent manner. The re-spective mean IC$_{50}$ values and maximal inhibition percentages are also shown in Table 11. The effects of 0.5 µM nitrendipine were tested on the equilibrium binding parameters as above. This 1,4-dihydropyridine channel blocker decreased the density of sites labeled by [^{3}H]D-*cis*-diltiazem at 2°C (Table 9).

In the absence of 1,4-dihydropyridines, [^{3}H]D-*cis*-diltiazem labeled more sites at 2 than at 30°C. It is therefore reasonable to conclude that the marked temperature dependence of [^{3}H]D-*cis*-diltiazem binding is reflecting the temperature dependence of the constant governing the equilibrium be-

Table 10. Pharmacological Profile of the [^{3}H]D-*cis*-Diltiazem Binding Sites Determined at 2°C[a]

Drug	IC$_{50}$ [nM]	nH
Ca^{2+}-channel drugs		
D-*cis*-Diltiazem	54.0 ± 1.4	0.99 ± 0.1
L-*cis*-Diltiazem	6680 ± 25.0	0.85 ± 0.04
(+)Gallopamil	42.1 ± 0.6	0.99 ± 0.06
(−)Gallopamil	17.5 ± 2.8	1.04 ± 0.04
(+)Verapamil	43.2 ± 0.6	1.02 ± 0.1
(−)Verapamil	54.0 ± 20.0	1.06 ± 0.14
Tiapamil	406.0 ± 45.0	1.19 ± 0.12
KB-944	358.0 ± 57.0	0.98 ± 0.03
La^{3+}	3.48 ± 0.82 × 10^5	1.09 ± 0.05
Na$^+$-channel drugs		
Tetrodotoxin	No effect	
Germitrine	No effect	
Seaanemonetoxin II	No effect	
Veratridine	No effect	

[a] (nH) Hill slope; (IC$_{50}$) concentration of drug causing 50% inhibition. IC$_{50}$ values and Hill slopes were derived from three or four binding-inhibition experiments in which seven to nine concentrations of drug were tested in duplicate. Na$^+$-channel drugs were tested at concentrations between 1 and 100 μM.

tween high-affinity (K_D = 39 nM) and low-affinity states ($K_D \geqslant$ 5 μM) of the Ca^{2+} channel D-*cis*-diltiazem binding sites.

Likewise, the same conclusion may be drawn for the 1,4-dihydropyridine labeling of Ca^{2+} channels, since we show that, as for [^{3}H]D-*cis*-diltiazem, maximal labeling occurs at low temperatures (<10°C). One of the actions of D-*cis*-diltiazem at temperatures of 20°C or more is the establishment of a new equilibrium of low- and high-affinity states for 1,4-dihydropyridine channel blockers, favoring the high-affinity state. In accord with this, the D-*cis*-diltiazem effect on the 1,4-dihydropyridine labeling of the channels was minimal or absent at 2°C and maximal at 37°C. In view of the Ca^{2+}-channel-blocking activity of D-*cis*-diltiazem and the 1,4-dihydropyridines nimodipine and nitrendipine, it is tempting to postulate that the high-affinity labeled channel for these radioligands is a "shut" channel, whereas the low-affinity state is equivalent to the "unshut" channel. Whether or not, for example, the hypothetical "shut" channel state in depolarized membrane fragments is comparable to the open (but drug-blocked), closed, or inactivated channel state, as they may occur in intact tissues, is an open question. On the basis of the aforestated assumptions, we provide the following hypothesis for the differential temperature effect of the 1,4-dihydropyridines and their different efficacies in stimulating (at, for example, 30°C) in comparison to their efficacy in inhibiting (at 2°C):

The 1,4-dihydropyridine Ca^{2+} channel blockers increase the fraction of channels in the "shut" state for [^{3}H]D-*cis*-diltiazem at 30°C, but because

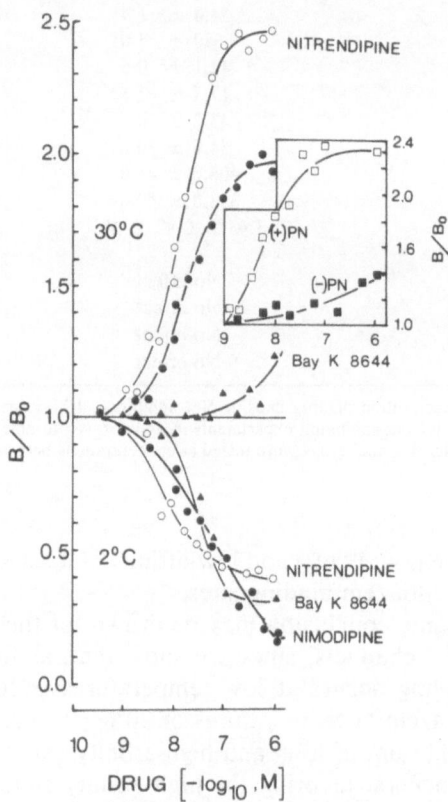

Figure 15.   Temperature-dependent regulation of [^{3}H]D-*cis*-diltiazem binding to guinea pig skel-etal-muscle microsomal membranes by 1,4-dihydropyridines. The concentration–effect curves were constructed by incubating 9–14 different concentrations of 1,4-dihydropyridines at either 2°C (*bottom*) (4 hr incubation) or 30°C (*top*) with [^{3}H]D-*cis*-diltiazem and guinea pig skeletal-muscle membranes. Each point is the mean from a duplicate determination for specific binding, and the results are expressed as the ratio between B (which is the concentration of [^{3}H]D-*cis*-diltiazem specifically bound in the presence of the respective 1,4-dihydropyridine) and B_o, which is the specifically bound [^{3}H]ligand concentration in the absence of the 1,4-dihydropyridine. *Insert:* An experiment with enantiomers of PN 200-110 is exemplified. [(+)PN] PN205-033; [(−)PN] PN205-034.

Table 11.   Effects of Various 1,4-Dihydropyridines on Ca^{2+}-Channel Labeling by [^{3}H]D-cis-Diltiazem at 2°C and 30°C

| | Temperature | | | |
| | 2°C | | 30°C | |
Drug	IC_{50} [nM]	Maximal inhibition	EC_{50} [nM]	Maximal stimulation
Nitrendipine	8.75 ± 2.8	59.8 ± 1.9	33.5 ± 14	250 ± 4
Nimodipine	34.0 ± 14.7	83.3 ± 2.0	24.5 ± 6.4	200 ± 6
Bay K 8644	47.0 ± 1.2	64.0 ± 3.5	500	123 ± 3
(+)205-033	7.8 ± 0.4	61.4 ± 0.4	6.1 ± 2.6	230 ± 14
(−)205-034	63.0 ± 11.0	81.0 ± 2.0	≥1000	144 ± 7
Vo 2605	N.D.		No effect up to 1 μM	
M 5579	No effect up to 1 μM		No effect up to 1 μM	

[a] For 2°C experiments, the average maximal inhibition data as percentages $(B_o - B) \times 100$ (at ≤1 μM) and the average IC_{50} values are given; for 30°C experiments, the EC_{50} values and the maximal stimulation values (at ≤1 μM). Stimulation is expressed as $(B/B_o) \times 100$; B is the concentration of [^{3}H]D-cis-diltiazem specifically bound in the presence of the 1,4-dihydropyridine and B_o that in the absence of the 1,4-dihydropyridine. (+)205-033 is the (+)enantiomer of PN 200-110 and (−)205-034 is the (−)enantiomer. Vo 2056 is the 7-bromo-substituted PN 200-110 and M 5579 an inactive nitrendipine derivative with a free carboxyl group. Data are means from two or from three or four (± S.E.M.) separate experiments. (N.D.) Not determined.

their relative affinities for "shut" and "unshut" channels differ, they vary in their intrinsic efficacy. The rank order of efficacies for the conversion into the "shut" state for these 1,4-dihydropyridines is, then: nitrendipine > (+)205-033 > nimodipine > (−)205-034 > Bay K 8644 ≫ Vo 2605, M 5579.

In contrast, at 2°C, where all the channels that can be labeled with [^{3}H]D-cis-diltiazem are "shut" channels, the rank order of efficacies for keeping channels in the "unshut" state is quite different: nimodipine = (−)205-034 > Bay K 8644 = (+)205-033 = nitrendipine. One must conclude that none of the 1,4-dihydropyridines investigated can be a pure Ca^{2+} channel agonist or antagonist. This is indeed the case. Bay K 8644 is only a partial agonist, and nimodipine, when compared to nitrendipine in classic pharmacological experiments, has stronger agonistic properties. Most interesting in this context is the behavior of the enantiomers of PN 200-110. The eudismic ratio of the EC_{50} values for the two enantiomers, which is 150 or more for stimulation, is reduced to approximately 10 when the IC_{50} values for inhibition are compared. Clearly, the interaction of Ca^{2+} channel drugs with their binding sites is of remarkable complexity and far from being understood. The concept of a continuum of Ca^{2+} channel drugs ranging from agonists to antagonists was proposed earlier, on the basis of a comparison of Ca^{2+}-channel labeling by different 1,4-dihydropyridines in skeletal-muscle microsomes. [^{3}H]D-cis-Diltiazem labeling of the allosteric regulatory site supports this concept. One important conclusion is that affinities of Ca^{2+}-channel drugs found in classic pharmacological or electrophysiological experiments may or may not be identical to the affinities measured by direct labeling of the channels. The partial agonism of the drugs, taken together with the possible existence of subtypes of Ca^{2+} channels, may be the molecular basis for the apparent tissue selectivity of Ca^{2+}-channel drugs, which is not yet understood but has considerable therapeutic implications.

SOLUBILIZATION AND PARTIAL PURIFICATION OF THE CALCIUM CHANNEL

High-affinity binding sites for the potent 1,4-dihydropyridine calcium channel blocker [^{3}H]nimodipine were solubilized from guinea pig skeletal-muscle microsomes with digitonin and CHAPS [3-(3-cholamidopropyl) dimethyl-ammonio-1-propanesulfonate]. Detergent-solubilized binding sites could not be sedimented by centrifugation (50,000g, 4 hr), passed freely through 0.2-μm nitrocellulose filters, and were stable at 4°C with half-lives of more than 60 hr. The solubilized 1,4-dihydropyridine drug receptors were precipitable with polyethyleneglycol 6000 on Whatman GF/C filters. Saturation analysis of solubilized microsomes with [^{3}H]nimodipine revealed a single class of binding sites (B_{max} = 0.5–1.7 pmoles/mg protein) with a K_D of 2.2–3.6 nM at 37°C. Specific binding of the 1,4-dihydropyridine calcium-channel label was fully reversible (k_{-1} = 1.5 min^{-1} at 37°C). The solubilized drug receptors discriminated between the optical enantiomers of chiral 1,4-dihydropyridine calcium-channel blockers, ($-$) and ($+$)D-600, as well as between L-cis- and D-cis-diltiazem. D-cis-Diltiazem stimulated the binding of [^{3}H]nimodipine (ED$_{50}$ = 3.6 μM) by increasing the B_{max} and slowed the dissociation rate of the labeled 1,4-dihydropyridine calcium-channel blocker.

The solubilized drug receptors were sensitive to pronase, chymotrypsin, and phospholipases A and C, indicating their protein nature as well as their lipid requirement. Chelation of endogenous divalent cations by EDTA, EGTA, or CDTA inhibits high-affinity [^{3}H]nimodipine binding, demonstrating that divalent cations are required for high-affinity [^{3}H]nimodipine binding.

Detergent-solubilized binding sites are adsorbed by several Sepharose-immobilized lectins, including concanavalin A, wheat germ agglutinin, and lentil-lectin, but not by *Helix pomatia* lectin. Preparative chromatography on concanavalin A–Sepharose was performed, and the adsorbed [^{3}H]nimodipine binding sites were selectively eluted by alpha-methylmannoside, NaCl (1 M) being completely ineffective as elutant. The purification factors by this method were 17- to 40-fold (Figure 16). The binding sites could be also purified (up to 10-fold) by sucrose-density centrifugation. The $S_{20,w}$ value of the drug receptors is 12.9 S (Figure 17).

It is concluded that the 1,4-dihydropyridine drug receptors of the putative calcium channel are intimately associated with carbohydrate-containing structures. Since the detergent-solubilized material shows allosteric reg-

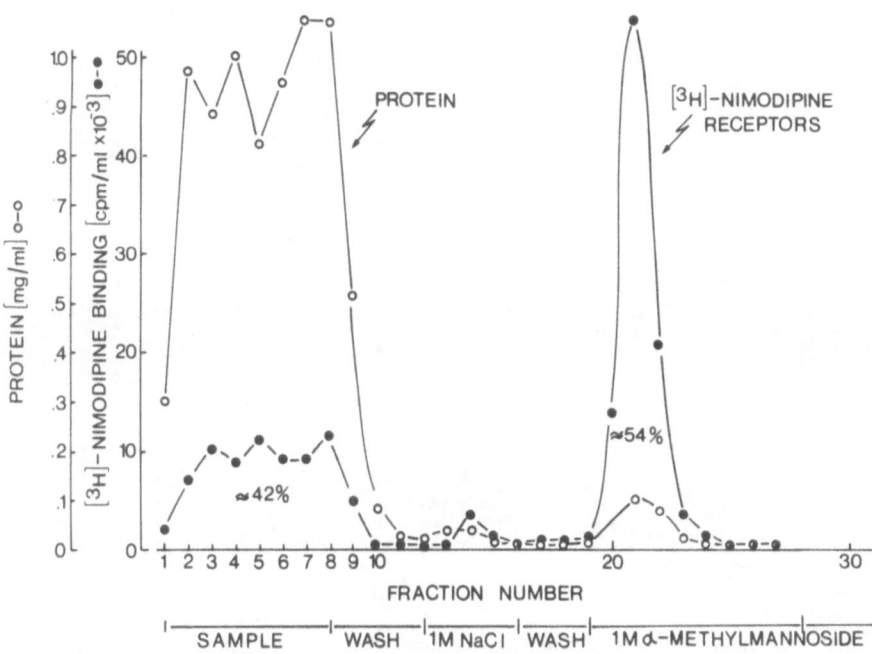

Figure 16.   Affinity chromatography of [³H]nimodipine binding sites on concanavalin A–Sepharose. Samples (25 ml) of digitonin-solubilized skeletal muscle membranes (21 mg protein) were applied by gravity flow to a concanavalin A–Sepharose column (7 ml packed gel) at 4°C. The column was previously washed with 50 mM Tris HCl, 0.1 mM PMSF, 0.1% (wt./vol.) digitonin, and 1 mM $CaCl_2$ (pH 7.4). The column was washed with this buffer (fractions of 2.5–3.5 ml were collected) after application of the sample, then with 1 M NaCl added to the afore-described buffer, subsequently with buffer, and left for 8 hr at 20°C with 1 M α-methylmannoside in buffer. The elution was then continued at 4°C as shown in the figure. Subsequently, 100-μl aliquots of the eluted fractions were tested for [³H]nimodipine binding (assay volume 300 μl; [³H]nimodipine concentration = 1.04 nM; = 62,300 cpm) and for protein. The overall recovery for protein was 126% and that for [³H]nimodipine binding sites was 92%. Aliquots of the starting material were kept under the same conditions. These control samples bound 22,200 cpm/ml, equivalent to 26,428 cpm/mg protein. The peak fraction (Fraction No. 21) bound 53,040 cpm/ml and contained 0.116 mg protein/ml, and its [³H]nimodipine binding was equivalent to 457,240 cpm/mg protein (purification factor 17.3-fold).

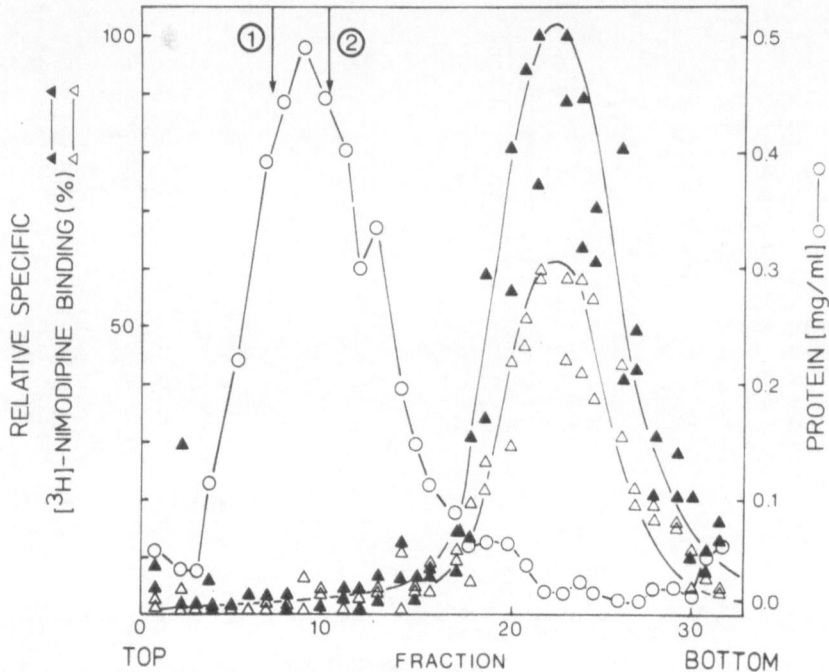

Figure 17.   Sucrose-density centrifugation of solubilized calcium channels. The figure shows pooled data from two gradients. A 5–20% linear sucrose gradient (11.5 ml) was overlaid with 0.65 or 1.0 ml of solubilized skeletal muscle, corresponding to 0.61 and 0.94 mg protein, respectively. [14C]-labeled ovalbumin (15,000 dpm) or rabbit gamma-globulin (10,000 dpm) was included in the overlays to serve as internal markers. Gradients were spun at 170,000 g in an SW 41 rotor for 16 hr. Gradients were dropped out into 25–28 fractions and 100-liter aliquots assayed for specific [3H]nimodipine (2.94 nM) binding in the absence (△) and presence (▲) of 10 μM D-*cis*-diltiazem. Peak binding in the presence of 10 μM D-*cis*-diltiazem was set at 100% and for the 1.0-ml overlay corresponds to 88,300 cpm of specifically bound [3H]nimodipine/ml and for the 0.65-ml overlay to 47,200 cpm/ml. The relative binding data for both overlays were then pooled and computer-fitted to the equation describing a normal distribution (using the error-sums-of-squares principle) to determine the peak position. The peak positions of specific [3H]nimodipine binding (± asymptotic standard deviation) were: in the absence of D-*cis*-diltiazem, fraction 21.98 ± 0.14; in the presence of 10 μM D-*cis*-diltiazem, 21.83 ± 0.14. The rabbit [14C]ovalbumin peak (arrow 1) was at fraction 10.1 ± 0.14 and the [14C]gamma-globulin peak (arrow 2) at fraction 7.36 ± 0.06. The purification factor for the specific binding of [3H]nimodipine in the presence of 10 μM D-*cis*-diltiazem in the 1.0-ml overlay was 9.4-fold (corresponding to 22,800 fmoles/mg protein) and for the 0.65-ml overlay 7.7-fold (corresponding to 18,475 fmoles/mg protein). The overall recovery of [3H]nimodipine binding sites in this experiment was 27% measured in the presence and 35% measured in the absence of D-*cis*-diltiazem, respectively.

ulation of 1,4-dihydropyridine binding, interaction with chemically different classes of calcium-channel blockers, metalloprotein nature, and a $S_{20,w}$ value that is indicative of structure large enough to span the membrane, we conclude that we have solubilized and partially purified the putative calcium channel.

ACKNOWLEDGMENTS

C. Auriga, B. Habermann, I. Seidel, A. Rücker, and M. Rombusch provided excellent technical assistance, and we are grateful to W. Nürnberger, who was in charge of typing the manuscript. We would also like to thank the chemists (Dr. Wehinger and Dr. Meyer) and our colleagues (Dr. Hoffmeister and Dr. Kazda) at BAYER AG for providing us with labeled and unlabeled 1,4-dihydropyridines, Dr. Traber and Dr. Dompert (TROPON AG) for constant advice and help, and our colleagues at SANDOZ AG, Basle, for the optically pure enantiomers of PN 200-110 as well as stimulating discussions. Special thanks are extended to Dr. Bahrmann and Dr. Satzinger at the GOEDECKE AG for [^{3}H]D-cis-diltiazem and to C.M. for support. Our research is funded by the Deutsche Forschungsgemeinschaft, Bonn-Bad Godesberg.

REFERENCES

1. Fleckenstein, A. 1977. Specific pharmacology of calcium in myocardium, cardiac pacemakers and vascular smooth muscle. *Annu. Rev. Pharmacol. Toxicol.* 17:149–166.
2. Bossert, F., and Vater, W. 1971. Dihydropyridine, eine Gruppe stark wirksamer Coronartherapeutika. *Naturwissenschaften* 58:578.
3. Vater, W., Kroneberg, G., Hoffmeister, F., Kaller, H., Meng, K., Oberdorf, A., Puls, W., Schlossmann, K., and Stoepel, K. 1972. Zur Pharmakologie von 4-(2-Nitrophenyl)-2,6,-dimethyl-1,4-dihydropyridin-3,5-dicarbonsäure-dimethylester (Nifedipine), BAY a 1040. *Arzneim.-Forsch.* 22:1–14.
4. Towart, R., Wehinger, E., and Meyer, H. 1981. Effects of unsymmetrical ester substituted 1,4-dihydropyridine derivatives and their optical isomers on contraction of smooth muscle. *Naunyn-Schmiedeberg's Arch. Pharmacol.* 317:183–185.
5. Stefani, E., and Chiarandani, D. J. 1982. Ionic channels in skeletal muscle. *Annu. Rev. Physiol.* 44:357–372.
6. Almers, W., Fink, R., and Palade P. T. 1981. Calcium depletion in frog muscle tubules: The decline of calcium currents under maintained depolarization. *J. Physiol.* 312:177–207.
7. Beaty, G. N., and Stefani, E. 1976. Inward calcium current in twitch muscle fibres of the frog. *J. Physiol.* 260:27p.
8. Gonzales-Serratos, H., Valle-Aguilera, R., Lathrop, D. A., and Garcia, M. del C. 1982. Slow inward calcium currents have no obvious role in muscle excitation–contraction coupling. *Nature (London)* 298:292–294.
9. Doble, A., and Iversen, L. L. 1982. Molecular size of benzodiazepine receptor in rat brain in situ: Evidence for a functional dimer? *Nature (London)* 295:522–523.
10. Chang, L. R., Barnard, E. A., Lo, M. M. S., and Dolly, J. O. 1981. Molecular sizes of benzodiazepine receptors and the interacting GABA receptors in the membrane. *FEBS Lett.* 126:309–312.
11. Paul, S. M., Kempner, E. S., and Skolnick, P. 1981. In situ molecular weight determination of brain and peripheral benzodiazepine binding sites. *Eur. J. Pharmacol.* 76:465–466.
12. Ferry, D. R., and Glossmann, H. 1983. Tissue-specific regulation of [^{3}H]-nimodipine binding to putative calcium channels by the biologically active isomer of diltiatem. *Br. J. Pharmacol.* 78:81p.

13. Janis, R., Maurer, S. C., Sarmiento, J. C., Bolger, G. T., and Triggle, D. J. 1982. Binding of [^{3}H]-nimodipine to cardiac and smooth muscle membranes. *Eur. J. Pharmacol.* 82:191.
14. Glossmann, H., Ferry, D. R., Lübbecke, F., Mewes, H., and Hofmann, F. 1983. Calcium channels: direct identification with radioligand binding studies. *J. Rec. Res.* 3:177–190.
15. Ferry, D. R., and Glossmann, H. Unpublished results.
16. Ferry, D. R., Kaumann, A. J., and Glossmann, H. Unpublished results.

The Measurement of Cardiac Membrane Channels following Their Incorporation into Phospholipid Bilayers

A. J. Williams

Department of Cardiac Medicine
Cardiothoracic Institute
University of London
London WIN 2DX, England

Abstract. This chapter describes the basic properties of integral membrane channels from both cardiac sarcoplasmic reticulum and sarcolemma. Channels are studied, under voltage-clamp conditions, following their incorporation into planar phospholipid bilayers by fusion of isolated native membrane vesicles with preformed membranes. The rate of fusion of vesicles may be influenced by a number of factors including divalent cations and negatively charged phospholipids in the preformed bilayer.

Mammalian cardiac sarcoplasmic reticulum contains a monovalent cation selective channel with a single-channel conductance of approximately 150 pico-Siemens in the presence of symmetrical solutions of 500 mM K^+ at holding potentials ranging from -60 to $+60$ mV. The probability of the channel being in the open state is high at positive holding potentials and low at negative holding potentials.

Mammalian cardiac sarcolemma contains at least three K^+-selective channels and one Cl^--selective channel.

INTRODUCTION

The electrical activity of excitable tissues, such as cardiac muscle, is dependent on the functioning of various ion-specific integral membrane protein channels. The opening of these channels allows the passive flux of ions across the membrane, producing either inward or outward currents and so depolarizing or repolarizing the cell.

Classically, these currents have been investigated macroscopically using the voltage-clamp technique [1]. Although this technique is difficult to apply to cardiac muscle, it has provided much useful information concerning the ionic currents underlying the cardiac action and resting potentials [2].

Our knowledge of the processes controlling tissue excitability has recently been extended by the introduction of patch-clamp techniques [3] that allow the measurement of the currents in single ionic channels of cultured or enzyme-disrupted cells. Application of this technique to cardiac-muscle cells has provided data on single sodium and calcium channels [4] (see also

H. Reuter, "Properties of single sodium and calcium channels," this volume) and calcium-activated monovalent cation channels [5].

The study of single-channel activity using the patch-clamp technique is, of course, limited to whole cells and hence channels located in the cell membrane. In this chapter, I will describe the attempts that have been made to monitor the channels from both cardiac sarcolemma and an intracellular organelle, the sarcoplasmic reticulum, using a "biochemical" approach. This has been done by incorporating isolated membrane vesicles, containing integral membrane channels, into planar phospholipid bilayers by fusion and then monitoring current flow under voltage-clamp conditions.

The monitoring of single-channel events in this way was introduced by Christopher Miller to study the activity of a monovalent cation channel of skeletal muscle sarcoplasmic reticulum [6]. This channel has now been extensively characterized by Miller and colleagues [7–11], and the technique has more recently been applied to a variety of channels from other membrane systems [12–15].

Incorporation of Cardiac Sarcoplasmic Reticulum Vesicles into Planar Phospholipid Bilayers

Rabbit ventricular muscle sarcoplasmic reticulum was extracted using an adaptation of the calcium oxalate loading procedure described by Jones et al. (Procedure 1) [16].

Planar phospholipid bilayers were formed across a small aperture (approximately 400 μm in diameter) in a polystyrene partition separating two chambers. The chambers contained 150 mM KCl, 0.1 mM EDTA, 5 mM Tris-HCl, pH 7.2. The bilayer was composed of 30 mM phospholipid (70% phosphatidylethanolamine, 30% phosphatidylserine) (Avanti Polar Lipids, Birmingham, Alabama) in decane. Formation of the bilayer is monitored by the increase in capacitance as the membrane thins. One chamber, designated trans, is held at virtual ground, while the other, cis, may be clamped at a range of holding potentials relative to ground.

Current flow through the bilayer is monitored using an operational amplifier as a current-to-voltage converter with a 1 GΩ feedback resistor and a 2.2 pF capacitor in parallel to provide extra compensation. The output of the amplifier is filtered at 500 Hz using a six-pole Bessel low-pass filter, displayed on an oscilloscope, and stored on FM tape for later analysis using a Z-80 based microcomputer (Figure 1).

The incorporation of cardiac sarcoplasmic reticulum membrane into preformed phospholipid bilayers by fusion requires an initial interaction between the bilayer and the native membrane vesicle. This interaction is enhanced by the presence of negatively charged phospholipids in the bilayer (provided in these experiments by phosphatidylserine) and divalent cations in the medium of the cis chamber to which the vesicles are added. The rate of fusion of native cardiac sarcoplasmic reticulum vesicles with the bilayer

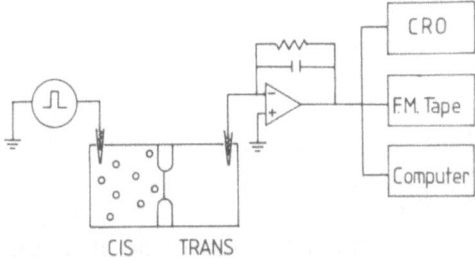

Figure 1. Schematic representation of the apparatus used to monitor single-channel activity following the incorporation of native membrane channels into planar phospholipid bilayers by fusion. The bilayer, formed as described in the text, separates the cis and trans chambers. Membrane vesicles are added only to the cis chamber.

is then further increased by imposing an osmotic gradient across the bilayer, with the cis chamber hyperosmotic to the trans chamber. This manipulation has been shown to increase the rate of fusion of liposomes with planar bilayers [17].

The generalized conditions that we have used to incorporate cardiac sarcoplasmic reticulum vesicles into phospholipid bilayers are shown in Figure 2. Vesicles of cardiac sarcoplasmic reticulum are added to the cis chamber, which is held 40 mV positive to the trans chamber, and the contents of the cis chamber are mixed using a small magnetic follower. Experiments are carried out at 25°C. The fusion of a vesicle of cardiac sarcoplasmic reticulum with the bilayer is accompanied by a sudden increase in membrane conductance. Additional fusion events are then inhibited by chelating the calcium in the cis chamber with EGTA, and unfused vesicles are perfused out.

Single-Channel Activity of Cardiac Sarcoplasmic Reticulum

Following fusion of a vesicle of cardiac sarcoplasmic reticulum with the bilayer, we observe discrete current fluctuations that correspond to the openings and closings of single channels (Figure 3). In Figure 3, we see examples of single-channel fluctuations in the presence of 250 mM K_2SO_4, 0.1mM

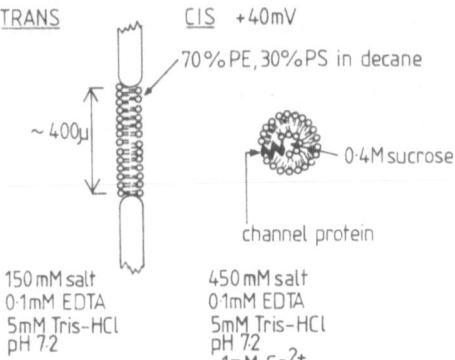

Figure 2. Requirements for fusion of cardiac sarcoplasmic reticulum vesicles with planar phospholipid bilayers. In most experiments, the salt used is KCl; however, fusion will also occur in other salts, for example, K_2SO_4.

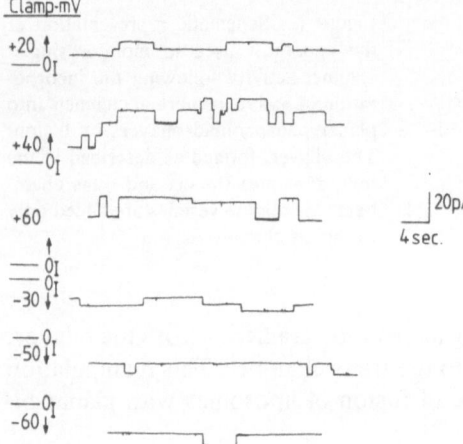

Figure 3. Single-channel fluctuations observed under voltage-clamp conditions following the fusion of a vesicle of cardiac sarcoplasmic reticulum with a preformed planar bilayer. Both cis and trans chambers contained 250 mM K_2SO_4, 0.1 mM EDTA, 10 mM Tris, 10 mM HEPES, pH 7.2. See the text for explanation.

EDTA, 10 mM Tris, 10 mM HEPES, pH 7.2, in both the cis and trans chambers. In this particular experiment, a single fusion event has incorporated a number of channels that randomly open and close with time. Recordings were made at a range of holding potentials as indicated in the figure. At positive holding potentials, an upward deflection corresponds to increasing current flow. At negative holding potentials, increased current flow is represented by a downward deflection. In each trace, the 0_I bar represents the conductance of the bilayer at zero holding potential.

The channel incorporated from cardiac sarcoplasmic reticulum appears to have three conductance states, one closed and two open. The probability of the channel being in the open conducting state is higher at positive holding potentials than at negative holding potentials. This is reflected by the higher mean conductance observed at positive holding potentials (cf. + 60 mV and − 60 mV in Figure 3) and confirmed by measurements of macroscopic conductance following the incorporation of large numbers of channels (data not shown).

The current flowing through the conducting channel varies with the holding potential, as can be seen in Figure 3. The relationship between single-channel current in the fully open state and holding potential is plotted in Figure 4. From these data it is clear that the single-channel current of the channel incorporated from the cardiac sarcoplasmic reticulum varies linearly with holding potential. Therefore, under the experimental conditions used here, the single-channel conductance (single-channel current/holding potential) remains constant, at approximately 150 pico-Siemens (pS), over this range of holding potentials.

The determination of the single-channel reversal potential in the presence of a KCl gradient across the membrane reveals that the cardiac sarcoplasmic reticulum channel is selective for potassium. Chloride ions do not pass through the channel.

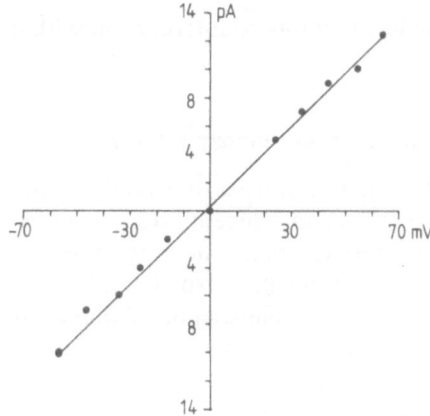

Figure 4.   Single-channel current–voltage relationship of the cardiac sarcoplasmic reticulum channel. Experimental conditions are as described in the Figure 3 caption.

From the findings outlined above, we conclude that cardiac-muscle sarcoplasmic reticulum contains an integral membrane channel that is selective for potassium ions. Recent work by Meissner and McKinley [18] supports this conclusion. These authors monitored macroscopic conductance for monovalent cations in canine cardiac sarcoplasmic reticulum vesicles using isotope flux, light-scattering, and membrane-potential measurements. They concluded that cardiac sarcoplasmic reticulum is permeable to a number of these ions.

In addition, Meissner and McKinley [18] suggested for this system a possible physiological role that is summarized in Figure 5. It is proposed that the channel allows a rapid flux of monovalent cations to counter electrogenic calcium movements across the sarcoplasmic reticulum membrane associated with excitation–contraction coupling. In the absence of such a system, the large electrogenic movement of calcium that occurs to initiate contraction would lead to the establishment of a considerable diffusion potential. The lumen of the sarcoplasmic reticulum would be at a negative potential with respect to the cytosol, which would in turn retard calcium efflux. A counterflux of monovalent cations would prevent the establishment of such a potential, allowing maximal rates of calcium movement. It is prob-

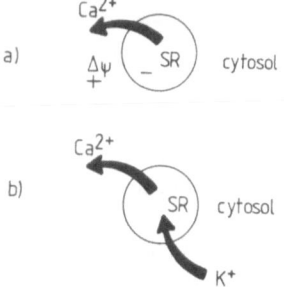

Figure 5.   Physiological role of the potassium channel of cardiac sarcoplasmic reticulum (based on the proposition of Meissner and McKinley [18]). (a) Calcium efflux from sarcoplasmic reticulum in the absence of a potassium countercurrent generates a diffusion potential ($\Delta\psi$) that would tend to retard calcium flux. (b) Potassium countercurrent flowing through the potassium channel would abolish the calcium-generated diffusion potential and allow maximal rates of calcium flux.

able that potassium will carry the vast majority of this countercurrent within the cell.

Incorporation of Cardiac Sarcolemmal Channels into Planar Bilayers

The techniques described above have also been used to investigate the channel activity of isolated cardiac sarcolemma. In a recent article, Coronado and Latorre [19] describe four species of ionic channel activity observed following the fusion of vesicles of calf cardiac sarcolemma, isolated following the method of Jones et al. (Procedure 2) [16] with planar phospholipid bilayers. These authors describe three of these channels as potassium-selective and the other as chloride-selective; their properties are summarized below.

95 pS Potassium Channel.   This channel is freely permeable to all the alkali cations. It is voltage-independent and has one open state and two closed states. The closed states are of very different duration. The existence of the longer of these closed states appears to be influenced by the calcium concentration in the cis chamber. It is not seen if the calcium concentration is reduced to less than 1 mM.

28 pS Potassium Channel.   This channel has a linear current–voltage relationship, is ideally selective for monovalent cations rather than anions, and has a potassium permeability/sodium permeability of 5. Coronado and Latorre [19] tentatively link this channel with the repolarizing i_x current [2].

15 pS Potassium Channel.   The potassium permeability/sodium permeability of this channel is 3, and the open-state conductance is described as "noisy."

55 pS Chloride Channel.   The chloride selective channel derived from the calf cardiac sarcolemma preparation appears to have several open states and at least two closed states. Mean single-channel current is not linearly related to holding potential. At negative holding potentials, current increase is hyperlinear, and with increasing positive holding potentials, it reaches a limiting value. Reversal-potential determinations suggest that the channel is ideally selective for chloride ions rather than potassium. Coronado and Latorre are unable to assign a physiological role to this channel.

CONCLUSIONS

The single-channel activity of cardiac muscle membranes may be monitored using the patch-clamp technique on whole cells or by incorporating membrane fragments into planar phospholipid bilayers.

The technique described here has the advantage that it may be applied to the study of channels derived from both the cell membrane and intracellular organelles. A limitation is that the membrane system used in the experiments must be as free as possible from contamination by other membrane fractions. We can be confident that the membrane fraction produced by the calcium oxalate loading technique is derived from the sarcoplasmic reticulum [16]. We observe only one species of channel following fusion of this fraction with planar phospholipid bilayers, and this channel shares a number of features with the monovalent-cation-selective channel found in skeletal-muscle sarcoplasmic reticulum.

The situation with sarcolemma is less clear-cut, and further work is required to fully establish the origin of the channel activities at present ascribed to this membrane. Comparison of the channel activities observed in phospholipid bilayers with those seen in patch-clamped whole cardiac cells will be of great help in resolving this issue.

ACKNOWLEDGMENTS

This work was supported by project grants from the Medical Research Council and the British Heart Foundation I am very grateful to Dr. Barbara Tomlins and Mr. Richard Montgomery for collaboration and useful discussions.

REFERENCES

1. Junge, D. 1981. *Nerve and Muscle Excitation*, 2nd ed. Sinauer Associates, Sunderland, Massachusetts.
2. Noble, D. 1979. *The Initiation of the Heart Beat*, 2nd ed. Clarendon Press, Oxford.
3. Hamill, O. P., Marty, A., Neher, E., Sakmann, B., and Sigworth, F. J. 1981. Improved patch-clamp techniques for high-resolution current recording from cells and cell-free membrane patches. *Pfluegers Arch.* 391:85–100.
4. Reuter, H., Stevens, C. F., Tsien, R. W., and Yellen, G. 1982. Properties of single calcium channels in cardiac cell culture. *Nature (London)* 297:501–504.
5. Colquhoun, D., Neher, E., Reuter, H., and Stevens, C. F. 1981. Inward current channels activated by intracellular calcium in cultured cardiac cells. *Nature (London)* 294:752–754.
6. Miller, C. 1978. Voltage-gated cation conductance channel from sarcoplasmic reticulum: Steady-state electrical properties. *J. Membr. Biol.* 40:1–23.
7. Coronado, R., and Miller, C. 1979. Voltage-dependent caesium blockade of a cation channel from fragmented sarcoplasmic reticulum. *Nature (London)* 280:807–810.
8. Labarca, P., Coronado, R., and Miller, C. 1980. Thermodynamic and kinetic studies of the gating behavior of a K^+-selective channel from the sarcoplasmic reticulum membrane. *J. Gen. Physiol.* 76:397–424.
9. Coronado, R., Rosenberg, R. L., and Miller, C. 1980. Ionic selectivity saturation and block in a K^+ channel from sarcoplasmic reticulum. *J. Gen. Physiol.* 76:425–446.
10. Coronado, R., and Miller, C. 1982. Conduction and block by organic cations in a K^+-selective channel from sarcoplasmic reticulum incorporated into planar phospholipid bilayers. *J. Gen. Physiol.* 79:529–547.
11. Miller, C. 1982. Bis-quaternary ammonium blockers as structural probes of the sarcoplasmic reticulum K^+ channel. *J. Gen. Physiol.* 79:869–891.
12. White, M. M., and Miller, C. 1981. Probes of the conduction process of a voltage gated Cl^- channel from *Torpedo electroplax*. *J. Gen. Physiol.* 78:1–18.
13. Miller, C. 1982. Open-state substructure of single chloride channels from *Torpedo electroplax*. *Philos. Trans. R. Soc. Lond. Ser. B* 299:401–411.

14. Latorre, R., Vergara, C., and Hidalgo, C. 1982. Reconstitution in planar lipid bilayers of a Ca^{2+}-dependent K^+ channel from transverse tubule membrane isolated from rabbit skeletal muscle. *Proc. Natl. Acad. Sci. U.S.A.* 79:805–809.
15. Krueger, B. C., Worley, J. F., and French, R. J. 1983. Single sodium channels from rat brain incorporated into planar lipid bilayer membranes. *Nature (London)* 303:172–175.
16. Jones, L. R., Besch, H. R., Fleming, J. W., McConnaughey, M. M., and Watanabe, A.M. 1979. Separation of vesicles of cardiac sarcolemma from vesicles of cardiac sarcoplasmic reticulum. *J. Biol. Chem.* 254:530–539.
17. Cohen, F. S., Zimmerberg, J., and Finkelstein, A. 1980. Fusion of phospholipid vesicles with planar phospholipid bilayer membranes. II. Incorporation of vesicular membrane marker into the planar membrane. *J. Gen. Physiol.* 75:251–270.
18. Meissner, G., and McKinley, D. 1982. Permeability of canine cardiac sarcoplasmic reticulum vesicles to K^+, Na^+, H^+ and Cl^-. *J. Biol. Chem.* 257:7704–7711.
19. Coronado, R., and Latorre, R. 1982. Detection of K^+ and Cl^- channels from calf cardiac sarcolemma in planar lipid bilayer membranes. *Nature (London)* 298:849–852.

CALMODULIN

The Calmodulin-Dependent Phosphorylation of Cardiac Myosin

Franz Hofmann and Manfred Zimmer

Pharmakologisches Institut der Universität Heidelberg
D-6900 Heidelberg
Federal Republic of Germany

Abstract. Cardiac myosin light chains are phosphorylated in vivo and in vitro. The enzyme, myosin light-chain kinase, has been purified and found to be very specific for cardiac myosin light chains. Experiments with skinned cardiac fibers suggest that phosphorylation of myosin light chain-2 decreases ATP consumption, presumably by lowering the cross-bridge cycle. These results are discussed in this chapter.

INTRODUCTION

Phosphorylation and dephosphorylation of enzymes have been recognized as an important mechanism by which many metabolic processes are regulated [1–3]. During the last decade, evidence has been accumulated that specific myofibrillar proteins are phosphorylated by protein kinases, and in some cases the contractile process may be affected by protein phosphorylation. In smooth muscle, calcium-dependent phosphorylation of myosin light chain-2 is closely associated with the initiation of contraction [4–6]. The calcium-dependent phosphorylation of myosin light chain-2 also occurs in striated muscle [7,8] and in nonmuscular cells [5,9]. This suggests that phosphorylation and dephosphorylation of myosin is a general phenomenon and that its state of phosphorylation may modulate the contractile properties of many cells [5]. This chapter will focus mainly on the properties and function of the phosphorylation of cardiac myosin by the calcium/calmodulin-dependent enzyme, myosin light-chain kinase.

Ca^{2+} BINDING TO THICK FILAMENTS AS A POTENTIAL REGULATION MECHANISM OF STRIATED-MUSCLE CONTRACTION

Activation of the contractile process in cardiac and skeletal muscle has been described as primarily under thin-filament control [10]. It is generally accepted that binding of Ca^{2+} to one of the troponin subunits, Tn-C, is a prerequisite for an increase in myofibrillar actin-activated myosin ATPase and the initiation of contraction in striated, vertebrate muscle. However,

87

evidence from several lines of investigation suggests the existence of a second control mechanism involving Ca^{2+} binding to the myosin thick filament and the Ca^{2+}-dependent phosphorylation of one of the light chains of myosin [11–13]. Ca^{2+} binding and phosphorylation occur on the same light chain of myosin, which several laboratories have referred to as "regulatory light chain," "P-light chain," or "myosin light chain-2." This light chain has been detected in myosin from vertebrates and invertebrates, and the molecular weight for these homologous proteins have been reported to be between 18,000 and 20,000 daltons. The binding of Ca^{2+} to myosin light chain-2 in molluscan myosin regulates the myofibrillar ATPase activity of this muscle [14]. This discovery led to the speculation that also in vertebrates, striated-muscle binding of Ca^{2+} to myosin light chain-2 regulates some properties of the contractile process. A physiological function of myosin Ca^{2+} binding is indicated from studies showing that vertebrate thick filaments undergo conformational changes in response to Ca^{2+} binding in the range of concentrations that activate myofibrils [15]. Further studies with cardiac myosin light chain-2 and intact myosin suggested that phosphorylation of myosin light chain-2 decreases about 2-fold the affinity for Ca^{2+} [16,17]. Other workers using equilibrium dialysis measurements did not observe any effect of myosin light chain-2 phosphorylation on the Ca^{2+} affinity [18]. It was calculated that 0.7 mole Ca^{2+}/mole myosin is bound in the presence of 10 μM Ca^{2+} and 2.5 mM Mg^{2+} [18]. From this result, it was inferred that in skeletal muscle, binding of Ca^{2+} to myosin may function as a tonic rather than a phasic control mechanism. It is unlikely that cation binding to myosin serves a similar function in cardiac muscle, since such high Ca^{2+} concentrations are achieved only during contracture, not during regular contraction–relaxation cycles [19]. It is therefore very questionable whether in cardiac muscle Ca^{2+} regulates some function of the contraction process by direct binding to myosin. On the other hand, Ca^{2+} may still exert some regulation on the contraction process via thick filament by the phosphorylation of the myosin light chain-2, since this reaction is under the direct control of Ca^{2+} and occurs during regular contraction–relaxation cycles.

IN VIVO PHOSPHORYLATION OF CARDIAC MYOSIN LIGHT CHAIN-2

In vivo phosphorylation of cardiac myosin light chain-2 has been studied in isolated perfused rabbit or rat hearts [20–25]. Basal levels of phosphorylation of the myosin light chain-2 in rabbit hearts beating in situ or in a perfusion chamber are between 0.3 and 0.5 mole phosphate/mole light chain-2 [20,23,24]. Similar basal values were obtained with rat hearts [21,22]. In both hearts, the alkali-labile phosphate content of the light chain-2 did not change with positive inotropic interventions such as adding isoproterenol or supraphysiological Ca^{2+} concentration to the perfusion medium [22–24].

These results suggested that light-chain phosphorylation occurred in vivo but was not correlated with an increase in cardiac contractility. In contrast, Kopp and Bárány [21] reported that in perfused rat hearts, incorporation of radioactive phosphate into light chain-2 increased and decreased with positive and negative inotropic interventions. Similarly, Resink et al. [25] reported that isoproterenol stimulates the phosphate content of myosin from 0.1 mole/mole light chain to 0.4 mole/mole light chain in the heart from trained rats. These latter workers were able to correlate the phosphate content of myosin light chain-2 with an increase in the V_{max} of the myosin Ca^{2+}-ATPase activity [25]. It is not clear why different results have been obtained with a positive inotropic intervention. It is quite conceivable that some of the results reported are artifactual. On the other hand, it was recently shown that the size of the increase in contractility due to the activation of the cAMP-regulated systems varies closely with the relative amount of the V_1 isozyme of rat myosin [26]. In skeletal muscle, phosphorylation of myosin light chain-2 occurs only in the myosin isozyme that is present in fast-twitch, glycolytic muscle, not in the isozyme present in slow-twitch muscle [27]. Furthermore, it is known that the relative amounts of the different rat cardiac myosin isozymes with the age of the animal [26]. It is therefore conceivable that a difference in the relative concentration in cardiac myosin isozymes is responsible for the reported discrepancies.

   The phosphate present in cardiac myosin is not stationary, but turns over. A slow decrease in light-chain-2-associated phosphate has been observed during arrest of cardiac contraction [23]. This indicates that cardiac myosin light-chain kinase requires micromolar Ca^{2+} for activity and that the phosphatase is not dependent on micromolar Ca^{2+} for activity. The latter point is of some importance, since it is at variance with the possibility that "calcineurin," a calcium/calmodulin-dependent phosphatase [28], dephosphorylates cardiac myosin light chain-2 in vivo. The nature and identity of the phosphatase responsible for the dephosphorylation of cardiac myosin light chains are unknown, whereas several properties of the cardiac myosin light-chain kinase have been established.

CARDIAC MYOSIN LIGHT-CHAIN KINASE

   Myosin light-chain kinase as purified from bovine muscle [29] contains a catalytic subunit of an apparent molecular weight (M_r) of 85,000–93,000 [30]. This value is similar to values reported for the enzyme from skeletal muscle [5], but is lower than those reported for the smooth-muscle enzymes [5]. The previously described enzyme of cardiac muscle that had a lower molecular weight and a low specific activity [32] was most likely a proteolytic fragment of the native enzyme. The native molecular weight of the cardiac enzyme has also been determined by immunological methods using antibodies raised against the smooth-muscle enzyme [33,34]. Apparent M_r's of

Table 1.   Substrate Specifity of Bovine Cardiac
Myosin Light-Chain Kinase

Substrate	Activity (%)[a]
Bovine cardiac myosin light chain-2	100.0
Chicken gizzard myosin light chain-2	10.0
Mixed histones	0.1
Bovine cardiac troponin	N.D.
Bovine cardiac sarcoplasmic reticulum	N.D.
Bovine cardiac sarcolemma	N.D.

[a] 100% equals 20–30 μmoles/min per mg; (N.D.) no detectable phosphate
incorporation.

130,000 [33] and 75,000 [34] were obtained for the native cardiac enzyme.
The higher value is identical to the M_r of the smooth-muscle enzyme. This
is no surprise, since (1) antibodies raised against the smooth-muscle enzyme
were used and (2) no precautions were used to prevent the extraction of the
smooth-muscle enzyme from the cardiac muscle mince. It is therefore likely
that these authors determined the M_r of the enzyme present in coronary
arteries. The second study [34] suggests that the rat heart enzyme has an
M_r of 75,000, which value is considerably lower than that of the bovine
cardiac enzyme. This may suggest that the reported variability for the molecular weight of the cardiac enzyme is due partially to species variability,
as evidenced by the different M_r's for the rat and beef heart enzymes.

As shown first for the smooth-muscle enzyme [35], the cardiac [30] and
skeletal-muscle [31] enzymes are phosphorylated by cAMP-dependent protein kinase in vitro. Slightly more than 1 mole phosphate/mole enzyme is
incorporated in vitro [29]. In contrast to the smooth-muscle enzyme, no
change in activity or in the apparent affinity for calmodulin is associated
with the phosphorylation of the enzymes from skeletal or cardiac muscle.
These results are consistent with the idea that the cardiac enzyme is distinct
from the smooth-muscle enzyme and that the cardiac enzyme is not regulated
by mechanisms that are similar to those observed with the smooth-muscle
enzyme.

The purified cardiac enzyme is inactive in the absence of Ca^{2+} and is
activated by the addition of Ca^{2+} and calmodulin [30]. The enzyme phosphorylates specifically cardiac myosin light chain-2 with a specific activity
of 20–30 μmoles phosphate transferred per min and mg enzyme. Smooth-
muscle light chain-2 is phosphorylated at approximately 1/10th this rate. The
enzyme does not phosphorylate membrane proteins present in bovine cardiac muscle sarcolemma or sarcoplasmic reticulum [36] and phosphorylates
mixed histones with a 1000-fold slower rate than light chain-2. This suggests
that the cardiac enzyme has a very narrow substrate specificity (Table 1).
The enzyme is activated half-maximally at 3 nM calmodulin in the presence

of saturating concentration of Ca^{2+}. Activation of the enzyme by Ca^{2+} at a fixed concentration of calmodulin shows positive cooperativity with an apparent Hill coefficient of 2.6 [30]. This number suggests that three or four of the Ca^{2+} binding sites of calmodulin have to be filled before the enzyme is activated by calmodulin. Similar conclusions have been reported by Blumenthal and Stull [37], who studied the requirement of skeletal-muscle myosin light-chain kinase for Ca^{2+} over a wide range of enzyme and calmodulin concentrations. Direct measurement of the binding of calmodulin by the skeletal-muscle enzyme indicated that only one of the four binding sites needed to be occupied to allow binding of calmodulin to the enzyme [38,39]. These authors used either tritiated calmodulin [38] or a calmodulin-induced increase in myosin light-chain kinase intrinsic tryptophan fluorescence [39]. It is possible that the different values reported for the stoichiometry of the activating complexes of Ca^{2+}/calmodulin reflect a different Ca^{2+} requirement for the binding of calmodulin to myosin light-chain kinase vs. for the activation of the enzyme by Ca^{2+}/calmodulin.

The basic mechanism by which Ca^{2+}/calmodulin increases the activity of the light-chain kinase has been extensively studied with the cardiac enzyme [40]. Of a number of principally possible mechanisms, two appear to be important for the in vivo function of the enzyme. In mechanism (1), Ca^{2+}/calmodulin will increase mainly the affinity of myosin light-chain kinase for its substrate myosin light chain-2 (an effect on K_m), whereas in mechanism (2), Ca^{2+}/calmodulin will increase the rate of phosphorylation (an effect on V_{max}) and has no effect on the K_m of the enzyme for its substrate. Mechanism (2) would imply that in vivo, the enzyme is always bound to its substrate myosin light chain-2. Immunocytochemical studies suggested, however, that in rat heart the enzyme is associated with the thin-filament protein actin [34]. Furthermore, activity measurements indicated that in bovine heart muscle, the concentration of the enzyme is about 0.02–0.05 μmoles enzyme/kg wet weight. Since the enzyme is present only in catalytic amount, an effect of Ca^{2+}/calmodulin on the catalytic rate was unlikely. With the use of highly purified components that were free of detectable amounts of calmodulin, it could be shown that Ca^{2+}/calmodulin lowered the apparent K_m for cardiac myosin light-chain kinase over 30-fold [40]. These results together with the finding that only catalytic concentrations of the enzyme are present in bovine cardiac muscle favor the idea that phosphorylation of cardiac-muscle myosin light chain is not primarily involved in beat-to-beat control of cardiac muscle contraction, but has a modulatory function on cardiac contractility.

FUNCTIONAL SIGNIFICANCE OF THE PHOSPHORYLATION OF CARDIAC MYOSIN LIGHT CHAIN-2

Phosphorylation of smooth-muscle myosin has been associated with the initiation of smooth-muscle contraction [5]. Phosphorylation of skeletal-mus-

Table 2.   Important Properties of Bovine Cardiac Myosin Light-Chain Kinase

Native molecular weight	89,000
Substrate specifity	Cardiac MLC-2
V_{max}	20–30 μmoles/min per mg
Activator	Calmodulin
Activation complex	$Ca^{2+}_{3-4} \cdot CaM$
Activation of MLCK by in vivo concentration of MLCK	Increase in K_a for MLC-2 0.02–0.05 μmole/kg wet wt.
Physiological effect of MLC-2 phosphorylation	Decrease in energy consumption during contraction

cle myosin occurs during tetanic stimulation of skeletal muscle and has been associated with posttetanic potentiation. More recently, it has been shown that phosphorylation of fast-twitch skeletal-muscle myosin light chain-2 is associated with a decrease in energy consumption [4,27]. Until recently, much less evidence was available concerning the function of light-chain phosphorylation of cardiac muscle. One report suggested that phosphory-lation of cardiac light chain-2 increased activated myosin ATPase [42]. The significance of this observation was unclear, since a proteolytic procedure was used to study the effect of light-chain phosphorylation.

More recently, we have studied the effect of addition of purified cardiac myosin light-chain kinase to skinned muscle fibers of pig hearts. Tension transients were studied in skinned right ventricular muscle fibers before and after incubation with ATPγS (2 mM), pure myosin light-chain kinase (0.1 μM), calmodulin (1 μM), and variable concentrations of Ca^{2+}. Isometric tension development elicited by 20 μMCa^{2+} in the presence of ATP was barely affected by addition of myosin light-chain kinase. However, ATPase activity measured in these fibers was decreased about 25% compared to unphosphorylated fibers. There was a marked decrease of about 50% in the contraction velocity determined by the recovery of tension following a quick release [43,44]. In addition, the velocity of tension rise following a quick stretch was decreased by approximately 30%. These results suggest that the cross-bridge cycling became slower after the phosphorylation of cardiac myosin light chains. These results are similar to those observed with skeletal muscle [27–41] and suggest that in cardiac muscle, tension maintenance becomes more economical after phosphorylation of the light chains, since energy consumption is reduced.

CONCLUSIONS

Some of the important properties of bovine cardiac myosin light-chain kinase are summarized in Table 2. The enzyme has a very narrow substrate specificity in vitro. None of the membrane-bound peptides known to be phosphorylated in vitro by calmodulin-dependent protein kinase was modified by myosin light-chain kinase. It is therefore anticipated that the enzyme phosphorylates only myosin light chain in vivo. Phosphorylation of the light chain lowers cross-bridge cycling and energy consumption in vitro and, presumably, also in vivo. Measurement of the in vivo phosphate content of myosin light chains indicated that under physiological conditions, this phosphate has a rather slow turnover, which is not changed to a great extent during manipulation of the inotropic state of the heart. These findings (1) are in line with the observation that in vitro, myosin light-chain kinase is active at micromolar concentrations of Ca^{2+}—a concentration of Ca^{2+} that is achieved during each contraction—but is present at a low concentration in vivo and (2) require that cardiac muscle have a very low myosin light-chain phosphatase activity. One may therefore speculate that complete phosphorylation of myosin light chains requires elevated intracellular Ca^{2+} concentrations for several minutes, which will completely activate myosin light-chain kinase. This speculation may suggest that complete phosphorylation of cardiac light chains is achieved only under some pathological conditions that increase the intracellular Ca^{2+} concentrations. Under such conditions, lowering of ATP consumption may be of invaluable help for the cell to survive. Although speculative, these considerations are supported by the observation that complete phosphorylation of skeletal-muscle myosin light chains occurs only after a prolonged tetanus, a condition that is not prevalent in normal muscle physiology.

ACKNOWLEDGMENTS

We are grateful to Mrs. K. Brandt for typing the manuscript. This research was supported by DFG and Fonds der Chemie.

REFERENCES

1. Krebs, E. G., and Beavo, J. A. 1979. Phosphorylation–dephosphorylation of enzymes. *Annu. Rev. Biochem.* 48:923–959.
2. Cohen, P. 1982. The role of protein phosphorylation in neural and hormonal control of cellular activity. *Nature (London)* 296:613–620.
3. Hofmann, F., and Schultz, G. 1980. Regulation of cellular functions by protein phosphorylation. *Arzneim.-Forsch.* 30(II):1991–1995.
4. Sparrow, M. P., Mrwa, W., Hofmann, F., and Rüegg, J. C. 1981. Calmodulin is essential for smooth muscle contraction. *FEBS Lett.* 125:141–145.
5. Adelstein, R. S. 1982. Calmodulin and the regulation of actin–myosin interaction in smooth muscle and nonmuscle cells. *Cell* 30:349–350.
6. Walsh, M. P., Bridenbaugh, R., Kerrick, W. G. L., and Hartshorne, D. J. 1983. Gizzard Ca^{2+}-independent myosin light chain kinase: Evidence in favor for the phosphorylation theory. *Fed. Am. Soc. Exp. Biol. Proc.* 42:45–50.

7. Perrie, W. T., Smillie, L. B., and Perry, S. V. 1973. A phosphorylated light-chain compound of myosin from skeletal muscle. *Biochem. J.* 135:151–164.

8. Stull, J. T., Blumenthal, D. K., and Cooke, R. 1980. Regulation of contraction of myosin phosphorylation: A comparison between smooth and skeletal muscles. *Biochem. Pharmacol.* 29:2537–2543.

9. Scholey, J. M., Smith, R. C., Drenckham, D., Groschel-Stewart, U., and Kendrick-Jones J. 1982. Thymus myosin. *J. Biol. Chem.* 257:7737–7745.

10. Weber, A., and Murray, J. M. 1973. Regulation of muscle contraction by calcium. *Physiol. Rev.* 53:612–673.

11. Lehmann, W. 1978. Thick-filament-linked calcium regulation in vertebrate striated muscle. *Nature (London)* 274:80–81.

12. Bárány, K., and Bárány, M. 1977. Phosphorylation of the 18,000-dalton light chain of myosin during a single tetanus of frog muscle. *J. Biol. Chem.* 252:4752–4754.

13. Bagishaw, C. R., and Kendrick-Jones, J. 1979. Characterization of homologous divalent metal ion binding sites of vertebrate and molluscan myosins using electron paramagnetic resonance spectroscopy. *J. Mol. Biol.* 130:317–336.

14. Kendrick-Jones, J., Szenthiralyi. E. M., and Szent-Gyorgyi, A. G. 1976. Regulatory light chains in myosins. *J. Mol. Biol.* 104:747–775.

15. Morimoto, K., and Harrington, W. F. 1974. Evidence for structural changes in vertebrate thick filament induced by calcium. *J. Mol. Biol.* 88:693–709.

16. Kardami, E., and Gratzer, W. B. 1982. Conformational effects of cation binding myosin and their relation to phosphorylation. *Biochemistry* 21:1186–1191.

17. Kardami, E., and Gratzer, W. B. 1982. Interaction of cardiac myosin and its light chains with calcium ions and regulation of binding by phosphorylation. *J. Mol. Cell. Cardiol.* 14:73–80.

18. Holroyde, M. J., Potter, J. D., and Solaro, R. J. 1979. The calcium binding properties of phosphorylated and unphosphorylated cardiac and skeletal myosins. *J. Biol. Chem.* 254:6478–6482.

19. Marban, E., Rink, T. J., Tsien, R. W., and Tsien, R. Y. 1980. Free calcium in heart muscle at rest and during contraction measured with Ca^{2+}-sensitive micro electrodes. *Nature (London)* 286:845–850.

20. Holroyde, M. J., Small, O. A. P., Howe, E., and Solaro, R. J. 1979. Isolation of cardiac myofibrils and myosin light chains with in vivo levels of light chain phosphorylation. *Biochem. Biophys. Acta* 587:628–637.

21. Kopp, S. J., and Bárány, M. 1979. Phosphorylation of the 19,000-dalton light chain of myosin in perfused rat heart under the influence of negative and positive inotropic agents. *J. Biol. Chem.* 254:12,007–12,012.

22. Jeacocke, S. A., and England, P. J. 1980. Phosphorylation of myosin chains in perfused rat hearts. *Biochem. J.* 188:763–768.

23. High, C. W., and Stull, J. T. 1980. Phosphorylation of myosin in perfused rabbit and rat hearts. *Am. J. Physiol.* 239:H756–H764.

24. Westwood, S. A., and Perry, S. V. 1981. The effect of adrenaline on the phosphorylation of the P light chain of myosin and troponin I in the perfused rabbit heart. *Biochem. J.* 197:183–185.

25. Resink, T. J., Gevers, V., Noakes, T. D., and Opie, L. H. 1981. Increased cardiac myosin ATPase activity as a biochemical adaptation to running training: Enhanced response to catecholamines and a role for myosin phosphorylation. *J. Mol. Cell. Cardiol.* 13:679–694.

26. Winegard, S., Mellellan, G., Tuchar, M. and Lis, L. E. 1983. Cyclic AMP regulation of myosin isozymes in mammalian cardiac muscle. *J. Gen. Physiol.* 81:749–765.

27. Crow, M. T., and Kushmerick, M. J. 1982. Myosin light chain phosphorylation is associated with a decrease in the energy cost for contraction in fast twitch mouse muscle. *J. Biol. Chem.* 257:2121–2124.

28. Stewart, A. A. Ingebritsen, T. S., Manalan, A., Klee, L. B. and Cohen, P. 1982. Discovery of a Ca^{2+}- and calmodulin-dependent protein phosphatase. *FEBS Lett.* 137:80–84.

29. Wolf, A., and Hofmann, F. 1980. Purification of myosin light chain kinase from bovine cardiac muscle. *Proc. Natl. Acad. Sci. U.S.A.* 77:5852–5855.
30. Hofmann, F., and Wolf, H. 1981. Basic properties of myosin light chain kinase from bovine cardiac muscle. *Cold Spring Harbor Conf. Cell Proliferation: Protein Phosphorylation* 8:841–847.
31. Edelman, A. M., and Krebs, E. G. 1982. Phosphorylation of skeletal muscle myosin light chain kinase by the catalytic subunit of cAMP-dependent protein kinase. *FEBS Lett.* 138:293–298.
32. Walsh, M. P., Vellet, B., Autric, F., and Demaille, J. G. 1979. Purification and characterization of bovine cardiac calmodulin-dependent myosin light chain kinase. *J. Biol. Chem.* 254:12,136–12,144.
33. Guerriero, V., Jr., Rowley, D. R., and Means, A. R. 1981. Production and characterization of an antibody to myosin light chain kinase and intracellular localization of the enzyme. *Cell* 27:449–458.
34. Cavadore, J. G., Molla, A., Harricane, M.-G., Gabrion, J., Benyamin, Y., and Demaille, J. G. 1982. Subcellular localization of myosin light chain kinase in skeletal, cardiac, and smooth muscles. *Proc. Natl. Acad. Sci. U.S.A.* 79:3475–3479.
35. Adelstein, R. S., Conti, M. B., Hathaway, D. R., and Klee, C. B. 1978. Phosphorylation of smooth muscle myosin light chain kinase by the catalytic subunit of adenosine 3':5'-monophosphate-dependent protein kinase. *J. Biol. Chem.* 253:8347–8350.
36. Flockerzi, V., Mewes, R., Ruth, P., and Hofmann, F. 1983. Phosphorylation of purified bovine cardiac sarcolemma and potassium stimulated calcium uptake. *Eur. J. Biochem.* 135:131–142.
37. Blumenthal, D. K., and Stull, J. T. 1980. Activation of skeletal muscle myosin light chain kinase by calcium (2+) and calmodulin. *Biochemistry* 19:5608–5614.
38. Crouch, T. H., Holroyde, M. J., Collins, J. H., Solaro, R. J., and Potter, J. D. 1981. Interaction of calmodulin with skeletal muscle myosin light chain kinase. *Biochemistry* 20:6318–6325.
39. Johnson, J. D., Holroyde, M. J., Crouch, T. H., Solaro, R. J., and Potter, J. D. 1981. Fluorescence studies of the interaction of calmodulin with myosin light chain kinase. *J. Biol. Chem.* 256:12,194–198.
40. Janko, P., Wolf, H., and Hofmann, F. 1982. On the activation mechanism of cardiac myosin light chain kinase. *Horm. Cell Regulation* 6:27–35.
41. Cooke, R., Franks, K., and Stull, J. T. 1982. Myosin phosphorylation regulates the ATPase activity of permeable skeletal muscle fibers. *FEBS Lett.* 144:33–37.
42. Bhan, A., Malhotra, A., Scheuer, J., Conti, M.-A., and Adelstein, R. S. 1981. Subunit function in cardiac myosin. *J. Biol. Chem.* 256:7741–7743.
43. Pfitzer, G., Hofmann, F., Eubler, D., and Rüegg, J. C. 1982. Contractility of skinned cardiac muscle may be modulated by cardiac myosin light chain kinase (MLCK). *Pfluegers Arch.* 392(Suppl.):R1.
44. Rüegg, J. C., Kuhn, H. J., Güth, K., Pfitzer, G., and Hofmann, F. 1984. Tension transients in skinned muscle fibres of insect flight muscle and mammalian cardiac muscle: Effect of substrate concentration and treatment with myosin light chain kinase. In: H. Suji and G. J. Pollack (eds.) *Contractile Mechanisms in Muscle*. pp. 605–615. Plenum Press, New York.

Calmodulin in the Regulation of Calcium Fluxes in Cardiac Sarcolemma

Ernesto Carafoli

Laboratory of Biochemistry
Swiss Federal Institute of Technology (ETH)
8092 Zurich, Switzerland

Abstract. Three systems mediate the fluxes of calcium across heart sarcolemma: the slow calcium channel (influx), the ATP-dependent calcium pump (efflux), and the Na^+/Ca^{2+} exchanger (efflux, but possibly also influx). Calmodulin regulates the pumping ATPase by direct interaction and also by activating a protein kinase. The Na^+/Ca^{2+} exchanger is modulated by calmodulin via a phosphorylation–dephosphorylation cycle. Both the kinase and the phosphatase are membrane-bound and calmodulin-sensitive. The kinase has higher Ca^{2+} affinity than the phosphatase.

INTRODUCTION

Of the three Ca^{2+}-transporting systems of heart sarcolemma, one, the slow Ca^{2+} channel, is apparently not influenced by calmodulin. Calmodulin influences the two other systems, which are the Ca^{2+}-pumping ATPase and the Na^+/Ca^{2+} exchanger. Since the ATPase and the exchanger are responsible for the ejection of Ca^{2+} from heart cells, it follows that calmodulin presides over the process of Ca^{2+} extrusion. It may, however, also influence the penetration of Ca^{2+}, since it is believed that the exchanger may also mediate the influx of Ca^{2+} into the cell during the plateau phase of the action potential [1].

Ca^{2+}-PUMPING ATPase

The existence of a Ca^{2+}-pumping ATPase in heart sarcolemma was conclusively documented by Caroni and Carafoli in 1980 [2]. Subsequent studies [3–5] have established the characteristics of the ATPase, purified it to virtual homogeneity, and reconstituted it in artificial phospholipid vesicles. The ATPase is a high-Ca^{2+}-affinity enzyme ($K_m \approx 0.5$ μM) that pumps Ca^{2+} with a rather low V_{max} (≈ 0.5 nmole/mg membrane protein per sec, at 30°C). Like all transport ATPases of the E_1–E_2 type, it forms an acyl-phosphate during the reaction cycle and is inhibited by low concentrations of vanadate ($K_{1/2} \approx 0.5$ μM). It is calmodulin-sensitive, as can be inferred indirectly from the inhibition by a number of anticalmodulin drugs [3]. Direct demonstration of calmodulin sensitivity by extraction of calmodulin from sarcolemma and readdition of the activator to it has been also obtained [3]. However, calmodulin is apparently bound to the ATPase in sarcolemma much more tightly than to the analogous enzyme in the plasma membrane of erythrocytes. This necessitates rather drastic extraction procedures, resulting in partial damage to the sarcolemmal vesicles, and thus in the incomplete recovery of Ca^{2+} pumping into the vesicles. At the time of the demonstration of the inhibitory effect of phenothiazines on the Ca^{2+}-ATPase of sarcolemma [3], it was generally assumed that such an inhibition automatically indicated calmodulin sensitivity. Later research [6] has proven, however, that the so called anticalmodulin drugs may interact directly with the Ca^{2+}-ATPase and has raised serious doubts concerning conclusions on calmodulin involvement in biochemical processes based solely on inhibition by drugs. In the case of the Ca^{2+}-ATPase of heart sarcolemma, the problem of whether the inhibition by phenothiazines does or does not reflect calmodulin involvement is fortunately irrelevant, since the enzyme can be isolated in a state of near homogeneity from calmodulin affinity columns [3–5]. This naturally proves that the ATPase interacts with calmodulin *directly*, and not, as so often is the case, through the activation of a protein phosphorylation process.

The purified enzyme has a molecular weight (M_r) of about 140,000 and repeats the functional properties of the ATPase in the membrane (e.g., high Ca^{2+} affinity, vanadate sensitivity, acyl-phosphate). It is very similar, if not identical, to the Ca^{2+}-pumping ATPase of erythrocytes, but differs considerably from the Ca^{2+}-pumping ATPase of sarcoplasmic reticulum. It can be reconstituted into liposomes, where it pumps Ca^{2+} with a 1:1 stoichiometry to ATP. As purified from calmodulin columns by EGTA elution, the enzyme displays low Ca^{2+} affinity (K_m about 10 μM) and is shifted to the appropriate submicromolar K_m (and also to a higher V_{max}) by calmodulin. The effect of calmodulin, however, is mimicked by the addition of any of a number of acidic phospholipids and/or long-chain polyunsaturated fatty acids, as already observed with the erythrocyte ATPase [7]. Since sarcolemma contains a considerable amount of phosphatidylserine, the effect of acidic phospholipids has potential regulatory implications, alternative to calmodulin, or additive to it.

In addition to interacting *directly* with the Ca^{2+}-pumping ATPase, calmodulin may also play an indirect role in its regulation. Caroni and Carafoli [8] have demonstrated that the enzyme is regulated by a phosphorylation–dephosphorylation process. The kinase, which activates Ca^{2+}-pumping, is membrane-bound and cAMP-dependent; the deactivating phosphatase has not been characterized as yet. In studying the properties of the activating, cAMP-dependent phosphorylation process, Caroni and Carafoli [8] observed that it was apparently depending on Ca^{2+} as well. Vetter et al. [9] have now demonstrated that the stimulation of Ca^{2+} pumping by the cAMP-dependent process is potentiated by a Ca^{2+}- and calmodulin-dependent protein kinase. According to recent studies of Lamers et al. [10], the latter phosphorylates a 9-kD protein, subunit of a 24-kD sarcolemmal protein, which is also the substrate of the cAMP dependent phosphorylation. The situation in heart sarcolemma is thus very similar to that of heart sarcoplasmic reticulum, where the Ca^{2+}-pumping ATPase is activated by the additive, cAMP- and calmodulin-dependent, phosphorylation of phospholamban [11]. The latter has now been separated into two components, having apparent M_r's of 26,000 and 28,000 [12], each consisting of two subunits of approximately 11 kD. Of the two components, one is the substrate of the cAMP-dependent, the other of the calmodulin-dependent, phosphorylation.

Na^+/Ca^{2+} EXCHANGER

The existence of a Na^+/Ca^{2+} exchange process in heart plasma membrane was demonstrated by Reuter and Seitz [13] in 1968. In 1979, Reeves and Sutko [14] succeeded in measuring Ca^{2+} uptake in Na^+-loaded heart sarcolemma vesicles. Sarcolemma vesicles are particularly convenient for the measurement of the Na^+/Ca^{2+} exchanger and have now become the standard tool for investigating the reaction. The exchanger operates electrogenically, with a probable 3 $Na^+/1$ Ca^{2+} stoichiometry [15–18], and has a lower affinity for Ca^{2+} than the pumping ATPase; depending on experimental conditions, K_m's between 1.5 and 18 μM have been determined [14,16]. The exchanger does not interact *directly* with calmodulin (the inhibition observed by Caroni et al. [14] at very high concentrations of phenothiazines could well be due to nonspecific membrane effects). Regulation by an ATP-dependent (phosphorylation) process is on the other hand suggested by the stimulation of the exchanger in squid axons by ATP [19] and hydrolyzable analogues of ATP [20]. Calmodulin could thus be involved in the exchange reaction indirectly, i.e., by phosphorylation–dephosphorylation. Work by Caroni and Carafoli [21] has now shown that the exchanger in heart sarcolemma is modulated by a phosphorylation–dephosphorylation process and has established that the activating and deactivating processes are indeed calmodulin-dependent.

In the experiments of Caroni and Carafoli [21], sarcolemmal vesicles are passively loaded with Na^+ to establish the Na^+-gradient and then exposed to phosphorylase phosphatase (to maximally dephosphorylate endogenous phosphoproteins), washed, and incubated in the presence of effectors that could, in principle, reverse the effects of the phosphatase. At the end of the two incubations (which are performed in the presence of Na^+ to maintain the Na^+ gradient), the vesicles are washed, and the initial rate of Na^+/Ca^{2+} exchange activity is measured. The results have shown that the treatment with phosphorylase phosphatase depresses the exchange activity. Phosphorylase phosphatase is a sarcoplasmic enzyme, which is unlikely to be responsible for dephosphorylating sarcolemmal proteins in vivo. Its effects, however, can be mimicked by incubating the vesicles with Ca^{2+}, Mg^{2+}, and calmodulin. Evidently, a membrane-bound, Ca^{2+}-$(+Mg^{2+})$-calmodulin-dependent phosphatase mediates the dephosphorylation of a sarcolemmal phosphoprotein (not necessarily the exchanger itself, however), which results in depressed Na^+/Ca^{2+} exchange activity. Phosphatase-inactivated vesicles (or vesicles treated with Ca^{2+}, Mg^{2+}, and calmodulin) are restored to full exchange activity on incubation with ATP and Mg^{2+}, providing compelling evidence for the existence of a membrane-bound protein kinase essential for the full expression of the exchanger. The kinase responsible for the reactivation reaction is not affected by protein kinase inhibitors, cAMP-dependent, and is thus not of the cAMP type. It does not require *added* calmodulin, but is inhibited by low concentrations of anticalmodulin drugs, which suggests regulation (dependence) by tightly bound calmodulin. A preliminary investigation of the kinetic properties of the phosphatase and the kinase has shown that the former has lower affinity for Ca^{2+} ($K_m > 1$ μM) than the latter ($K_m < 1$ μM). An integrated picture can thus be attempted, in which the exchanger would become activated, via stimulation of the Ca^{2+}-calmodulin-dependent kinase, as Ca^{2+} increases in heart sarcoplasm. Further increases in cell Ca^{2+} would then activate the Ca^{2+}-calmodulin-dependent phosphatase and thus depress the exchange activity. Whether the result of the activating and of the deactivating portion of this regulatory process will be the potentiation of contraction or of relaxation of heart myofibrils will depend on which assumptions are made concerning the direction of Ca^{2+} transport on the Na^+/Ca^{2+} exchanger.

REFERENCES

1. Langer, G. A., Frank, J. B., and Brady, A. J. 1976. In: A. C. Guyton and A. W. Cowley (eds.), *International Review of Physiology II*. Vol. 9, pp. 191–226. University Park Press, Baltimore.
2. Caroni, P., and Carafoli, E. 1980. An ATP-dependent calcium pumping system in dog heart sarcolemma. *Nature (London)* 283:765–767.
3. Caroni, P., and Carafoli, E. 1981. The Ca^{2+}-pumping ATPase of heart sarcolemma: Characterization, calmodulin dependence, and partial purification. *J. Biol. Chem.* 256:3263–3270.
4. Caroni, P., Zurini, M., and Clark, A. 1982. The calcium pumping ATPase of heart sarcolemma. *Ann. N. Y. Acad. Sci.* 402:402–421.
5. Caroni, P., Zurini, M., Clark, A., and Carafoli, E. 1982. Further characterization and reconstitution of the purified Ca^{2+}-pumping ATPase of heart sarcolemma. *J. Biol. Chem.* 258:7305–7310.
6. Adunyah, E. S., Niggli, V., and Carafoli, E. 1982. The anticalmodulin drugs trifluoperazine and R24571 remove the activation of the purified erythrocyte Ca^{2+} ATPase by acidic phospholipids and by controlled proteolysis. *FEBS Lett.* 143:65–68.
7. Niggli, V., Adunyah, E. S., and Carafoli, E. 1981. Acidic phospholipids, unsaturated fatty acids, and limited proteolysis mimic the effect of calmodulin on the purified erythrocyte Ca^{2+} ATPase. *J. Biol. Chem.* 256:8688–8592.

8. Caroni, P., and Carafoli, E. 1981. Regulation of Ca^{2+}-pumping ATPase of heart sarcolemma by a phosphorylation–dephosphorylation process. *J. Biol. Chem.* 256:9371–9373.

9. Vetter, R., Haase, H., and Will, H. 1982. Potentiating effect of calmodulin and catalytic subunit of cyclic-AMP-dependent protein kinase on ATP-dependent Ca^{2+} transport by cardiac sarcolemma. *FEBS Lett.* 148:326–330.

10. Lamers, J. M. J., Stinis, J. T., and De Jonge, H. R. 1981. On the role of cyclic AMP and Ca^{2+}-calmodulin-dependent phosphorylation in the control of $(Ca^{2+} + Mg^{2+})$-ATPase of cardiac sarcolemma. *FEBS Lett.* 127:139–143.

11. Le Peuch, C. J., Haiech, J., and Demaille, J. G. 1979. Concerted regulation of cardiac sarcoplasmic reticulum: Ca^{2+} transport by cyclic adenine monophosphate-dependent and Ca^{2+}-calmodulin-dependent phosphorylation. *Biochemistry* 18:5110–5117.

12. Chiesi, M., Gasser, J., and Carafoli, E. 1983. Phospholamban of cardiac sarcoplasmic reticulum consists of two functionally distinct proteolipids. *FEBS Lett.* 160:61–66.

13. Reuter, H., and Seitz, N. 1968. The dependence of Ca^{2+} efflux from cardiac muscle on temperature and external ion composition. *J. Physiol. (London)* 195:451–470.

14. Reeves, J. P., and Sutko, J. L. 1979. Sodium–calcium exchange in cardiac membrane vesicles. *Proc. Natl. Acad. Sci. U.S.A.* 76:590–594.

15. Pitts, B. J. R. 1979. Stoichiometry of sodium calcium exchange in cardiac sarcolemmal vesicles. *J. Biol. Chem.* 254:6232–6235.

16. Caroni, P., Reinlib, L., and Carafoli, E. 1980. Charge movements during $Na-Ca^{2+}$ exchange in heart sarcolemmal vesicles. *Proc. Natl. Acad. Sci. U.S.A.* 77:6354–6358.

17. Reeves, J. P., and Sutko, J. L. 1980. Sodium–calcium exchange activity generates a current in cardiac membrane vesicles. *Science* 208:1461–1464.

18. Philipson, K. D., and Nishimoto, A. Y. 1980. $Na^{+}-Ca^{2+}$ exchange is affected by membrane potential in cardiac sarcolemmal vesicles. *J. Biol. Chem.* 255:6880–6882.

19. Di Polo, R. 1974. Effect of ATP on the calcium efflux in dialyzed squid giant axons. *J. Gen. Physiol.* 64:503–517.

20. Di Polo, R. 1977. Characterization of the ATP-dependent calcium efflux in dialyzed squid giant axons. *J. Gen. Physiol.* 69:795–813.

21. Caroni, P., and Carafoli, E. 1983. The regulation of the $Na^{+}-Ca^{2+}$ exchanger of heart sarcolemma. *Eur. J. Biochem.* 132:451–460.

PROTEIN SYNTHESIS AND DEGRADATION

The Effects of Hormonal Factors on Cardiac Protein Turnover

Peter H. Sugden

Department of Cardiac Medicine
Cardiothoracic Institute
London W1N 2DX, England

INTRODUCTION

The purpose of this chapter is to describe some of the hormonal factors that have been suggested to influence cardiac protein turnover. Because it is easier technically and interpretatively to carry out experiments in vitro, much of the work described here is based on this approach. It is important, however, to attempt to relate phenomena observed in vitro to the in vivo situation. This can be done by attempting to simulate in vivo conditions (e.g., hormone and fuel concentrations, cardiac workload) in experiments in vitro or by examining the effects in vivo of substances known to have effects in vitro. In many cases, there has not yet been sufficient time for all these experiments to have produced conclusive results, although this omission should be rectified in the future.

DEFINITIONS OF TERMS USED

To assist those unfamiliar with the terminology used, I have decided to provide some definitions at the outset. Protein *synthesis* is the incorporation of amino acids into proteins by ribosomally mediated peptide bond formation encoded by messenger RNA (mRNA). Protein *degradation* is the process of intracellular hydrolysis of proteins to their constituent amino acids by as yet ill-defined proteolytic enzymes. Rates of these two processes are normally expressed relative to tissue protein content or to tissue wet or dry weight. Protein *turnover* is the cyclical process that has as its constituents the simultaneously active processes of protein synthesis and degradation. Because of the cyclical nature of protein turnover, changes in tissue protein content are brought about by imbalances between the rates of protein synthesis and degradation. In the steady state, the ratio of the rates of protein synthesis to degradation is unity. Any decrease in this ratio, however caused, will result in tissue protein loss, and any increase will result in tissue protein accretion. It is thus important when considering changes in total tissue protein content to consider both the processes involved in protein turnover.

Efficiency of protein synthesis (sometimes called *RNA activity*) is the rate of protein synthesis expressed relative to tissue total RNA. Most of the tissue RNA is ribosomal (80–90%), with transfer RNA (tRNA) the next most abundant species, followed by mRNA. Changes in the efficiency of protein synthesis are caused by altering the activity of one or more processes involved in transcription or translation, although the molecular mechanisms whereby changes are produced are still ill-defined. Efficiency of protein synthesis is thus a rather nebulous term. However, since in the absence of perturbing factors the rate of protein synthesis is a function of tissue total RNA content, calculation of the efficiency of protein synthesis is useful in normalizing rates of protein synthesis and is also particularly useful in detecting perturbing factors that affect the mRNA translation rate or content.

Lysosomal *latency* is another term often encountered. A number of methods have been used to measure this ratio. It can be expressed as the ratio of activity of a lysosomal marker enzyme (usually the endoprotease cathepsin D or β-acetylglucosaminidase) that is sedimentable following tissue extraction in isotonic media to the total tissue activity of the enzyme measured after lysosomal rupture by Triton X-100. A decrease in the ratio expressed as described possibly indicates an increase in the fraction of lysosomal enzyme activity present in the cell in large autophagic vacuoles, which are supposedly more easily ruptured than primary lysosomes during homogenization. The suggestion is that a decrease in lysosomal latency should be associated with an increase in protein degradation rate. Unfortunately, the several unproven assumptions implicit in this hypothesis (e.g., that lysosomal proteases are wholly responsible for protein degradation in vivo, that latency in vitro is representative of autophagic vacuole formation in vivo) make measurements of lysosomal latency somewhat uninterpretable. Changes in lysosomal latency do not always correlate well with changes in rates of protein degradation. Work using this approach is, however, described in this review.

GENERAL COMMENTS ON THE MEASUREMENT OF PROTEIN TURNOVER IN VITRO AND IN VIVO

Methods used in measurement of protein turnover in vitro have been reviewed recently [1–3] and problems discussed. In the heart, protein synthesis is probably best measured by the incorporation of [14C]phenylalanine into protein in the presence of the other plasma amino acids. Similarly, protein degradation is probably best measured by the release of phenylalanine into the perfusate in the presence of cycloheximide to prevent reutilization of the amino acid by protein synthesis, or by the dilution of the specific radioactivity of radiolabeled phenylalanine added to the perfusate. Three general points should be mentioned briefly: First, most isolated muscle preparations are in negative nitrogen balance and may therefore be unphysiological to varying extents. This is obviously true in protein-degradation experiments in the presence of cycloheximide. Cardiac work and hormones or noncarbohydrate fuels improve nitrogen balance [4,5]. Second, care must be exercised if side-chain-labeled [^{3}H]phenylalanine or [^{3}H]tyrosine is used to measure protein synthesis rates because tritium is rapidly lost by exchange reactions, thereby altering precursor specific radioactivities [6,7]. Third, there is evidence that cycloheximide inhibits protein degradation [1,8], and its inhibition of protein synthesis is probably never more than 95%.

In vivo measurements of protein synthesis have until recently involved prolonged intravenous infusions of radiolabeled amino acids. Tissues are thus exposed to normal plasma concentrations of amino acids of which one is of theoretically (but rarely practically) constant specific radioactivity [9]. It is difficult, however, to assess the specific radioactivity of the amino acid at the site of protein synthesis throughout the time course of the experiment. A "large-dose" method based on earlier work [10] has recently been introduced [11,12] in which plasma and tissue pools of a given plasma amino acid are flooded by a single intravenous injection of a large quantity of an amino acid (usually [^{3}H]leucine or [^{3}H]phenylalanine) at high specific radioactivity. This approach appears to be reliable and overcomes the problems of prolonged infusions. Measurements can be made 10 min after injection. Changes in the specific radioactivity of the administered amino acid during the experiment are negligible (because body pools are flooded) and high plasma concentrations of radiolabeled amino acid ensure rapid equilibration of the amino acid with amino acyl tRNA. This method promises to be widely and easily applicable.

In vivo measurement of protein degradation is much more difficult. Decay in radioactivity of protein following prelabeling suffers from the problem of amino acid reincorporation except under rare specific circumstances [9]. This problem is not insuperable, since, by use of double-labeling, corrections can be made for reincorporation [9]. Subtraction of the rate of protein synthesis from the rate of accretion of tissue protein mass gives the rate of protein degradation, but this is a relatively insensitive method. Measurement of 3-methylhistidine excretion in vivo was once purported to be an index of skeletal-muscle breakdown (since this post translationally modified amino acid is present mainly in skeletal-muscle actin and myosin), but there is now good evidence that much of the 3-methylhistidine excreted is derived from the rapid turnover of smaller pools of contractile protein in, for example, the digestive tract [13,14]. Reliable methods of measuring in vivo protein degradation are thus sadly lacking. Data on the effects of interventions on cardiac protein degradation therefore rely more heavily on the in vitro approach than experiments on cardiac protein synthesis.

LABILITY OF CARDIAC MASS

It is well established that in vivo the heart can increase its size rapidly in response to an increase in cardiac workload [15,16]. This phenomenon of cardiac hypertrophy occurs clinically where large increases in cardiac mass may occur over several years in, for example, response to chronic systemic hypertension. In experimental animals, removal of the hypertrophic stimulus leads to the heart reverting to its original size. Atrophy of the normal-sized heart is less well characterized. The heart will lose protein mass in response to prolonged starvation, but this probably occurs only dramatically immediately before death. It seems that there is a differential lability of protein in tissues in response to wasting conditions. Thus, the liver decreases its protein mass very rapidly on starvation, and it is rapidly repleted on refeeding. White skeletal muscle is probably of intermediate lability. The mass of muscles that perform vital function such as the heart and the diaphragm is considerably less labile. Consideration of factors that play a physiological role in tissue protein conservation or loss must take the differential sensitivity into account. However, mechanisms by which differential tissue loss is effected are not understood.

INSULIN AND CARDIAC PROTEIN TURNOVER

The importance of insulin in maintaining whole-body nitrogen balance has been known for many years. Diabetic animals exhibit muscle wasting that can be reversed by administration of insulin. Insulin stimulated the incorporation of radiolabeled amino acids into bulk protein in perfused heart [17–19], incubated fetal hearts [20], incubated atrial strips [21], and cultured cardiac-muscle cells [22]. Although insulin promotes the uptake of amino acids into cells [23,24] and charging of tRNA [25–27], its effects on protein synthesis are independent of these effects because the hormone stimulates protein synthesis despite unchanged or decreased intracellular amino acid concentrations [8]. The effects of insulin on cardiac protein synthesis are probably independent of the well-established stimulatory effects of the hormone on cardiac glucose uptake [28,29]. In hearts that were initially preperfused in the absence of substrate (to deplete carbohydrates), insulin still stimulated [14C]glycine incorporation into protein when the hearts were subsequently perfused with pyruvate [29].

The short-term effects of insulin on protein synthesis are not blocked by the inhibitor of RNA synthesis actinomycin D [18]. The hormone appears to affect the initiation step in protein synthesis, i.e., the binding of ribosomal subunits to mRNA. This conclusion is based on the finding that hearts retrogradely perfused with glucose in the absence of insulin [1,18] develop a "perfusion-induced block" in protein synthesis (i.e., a decrease in protein synthesis rates) after about 1 hr of perfusion, with a simultaneous accumulation of ribosomal subunits. The perfusion-induced block is prevented by insulin. The lag period has been attributed to the time taken for the heart to release/degrade insulin bound prior to its removal from the animal and for utilization of endogenous fatty fuels [1] that also prevent the perfusion-induced block when provided in the perfusate [1,30]. Although the existence of the perfusion-induced block is well established in the retrogradely (Langendorff) perfused heart with glucose as sole fuel, we did not observe any such block in anterogradely perfused (working) rat hearts [31]. This may have been a consequence of the amino acid concentrations used, since increased concentrations can overcome the perfusion-induced block [30], or of insulin remaining bound to the hearts. Alternatively, the response of the two heart preparations may differ in this regard. When raised amino acid concentrations are used to overcome the perfusion-induced block, the stimulatory effects of fatty fuels on protein synthesis are reduced [30]. It is probably worthwhile to reexamine the interplay of effects of insulin workload and fuels on protein synthesis. This is especially the case since Rannels et al. [30] have reported a similar stimulation of protein synthesis by glucose–pyruvate and glucose–insulin compared with hearts perfused with glucose alone, yet Chain and Sender [29] have reported stimulatory effects of insulin on protein synthesis when pyruvate is the sole fuel for contraction.

The concentration dependence of the stimulation of cardiac protein synthesis by insulin has been relatively ignored, perhaps because of the difficulties of interpretation engendered by the phenomena described above. Physiological concentrations of insulin stimulate protein synthesis in the diaphragm [32,33], the soleus, and the extensor digitorum longus muscles [34] in vitro. In cultured chick cardiac-muscle cells, insulin stimulated protein synthesis by about 13% at concentrations as low as 11 μU/ml, (0.08 nM), i.e., well within the the physiological range, although the maximal stimulation was not achieved until 1100 μU/ml, which is grossly superphysiological [22]. No insulin stimulation of protein synthesis could be detected until after the first hour of exposure of the cells to the hormone. It is still not known whether physiological concentrations of insulin regulate cardiac protein synthesis in vivo. Experiments analogous to those in which the in vivo stimulatory effect of insulin on skeletal muscle protein synthesis was established using physiological hormone concentrations [35] should soon clarify the situation.

The role of insulin in regulation of cardiac protein degradation has also been studied. Rannels et al. [8] established some years ago that insulin inhibited this process in the retrogradely perfused heart, albeit with a somewhat superphysiological concentration dependence. The hormone also increased the latency of the lysosomal enzymes cathepsin D and β-acetylglucosaminidase compared with perfusions with glucose alone [8], with which increases in autophagic vacuole content within the cardiac myocyte are known to occur. We recently reexamined the concentration dependence of the inhibitory effects of insulin on protein degradation in the perfused working rat heart [36]. We showed that there was significant inhibition at hormone concentrations of 50 μU/ml and that maximal inhibition of about 30% occurred at concentrations of 100 μU/ml. These concentrations refer to the insulin concentrations added to the perfusate. Since the tendency of insulin to bind to glass is widely recognized, the actual concentrations in the perfusate may be considerably lower than the added concentrations. We sought to control these problems simply by comparing the effects of insulin on protein degradation with its effects on the well-established insulin-influenced processes of glucose uptake and lactate output. We found that the insulin-concentration dependence of all three processes was similar. Since insulin concentrations used in this study were within the physiological range, it is possible that insulin might act to restrain cardiac protein degradation in vivo. The effect of insulin on protein degradation was exerted rapidly, certainly by less than 1 hr after initiation of perfusion. In all these experiments, overnight-fasted rats were used and time courses of protein degradation were linear throughout the perfusions. Thus, no lag period for the effects of insulin on protein degradation could be detected. In this respect, protein synthesis and degradation may differ, although the difference may be related to differences in technique among investigators.

We have also shown that insulin inhibited cardiac protein degradation when acetate or lactate were sole fuels for contraction, but that the inhibition was proportionally less than when glucose was sole fuel [36]. We were unable to demonstrate any inhibition of protein degradation by acetate or lactate compared with perfusions with glucose, a result that was at variance with the results of other workers [37,38]. Provision of glucose may therefore be necessary for insulin to exert maximal inhibitory effects on protein degradation. Increased pressure development may also increase the inhibitory action of maximally effective insulin concentrations [39].

In summary, insulin is probably physiologically important in maintaining cardiac nitrogen balance, exerting its effects at the levels of both protein synthesis and degradation. The actions of insulin represent one way in which cardiac nitrogen balance is coupled to the nutritional state of the animal. However, effectors other than insulin couple cardiac nitrogen balance to other requirements, e.g., the hypertrophic response to increased workload.

DIABETES AND CARDIAC PROTEIN TURNOVER

Although untreated diabetes mellitus is associated with skeletal-muscle wasting, there is no evidence in man that the disease causes significant deleterious cardiac atrophy. In humans with long-standing disease, cardiac hypertrophy may sometimes be observed [40], presumably as a result of vascular complications of the disease. There have, however, been reports of changes in cardiac performance characteristics induced by diabetes in man [41,42] and animals [43–47] that could be reversed by insulin. In prolonged (6-months) alloxan diabetes in rats, heart/body weight ratios were increased initially because of the lesser sensitivity of the heart to the disease compared with skeletal muscle and subsequently because of cardiac hypertrophy [48]. However, cardiac wet weight and cardiac protein mass of young streptozotocin-diabetic rats increased less rapidly than controls and heart/body weight ratio was less than controls after 14 days of streptozotocin diabetes [49].

With the use of perfused hearts from 2-day alloxan-diabetic rats, protein synthesis was shown to be relatively unaffected compared with controls during the first hour of perfusion [30,50]. After 1 hr of perfusion, the proportion of ribosomes as subunits was less in hearts from diabetic animals compared with controls. This finding reflects the perfusion-induced block in peptide-chain initiation in control hearts. After 3 hr of perfusion, ribosomal subunit contents relative to total RNA were similar in hearts from control and diabetic animals, but protein synthesis rates were less in the latter, possibly as a consequence of the decreased total RNA content in the hearts of diabetic animals. In unperfused hearts removed from diabetic animals, 60 S ribosomal subunit levels were not significantly different from controls, although 40 S subunit levels were increased. In contrast, in the psoas, diabetes induced a doubling of ribosomal subunit levels [30]. It should be emphasized that ribosomal subunit populations are usually expressed relative to total RNA, and thus changes in total ribosomal content would not be detected. It was concluded [30] that 2-day alloxan diabetes does not significantly affect cardiac protein synthesis and that maintenance of the rates of protein synthesis (despite the absence of plasma insulin) could be ascribed to the utilization by the heart of noncarbohydrate fuels. (The plasma concentrations of long-chain fatty acids, lactate, and ketone bodies are increased during diabetes and starvation.) Although utilization of these fuels does not affect cardiac adenine nucleotide concentrations, they (and insulin plus glucose [8]) are known to maintain creatine phosphate concentrations [30]. As yet, however, there is no established role for creatine phosphate in regulation of protein synthesis. A variety of factors associated with maintenance of protein synthesis rates (insulin, fatty fuels, diabetes, starvation, pressure development) are associated with increased intracellular concentrations of glucose-6-phosphate [5,51], a known stimulator of reticulocyte lysate protein synthesis [52]. Involvement of the pentose phosphate pathway, for which glucose-6-phosphate is an intermediate (in addition to being a glycolytic intermediate), has been suggested in the regulation of protein synthesis in cultured heart cells [53]. At the moment, evidence of the importance of creatine phosphate and glucose-6-phosphate in the regulation of cardiac protein synthesis is exiguous. Cell-free preparations of heart analogous to reticulocyte lysates are required for investigation of the roles of these putative regulators.

In vivo experiments in 5-day streptozotocin-diabetic rats showed a 40% decrease in cardiac protein synthesis [54]. There was a decrease in cardiac

RNA content in these animals, but this could account for only about half the observed inhibition, suggesting a decrease in the efficiency of protein synthesis. Insulin treatment only partially restored cardiac protein synthesis [54], presumably because of the loss of cardiac RNA. Skeletal-muscle protein synthesis was more severely inhibited than cardiac protein synthesis [54]. The view that in some circumstances diabetes may inhibit cardiac protein synthesis was reinforced by the finding of a progressive inhibition (with length of alloxan diabetes) of peptide synthesis in ribosomes prepared from hearts of diabetic rats [55].

The effects of longer-term diabetes have recently been examined in perfused hearts [56]. Following 2 days of alloxan diabetes, rats were maintained by 5 days of intramuscular insulin injections and were then withdrawn from insulin for 3 days before experimentation. Cardiac protein synthesis was depressed when hearts from diabetic animals were perfused with media simulating control (containing 100 μU/ml of insulin) or diabetic sera (the latter containing raised concentrations of palmitate, glucose, ketone bodies, lactate, glucagon, and branched-chain amino acids and altered concentrations of other amino acids). Neither control (+ insulin) nor "diabetic" perfusate restored protein synthesis in hearts of diabetic animals, but the rates of protein synthesis were not significantly different, suggesting maintenance of protein synthesis by "diabetic" perfusate [56]. Higher concentrations of insulin (25 mU/ml) only partially restored protein synthetic rates in hearts from diabetic animals [56], as was found in vivo [54]. The reasons for this were a decrease in cardiac RNA content [56] and a decrease in efficiency of protein synthesis, the latter being only partially reversed by high concentrations of insulin. The decreased efficiency of protein synthesis in the hearts of the diabetics was the result of decreased elongation/termination of peptide chains because the proportion of ribosome subunits relative to total RNA was the same as or less than controls, indicating similar (or even increased) rates of peptide-chain initiation in diabetic hearts. Effects of diabetes and insulin were similar to the whole heart when isolated heart cells were used [56]. It has been suggested using an in vitro protein synthetic model that effects of diabetes in skeletal muscle are exerted at the elongation-factor level [57].

Specific alterations in cardiac myosin isoenzymes have been observed in the streptozotocin- or alloxan-diabetic rat [58–60]. A decrease in actomyosin Ca^{2+}-dependent ATPase specific activity corresponded with a shift in myosin isoenzyme profile from the V_1 to the V_3 form (see Cummins [61] for a review). These alterations could be partly the result of the depressed plasma thyroid hormone concentrations seen in diabetic animals [59,60]. They myosin isoenzyme pattern of the diabetic reverted to the control on treatment with insulin [58,60], but was only partly reversed by triiodothyronine [60]. Diabetes-induced changes in cardiac performance may be related to alterations in the myosin isoenzyme profile [43–46].

The effects of diabetes on protein degradation have not been fully explored. In the Langendorff-perfused heart perfused with buffer simulating control serum, the rates of protein degradation in hearts from the alloxan-diabetic/insulin-maintained and withdrawn rats were not significantly different from controls [56]. Perfusion with buffer simulating diabetic serum decreased protein degradation in control hearts compared with control serum buffer, but increased protein degradation in diabetic hearts compared with control hearts/control serum buffer. These findings suggest the possibility of an increased rate of protein degradation in hearts from diabetic animals. Insulin reduced rates of protein degradation in hearts from either control or diabetic rats. More prolonged (2-hr) perfusions were dogged by nonlinearity of the time course of protein degradation, but the suggestion was that the stimulation of protein degradation by diabetes could be more readily observed in anterogradely (working) heart perfusions [56].

Increases in alkaline proteolytic (chymotryptic) activity have been observed in hearts of streptozotocin-diabetic rats [62], although this finding has been contradicted recently [49]. Although increases in alkaline proteolytic activity occur in skeletal muscle during wasting conditions [63,64], this activity is not thought to be important in intracellular cardiac (or skeletal) myocytic protein degradation, since it is primarily of mast-cell origin [65,66].

In conclusion, the effects of diabetes on cardiac protein synthesis depend partly on the animal model used. In short-term diabetes, protein synthesis is apparently maintained, and this may be attributable to the stimulatory effects of fatty fuels on protein synthesis. In longer-term diabetes, there is an inhibition of cardiac protein synthesis both in vitro and in vivo. Decreases in cardiac RNA content and efficiency of protein synthesis are probably the cause. Degradation of cardiac protein is probably increased by diabetes. This finding is surprising, since in most circumstances, the effects of diabetes and starvation are similar. The work of several groups has established that cardiac protein degradation is reduced in vitro by starvation (see below), although variations in perfusate contents among various laboratories may account for this difference.

STARVATION AND CARDIAC PROTEIN TURNOVER

The effects of starvation on cardiac protein turnover have not been extensively investigated. In the rat, 2 days of starvation reduced in vitro cardiac protein synthesis rates by about 16% [67]. Psoas protein synthesis was inhibited much more (by about 50%). The protein-synthesis machinery therefore appears to be partially protected against the effects of starvation, as is the case in diabetes. Decreased cardiac protein synthetic rates after 2 days' starvation were directly attributable to a 13% decrease in cardiac RNA content [67], probably in the absence of any change in the proportion of

RNA present as ribosomal subunits. Although starvation caused significant decreases in initiation factor eIF-2 binding activity for [^{35}S]met-tRNA$_f^{met}$ in both heart and psoas muscles, these changes were not well correlated with changes in protein-synthesis rates [67].

In vivo, in the rat, 2 days of starvation caused a decrease in the fractional synthesis rate of cardiac protein from 20% per day to 12% per day, a decrease of 40% [68]. There was also a 27% decrease in the efficiency of protein synthesis from 12.5 to 9.1 mg protein/mg RNA per day. Thus, although a proportion of the decrease in protein synthesis could be attributed directly to a decrease in cardiac RNA content, a greater proportion could be attributed to a decrease in protein-synthesis efficiency. At first sight, these results are at variance with in vitro experiments [67]. However, rats used in the in vivo experiments were smaller than those used in the in vitro studies. The younger rats could be expected to be more deleteriously affected by 2 days of starvation. It is unfortunate that cardiac protein-synthesis rates in vitro were not measured using the larger animals starved for periods of longer than 2 days, when a decrease in the efficiency of protein synthesis might have been apparent. In 4-day-starved rats, the proportion of RNA as 60 S ribosomal subunits was decreased in hearts, hinting at changes in protein-synthesis efficiency [67]. It is worth commenting that in in vivo experiments [68], gastrocnemius-muscle protein-synthesis rates and efficiencies were proportionally decreased to a greater extent than in the heart, suggesting the greater resistance to starvation of cardiac protein synthesis compared with skeletal-muscle protein synthesis. These results concur with in vitro experiments [67] and may reflect the maintenance of cardiac protein synthesis by raised serum concentrations of noncarbohydrate fuels [30] in the face of a decreased plasma insulin concentration.

Turning now to the effects of starvation on protein degradation, Crie et al. [69] showed that in glucose-perfused hearts, rates of protein degradation decreased by 18% after 1 day of starvation and by 29% after 5 days of starvation. Degradation was still depressed by 29% after 5 days of starvation followed by 1 day of refeeding. Curfman et al. [70], using incubated rat left atria, showed a 29% decrease in protein degradation after only 1 day of starvation. Insulin further inhibited protein degradation in incubated left atria from 2-day-starved rats [70]. The rate of protein degradation in these incubations was significantly less than in atria from fed animals incubated in the presence of insulin, showing additivity of the two effects [70]. In the glucose-perfused heart, we have also observed significant decreases in rates of protein degradation after 2 or 3 days of starvation, with a 30% inhibition after 3 days. No significant inhibition of starvation could be detected after 1 day of starvation (P. H. Sugden and D. M. Smith, unpublished results).

The inhibitory effects of starvation do not correlate with specific-activity changes of cathepsin D in the heart. In the 3-day-starved mouse, ventricular weight decreased by 16% and the ventricular specific activity (relative to protein) of cathepsin D increased by 26%. Since there was no change in cardiac protein/wet ratio, the total tissue activity of the enzyme was increased. The specific activities of two other lysosomal enzymes (acid phosphatase and β-acetylglucosaminidase) were unchanged [71]. Latency of cathepsin D decreased from 76% in the fed mouse to 53% in the 3-day-starved animal. Latency of acid phosphatase was unaltered and that of β-acetylglucosaminidase was only slightly altered. Qualitatively similar results were obtained in the starved rabbit [71]. Increases in cathepsin D specific activity of 19% have been observed in hearts of 6-day-starved rats in which ventricular weight had fallen by 34% [62]. These rats must have been very close to death. Increases in the specific activity of "myofibrillar" alkaline protease were found in the hearts of these animals, but again it is considered unlikely that this chymotryptic enzyme is involved in intramyocytic protein degradation, being primarily of mast-cell origin [65,66].

When one attempts to collate the disparate findings on the effects of starvation on cardiac protein turnover, the results are confusing. In in vitro experiments, cardiac protein synthesis [67] and degradation [68,69] are both inhibited, with the latter possibly being slightly more inhibited. Logically, this should lead to a conservation of cardiac mass. However, experimental findings point to a decrease in cardiac mass on starvation [62,71] Increases in heart total cathepsin D activity, and a decrease in cathepsin D lysosomal latency [71], should increase the rate of cardiac protein degradation if the rate of the process is limited by the activity and/or latency of cathepsin D. One problem is that so far there has not been a single consistent study of the effects of starvation on cardiac protein turnover, and conclusions must of necessity be based on the findings of several groups of workers.

A comparison of the effects of insulin and starvation on skeletal- and cardiac-muscle processes is interesting. In skeletal muscle, the effects of insulin and starvation are antagonistic. Thus, insulin stimulates skeletal-muscle glycogen accumulation [72] and starvation depletes it [73]. Insulin stimulates skeletal-muscle protein synthesis and inhibits degradation [74,75]. In the starved 400-g rat, skeletal-muscle protein degradation may be slightly inhibited after 2 days of starvation, but is increased after 4 days of starvation compared with controls [76]. Protein synthesis is decreased in both instances. Presumably, some of the effects of starvation in skeletal muscle are brought about by decreases in plasma insulin concentrations. In the heart, although the effects of insulin and starvation on protein synthesis are antagonistic (but perhaps less dramatically so than in skeletal muscle), starvation promotes cardiac glycogen accumulation [77] and inhibits cardiac protein degradation, as does insulin. Thus, in the heart, factors other than the fall in plasma insulin concentration (e.g., increased plasma concentrations of noncarbohydrate fuels) must affect these processes.

OTHER HORMONAL EFFECTS (GLUCOCORTICOIDS, THYROID HORMONES, HYPOPHYSECTOMY, GLUCAGON)

The glucocortoids are involved in the maintenance of blood glucose concentrations during starvation. At least part of this effect is thought to be exerted by promoting intracellular protein loss from tissues such as skeletal muscle with the resultant amino acids being utilized in gluconeogenic tissues for glucose synthesis. Glucocorticoids inhibit skeletal-muscle protein synthesis (see Young [78]), induce insulin resistance [79], and possibly stimulate muscle protein degradation (although this is controversial) [80]. Plasma glucocorticoid concentrations are increased in diabetes, when skeletal-muscle wasting also occurs. The heart appears to be relatively insensitive to glucocorticoids. Administration of cortisone acetate to rats for 5 days did not alter the rate of in vitro cardiac protein synthesis, although skeletal-muscle protein synthesis was inhibited [81]. In cultured fetal mouse hearts, hydrocortisone stimulated protein degradation in the absence of insulin, but inhibited it in the presence of insulin [82].

Thyrotoxicosis is a well-established manipulation for inducing cardiac hypertrophy. Administration of triiodothyronine can produce a 30% increase in heart weight in 3 days. Relatively little work has been done on protein turnover in thyrotoxocosis in vivo. In vitro, thyroid hormone preadministration increases rates of protein synthesis and decreases rates of protein degradation, albeit transiently [83]. During the regression of thyrotoxic cardiac hypertrophy, rates of protein synthesis and degradation were both depressed, with the latter being proportionally less depressed than the former [83]. Cathepsin D activity in the heart was decreased during thyrotoxic hypertrophy and was increased during regression [84], although the importance of these activity changes is open to question [83]. As with the glucocorticoids, cardiac and skeletal muscle differ in their response to thyrotoxicosis, since this condition induces skeletal-muscle wasting.

Thyroid hormone modifies the myosin isoenzyme profile in the heart (see Cummins [61] for a review). Actomyosin ATPase specific activity is stimulated by thyrotoxicosis [85] (see Morkin [86] for a review). Hypophysectomy in rats leads to a decrease in cardiac myosin V_1 isoenzyme (high ATPase specific activity) content and a corresponding increase in V_3 (low ATPase specific activity) content. These changes are prevented or reversed by administration of thyroid hormone [87,88]. It should be noted that changes in cardiac myosin isoenzymes and cardiac hypertrophy during thyrotoxicosis are not necessarily interdependent. Changes in tension–velocity relationships indicative of increased myosin ATPase specific activity (and therefore altered myosin isoenzyme profiles) are seen in nonhypertrophied hearts [89,90]. The hypertrophic response of the heart in thyrotoxicosis may be dependent on the increased cardiac output and myocardial oxygen uptake. The increase in cardiac output is presumably necessitated by the raised basal metabolic rate in thyrotoxicosis.

Hypophysectomy prevents growth and induces a decrease in the heart/body weight ratio [90,91]. Rates of cardiac protein synthesis are depressed, but the efficiency of protein synthesis is unchanged [92]. Other work has shown that after hypophysectomy, although total cardiac RNA content falls, polysome content also decreases and ribosomal subunits accumulate [30,92,93]. This indicates an inhibition of initiation of protein synthesis relative to elongation/termination that might have been expected to be reflected in a decrease in efficiency of protein synthesis. Induction of diabetes in hypophysectomized rats decreased the proportion of RNA present as ribosomal subunits [30]. Administration of growth hormone and thyroid hormone restored body and heart growth [92]. Changes in myosin isoenzyme profiles after hypophysectomy were described above. No changes were observed in rates of protein degradation after hypophysectomy [91]. Although cathepsin D specific activities were increased, lysosomal latency was unchanged [91].

Glucagon and dibutyryl-cyclic AMP have been reported to inhibit protein synthesis in rabbit atria incubated in vitro [21]. The significance of these findings is obscure, since catecholamine administration in vivo causes cardiac hypertrophy. Although the catecholamine-induced hypertrophy is probably the result of an increased cardiac workload, the effect of cardiac work on cardiac protein accretion would apparently be opposed by the inhibitory effects of catecholamine-induced rises in cardiac cyclic AMP (cAMP) concentration on protein synthesis. It is, possible, however that cAMP could inhibit protein degradation to a proportionally greater extent than protein synthesis, in which case cardiac protein accretion could still be stimulated.

ACKNOWLEDGMENTS

The author's work was supported by grants from the British Heart Foundation and the British Diabetic Association.

REFERENCES

1. Morgan, H. E., Rannels, D. E., and McKee, E. E. 1979. Protein metabolism of the heart. *Handb. Physiol. Sect. 2: Cardiovasc. Syst.* 1:845-871.
2. Schreiber, S. S., Evans, C. D., Oratz, M., and Rothschild, M. A. 1981. Protein synthesis and degradation in cardiac stress. *Circ. Res.* 48:601-611.
3. Rannels, D. E., Wartell, S. A., and Watkins, C. L. 1982. The measurement of protein synthesis in biological systems. *Life Sci.* 30:1679-1690.
4. Chua, B. H. L., Siehl, D. L., and Morgan, H. E. 1980. A role for leucine in regulation of protein synthesis in working rat hearts. *Am. J. Physiol.* 239:E510-E514.
5. Morgan, H. E., Chua, B. H. L., Fuller, E. O., and Siehl, D. 1980. Regulation of protein synthesis and degradation during in vitro cardiac work. 1980. *Am. J. Physiol.* 238:E431-E442.
6. Sugden, P. H. 1980. Metabolism of aromatic amino acids by the rat heart and diaphragm. *FEBS Lett.* 114:127-131.
7. Williams, I. H., Sugden, P. H., and Morgan, H. E. 1981. Use of aromatic amino acids as monitors of protein turnover. *Am. J. Physiol.* 240:E677-E681.
8. Rannels, D. E., Kao, R., and Morgan, H. E. 1975. Effect of insulin on protein turnover in heart muscle. *J. Biol. Chem.* 250:1694-1701.
9. Waterlow, J. C., Garlick, P. J., and Millward, D. J. 1978. *Protein Turnover in Mammalian Tissues and the Whole Body.* North-Holland, Amsterdam.

10. Henshaw, E. C., Hirsch, C. A., Morton, B. E., and Hiat, H. H. 1971. Control of protein synthesis in mammalian tissues through changes in ribosome activity. *J. Biol. Chem.* 246:436–446.

11. McNurlan, M. A., Tomkins, A. M., and Garlick, P. J. 1979. The effect of starvation on the rate of protein synthesis in rat liver and small intestine. *Biochem. J.* 178:373–379.

12. Garlick, P. J., McNurlan, M. A., and Preedy, V. R. 1980. A rapid and convenient technique for measuring the rate of protein synthesis in tissues by injection of [^{3}H]phenylalanine. *Biochem. J.* 192:719–723.

13. Millward, D. J., Bates, P. C., Grimble, G. K., Brown, J. G., Nathan, M., and Rennie, M. J. 1980. Quantitative importance of non-skeletal muscle sources of N^τ-methylhistidine in urine. *Biochem. J.* 190:225–228.

14. Wassner, S. J., and Li, J. B. 1982. N^τ-Methylhistidine release: Contributions of rat skeletal muscle, GI tract and skin. *Am. J. Physiol.* 243:E293–E297.

15. Rabinowitz, M., and Zak, R. 1972. Biochemical and cellular changes in cardiac hypertrophy. *Annu. Rev. Med.* 23:245–261.

16. Zak, R., and Rabinowitz, M. 1979. Molecular aspects of cardiac hypertrophy. *Annu. Rev. Physiol.* 41:539–552.

17. Manchester, K. L., and Wool, I. G. 1963. Insulin and incorporation of amino acids into protein. 2. Accumulation and incorporation studies with the perfused rat heart. *Biochem. J.* 89:202–209.

18. Morgan, H. E., Jefferson, L. S., Wolpert, E. B., and Rannels, D. E. 1971. Regulation of protein synthesis in heart muscle. II. Effect of amino acid levels and insulin on ribosomal aggregation. *J. Biol. Chem.* 246:2163–2170.

19. Sender, P. M., and Garlick, P. J. 1973. Synthesis rates of protein in the Langendorff perfused rat heart in the presence and absence of insulin, and in the working heart. *Biochem. J.* 132:603–608.

20. Clarke, C. M., Jr. 1971. The stimulation by insulin of amino acid uptake and protein synthesis in the isolated fetal rat heart. *Biol. Neonate.* 19:379–388.

21. Hait, G., Kypson, J., and Massih, R. 1972. Amino acid incorporation into myocardium: Effect of insulin, glucagon, and dibutyryl 3′,5′-AMP. *Am. J. Physiol.* 222:404–408.

22. Airhart, J., Arnold, J. A., Stirewalt, W. S., and Low, R. B. 1982. Insulin stimulation of protein synthesis in cultured skeletal and cardiac muscle cells. *Am. J. Physiol.* 248:C81–C86.

23. Kipnis, D. M., and Noall, M. W. 1958. Stimulation of amino acid transport by insulin in the isolated rat diaphragm. *Biochim. Biophys. Acta* 28:226–227.

24. Wool, I. G., and Krahl, M. E. 1959. Incorporation of C^{14}-amino acids into protein of isolated diaphragms: An effect of insulin independent of glucose entry. *Am. J. Physiol.* 196:961–964.

25. Davey, P. J., and Manchester, K. L. 1969. Isolation of labelled aminoacyl transfer RNA from muscle: Studies of the entry of labelled amino acids into acyl transfer RNA linkage in situ and its control by insulin. *Biochim. Biophys. Acta* 182:85–97.

26. Manchester, K. L. 1970. The control by insulin of amino acid accumulation by muscle. *Biochem. J.* 117:457–465.

27. Manchester, K. L. 1970. Insulin and protein synthesis. *Biochem. Actions Horm.* 1:267–320.

28. Morgan, H. E., Henderson, M. J., Regen, D. M., and Park, C. R. 1961. Regulation of glucose uptake in muscle. I. The effects of insulin and anoxia on glucose transport and phosphorylation in the isolated, perfused heart of normal rats. *J. Biol. Chem.* 236:253–261.

29. Chain, E. B., and Sender, P. M. 1973. Protein synthesis by perfused hearts from normal and insulin-deficient rats. Effects of insulin in the presence of glucose and after depletion of glucose, glucose-6-phosphate and glycogen. *Biochem. J.* 132:593–601.

30. Rannels, D. E., Hjalmarson, Å. C., and Morgan, H. E. 1974. Effects of noncarbohydrate substrates on protein synthesis in muscle. *Am. J. Physiol.* 226:528–539.

31. Smith, D. M., and Sugden, P. H. 1983. Differential rates of protein synthesis in vitro and RNA contents in rat heart ventricular and atrial muscle. *Biochem. J.* 214:497–502.

32. Manchester, K. L., and Young, F. G. 1959. Hormones and protein synthesis in isolated rat diaphragm. *J. Endocrinol.* 18:381–394.

33. Manchester, K. L., Randle, P. J., and Young, F. G. 1959. An insulin assay based on the incorporation of labelled glycine into protein of isolated rat diaghragm. *J. Endocrinol.* 19:249–262.

34. Frayn, K. N., and Maycock, P. F. 1979. Regulation of protein metabolism by a physiological concentration of insulin in mouse soleus and extensor digitorum longus muscles: Effect of starvation and scald injury. *Biochem. J.* 184:323–330.

35 Garlick, P. J., Fern, M., and Preedy, V. R. 1983. The effect of insulin infusion and food intake on muscle protein synthesis in postabsorptive rats. *Biochem. J.* 210:669–676.

36. Sugden, P. H., and Smith, D. M. 1982. The effects of glucose, acetate, lactate and insulin on protein degradation in the perfused rat heart. *Biochem. J.* 206:467–472.

37. Chua, B., Siehl, D. L., and Morgan, H. E. 1979. Effect of leucine and metabolites of branched chain amino acids on protein turnover in heart. *J. Biol. Chem.* 254:8358–8362.

38. Chua, B., Kao, R. L., Rannels, D. E., and Morgan, H. E. 1979. Inhibition of protein degradation by anoxia and ischemia in perfused rat hearts. *J. Biol. Chem.* 254:6617–6623.

39. Smith, D. M., and Sugden, P. H. 1983. Effect of insulin and lack of effect of workload and hypoxia on protein degradation in the perfused working rat heart. *Biochem. J.* 210:55–61.

40. Farah, A. E., and Alousi, A. A. 1981. The actions of insulin on cardiac contractility. *Life Sci.* 29:975–1000.

41. Regan, T. J., Lyons, M. M., Ahmed, S. S., Levinson, G. E., Oldewurtel, H. A., Ahmad, M. R., and Haider, B. 1977. Evidence of cardiomyopathy in familial diabetes mellitus. *J. Clin. Invest.* 60:885–899.

42. Sanderson, J. E., Brown, D. J., Rivellese, A., and Kohner, E. 1978. Diabetic cardiomyopathy? An echocardiographic study of young diabetics. *Br. Med. J.* 1:404–407.

43. Regan. T. M., Ettinger, P. O., Khan, M. I., Jesrani, M. U., Lyons, M. M., Oldewurtel, H. A., and Weber, M. 1974. Altered myocardial function and metabolism in chronic diabetes mellitus without ischemia in dogs. *Circ. Res.* 35:222–237.

44. Miller, T. B. 1979. Cardiac performance of isolated perfused hearts from alloxan diabetic rats. *Am. J. Physiol.* 236:H808–H812.

45. Fein, F. S., Kornstein, L. B., Strobeck, J. E, Capasso, J. M., and Sonnenblick, E. H. 1980. Altered myocardial mechanics in diabetic rats. *Circ. Res.* 47:922–933.

46. Penpargkul, S., Schiable, T., Yipintsoi, T., and Scheuer, J. 1980. The effects of diabetes on performance and metabolism of rat hearts. *Circ. Res.* 47:911–921.

47. Schiable, T. F., Malhotra, A., Bauman, W. A., and Scheuer, J. 1983. Left ventricular function after chronic insulin treatment in diabetic and normal rats. *J. Mol. Cell. Cardiol.* 15:445–458.

48. Goodman, M. N., and Hazelwood, R. L. 1971. Influence of fasting and alloxan diabetes on rat cardiac actomyosin and subcellular phosphorus levels. *Proc. Soc. Exp. Biol. Med.* 137:614–618.

49. Dahlmann, B., Metzinger, H., and Reinauer, H. 1982. Studies on proteolytic activities in heart muscle of diabetic rats. *Diabete Metab.* 2:129–135.

50. Rannels, D. W., Jefferson, L. S., Hjalmarson, Å. C., Wolpert, E. B., and Morgan, H. E. 1970. Maintenance of protein synthesis in hearts of diabetic animals. *Biochem. Biophys. Res. Commun.* 40:1110–1116.

51. Jefferson, L. S. 1980. Role of insulin in the regulation of protein synthesis. *Diabetes* 29:487–496.

52. Ernst, V., Levin, D. H., and London, I. M. 1978. Evidence that glucose-6-phosphate regulates protein synthesis initiation in reticulocyte lysates. *J. Biol. Chem.* 253:7163–7172.

53. Ravid, K., Diamant, P., and Avi-Dor, Y. 1980. Glucose dependent stimulation of protein synthesis in cultured heart cells: Possible involvement of the pentose phosphate pathway. *FEBS Lett.* 119:20–24.

54. Pain, V. M., and Garlick, P. J. 1974. Effect of streptozotocin diabetes and insulin treatment on the rate of protein synthesis in tissues of the rat in vivo. *J. Biol. Chem.* 249:4510–4514.

55. Wool, I. G., Stirewalt, W. S., Kurihara, K., Low, R. B., Bailey, P., and Oyer, D. 1968. Mode of action of insulin in the regulation of protein biosynthesis in muscle. *Recent Prog. Horm. Res.* 24:139–208.

56. Williams, I. H., Chua, B. H. L., Sahms, R. H., Siehl, D., and Morgan, H. E. 1980. Effects of diabetes on protein turnover in cardiac muscle. *Am. J. Physiol.* 239:E178–E185.

57. Pain, V. M. 1973. Effect of streptozotocin diabetes on the ability of muscle cell sap to support protein synthesis by ribosomes in cell-free systems. *Biochim. Biophys. Acta* 308:180–187.

58. Dillman, W. H. 1980. Diabetes mellitus induces changes in cardiac myosin of the rat. *Diabetes* 29:579–582.

59. Garber, D. W., and Neely, J. R. 1983. Decreased myocardial function and myosin ATPase in hearts from diabetic rats. *Am. J. Physiol.* 244:H586–H591.

60. Garber, D. W., Everett, A. W., and Neely, J. R. 1983. Cardiac function and myosin ATPase in diabetic rats treated with insulin, T_3 and T_4. *Am. J. Physiol.* 244:H592–H598.

61. Cummins, P. 1983. Contractile proteins in muscle disease. *J. Muscle Res. Cell Motil.* 4:5–24.

62. Griffin, W. S. T., and Wildenthal, K. 1978. Myofibrillar alkaline protease activity in rat heart and its responses to some interventions. *J. Mol. Cell. Cardiol.* 10:669–676.

63. Mayer, M., Amin, R., Milholland, R. M., and Rosen, F. 1976. Possible significance of myofibrillar protease in muscle catabolism: Enzyme activity in dystrophic, tumor-bearing, and glucocorticoid-treated animals. *Exp. Mol. Pathol.* 25:9–19.

64. Mayer, M., Amin, R., and Shafrir, E. 1974. Rat myofibrillar protease: Enzyme properties and adaptive changes in conditions of muscle protein degradation. *Arch. Biochem. Biophys.* 161:20–25.

65. Clark, M. G., Beinlich, C. J., McKee, E. E., Lins, J. A., and Morgan, H. E. 1980. Relationship between alkaline proteolytic activity and protein degradation in rat heart. *Fed. Proc. Fed. Am. Soc. Exp. Biol.* 39:26–30.

66. McKee, E. E., Clark, M. G., Beinlich, C. J., Lins, J. A., and Morgan, H. E. 1979. Neutral-alkaline proteases and protein degradation in rat heart. *J. Mol. Cell. Cardiol.* 11:1033–1051.

67. Rannels, D. E., Pegg, A. E., Rannels, S. R., and Jefferson, L. S. 1978. Effect of starvation on initiation of protein synthesis in skeletal muscle and heart. *Am. J. Physiol.* 235:E126–E133.

68. McNurlan, M. A., Fern, E. B., and Garlick, P. J. 1982. Failure of leucine to stimulate protein synthesis in vivo. *Biochem. J.* 204:831–838.

69. Crie, J. S., Sanford, C. F., and Wildenthal, K. 1980. Influence of starvation and refeeding on cardiac protein degradation in rats. *J. Nutr.* 110:22–27.

70. Curfman, G. D., O'Hara, D. S., Hopkins, B. E., and Smith, T. W. 1980. Suppression of myocardial protein degradation in the rat during fasting: Effects of insulin, glucose and leucine. *Circ. Res.* 46:581–589.

71. Wildenthal, K., Poole, A. R., and Dingle, J. T. 1975. Influence of starvation on the activities and localization of cathepsin D and other lysosomal enzymes in hearts of rabbits and mice. *J. Mol. Cell. Cardiol.* 7:841–855.

72. Soderling, T. R., and Park, C. R. 1974. Recent advances in glycogen metabolism. *Adv. Cyclic Nucleotide Res.* 4:283–333.

73. Sugden, M. C., Sharples, S. C., and Randle, P. J. 1976. Carcass glycogen as a potential source of glucose during short-term starvation. *Biochem. J.* 160:817–819.

74. Jefferson, L. S., Rannels, D. E., Munger, B. L., and Morgan, H. E. 1974. Insulin in the regulation of protein turnover in heart and skeletal muscle. *Fed. Proc. Fed. Am. Soc. Exp. Biol.* 33:1098–1104.

75. Jefferson, L. S., Li, J. B., and Rannels, S. R. 1977. Regulation by insulin of amino acid release and protein turnover in the perfused rat hemicorpus. *J. Biol. Chem.* 252:1476–1483.

76. Millward, D. J., Garlick, P. J., Nnanyelugo, D. O., and Waterlow, J. C. 1976. The relative importance of muscle protein synthesis and breakdown in the regulation of muscle mass. *Biochem. J.* 156:185–188.

77. Randle, P. J., and Tubbs, P. K. 1979. Carbohydrate and fatty acid metabolism. *Handb. Physiol. Sect. 2: Cardiovasc. Syst.* 1:805–844.

78. Young, V. R. 1970. The role of skeletal and cardiac muscle in the regulation of protein metabolism. *Mamm. Protein Metab.* 4:585–674.

79. Odedra, B. R., Dalal, S. S., and Millward, D. J. 1982. Muscle protein synthesis in the streptozotocin-diabetic rat: A possible role for corticosterone in the insensitivity to insulin infusion in vivo. *Biochem. J.* 202:363–368.

80. Tomas, F. M., Munro, H. N., and Young, V. R. 1978. Effect of glucocorticoid administration on the rate of muscle protein breakdown in vivo in rats, as measured by urinary excretion of N^τ methylhistidine. *Biochem. J.* 178:139–146.

81. Rannels, S. R., Rannels, D. E., Pegg, A. E., and Jefferson, L. S. 1978. Glucocorticoid effects on peptide chain initiation in skeletal muscle and heart. *Am. J. Physiol.* 235:E134–E139.

82. Griffin, E. E., and Wildenthal, K. 1978. Regulation of cardiac protein balance by hydrocortisone: Interaction with insulin. *Am. J. Physiol.* 234:E306–313.

83. Sanford, C. F., Griffin, E. E., and Wildenthal, K. 1978. Synthesis and degradation of myocardial protein during the development and regression of thyroxine-induced cardiac hypertrophy in rats. *Circ. Res.* 43:688–694.

84. Wildenthal, K., and Mueller, E. A. 1974. Increased myocardial cathepsin D activity during regression of thyrotoxic cardiac hypertrophy. *Nature (London)* 249:478–479.

85. Goodkind, M. J., Damback, G. E., Thyrum, P. T., and Luchi, R. J. 1974. Effect of thyroxine on ventricular myocardial contractility and ATPase activity in guinea pigs. *Am. J. Physiol.* 226:66–72.

86. Morkin, E. 1979. Stimulation of cardiac myosin adenosine triphosphatase in thyrotoxicosis. *Circ. Res.* 44:1–7.

87. Hoh, J. F. Y., McGrath, P. A., and Hale, P. T. 1978. Electrophoretic analysis of multiple forms of rat cardiac myosin: Effects of hypophysectomy and thyroxine replacement. *J. Mol. Cell. Cardiol.* 10:1053–1076.

88. Hoh, J. F. Y., and Egerton, L. J. 1979. Action of triiodothyronine on the synthesis of rat ventricular myosin isoenzyme. *FEBS Lett.* 101:143–148.

89. Buccino, R. A., Spann, J. F., Pool, P. E., Sonnenblick, E. H., and Braunwald, E. 1967. Influence of the thyroid state on the intrinsic contractile properties and energy stores of the myocardium. *J. Clin. Invest.* 46:1669–1682.

90. Taylor, R. R., Covell, J. W., and Ross, R. J. 1969. Influences of the thyroid state on left ventricular tension–velocity relations in the intact sedated dog. *J. Clin. Invest.* 48:775–784.

91. Iljalmarson, Å. C., Rannels, D. E., Kao, R., and Morgan, H. E. 1975. Effects of hypophysectomy, growth hormone and thyroxine on protein turnover in heart. *J. Biol. Chem.* 250:4556–4561.

92. Kao, R., Rannels, D. E., Whitman, V., and Morgan, H. E. 1978. Factors accounting for the growth and atrophy of the heart. *Recent Adv. Stud. Cardiac Struct. Metab.* 12:105–113.

93. Earl, D. C. N., and Korner, A. 1966. Effect of rat hypophysectomy and growth hormone treatment on cardiac polysomes and ribonucleic acid. *Arch. Biochem. Biophys.* 115:445–449.

Ethanol and Cardiac Protein Synthesis

Sidney S. Schreiber, Carole D. Evans, Murray Oratz, and Marcus A. Rothschild

Department of Nuclear Medicine
Veterans Administration Medical Center
and
Department of Medicine
New York University School of Medicine
New York, New York 10016

Abstract. Acute exposure of the heart to ethanol does not appear to alter the rate of young guinea pig cardiac protein synthesis when assayed in vitro. In contrast, the primary metabolite of ethanol, acetaldehyde, markedly diminishes synthesis despite its chronotropic and inotropic effects. On the other hand, after 11–13 weeks of ethanol-drinking during growth and maturation, the synthetic capacity of the working right ventricle was decreased when measured in vitro with normal perfusate. Assay of synthesis of the contractile proteins myosin heavy and light chains, actin and tropomyosin suggests a change in synthesis or pool size of actin reflected in an alteration of relative synthesis of this protein compared to that of heavy chains. The relative synthesis of the other proteins remained at control levels. When hearts from ethanol-drinking and matched control animals were perfused under conditions of severe ischemia, there was a profound fall in protein synthesis in all hearts, and ethanol did not enhance the inhibition of synthesis. However, the hearts from ethanol-drinking animals showed a more marked and significant impairment of maintaining ejection pressure with a marked increase in coronary resistance as the perfusion progressed. It is postulated that some impairment of protein metabolism may occur during prolonged ethanol exposure, which may influence the cardiac response of another induced stress, e.g., ischemia.

In the last decade, studies of alcoholic cardiac disease have demonstrated a wide variety of metabolic alterations following chronic ethanol abuse. The cardiac changes appear to be independent of associated liver malfunction or malnutrition. Animal studies have not produced consistent data. The cardiac physiological and metabolic changes have varied with the model used, but there has been a general flow of data suggesting that while contractile function of hearts from ethanol-exposed animals (and in chronic alcoholic humans) may be within normal limits under control conditions, the addition of another stress may demonstrate some impairment in cardiac function. Thus, little impairment of contraction in vivo has been reported after ethanol exposure unless there is elevation of pressure with hypertension [1], with increased afterload [2], or after ischemia [3] or fast electrical pacing [4].

Since the contractile elements are proteins, our interest was focused on synthesis of cardiac proteins with acute or chronic exposure to ethanol to

123

see whether any correlation can be established between altered function and protein synthesis. Our approach may be divided into two categories: Our initial studies were directed toward acute exposure of the heart to ethanol, and our more recent experiments concerned assay of protein synthesis after chronic ethanol ingestion. Some time ago, we found that acute perfusion in vitro with ethanol did not impair cardiac synthesis of proteins in the hearts of young guinea pigs even at levels (250 mg/100 ml) that blocked hepatic synthesis of albumin [5]. This ethanol level produced no alteration in contractility of the left ventricle, which performed work against a normal afterload, and incorporation of [^{14}C]lysine was the same as in controls in both the working left ventricle and the nonworking but beating right ventricle. In this early work, synthesis, expressed as incorporation of labeled lysine, was calculated using both the extracellular-space (ECS) and intracellular-space (ICS) specific activities as estimates of the precursor-pool specific activity. In either case, ethanol (250 mg/100 ml) produced no effect on this incorporation [5]. When ethanol in acute perfusion studies was drastically increased to levels of 1500 mg/100 ml, there was decreased function of the left ventricle, diminished incorporation of labeled amino acids into protein of both ventricles, and a significant decrease in protein N without change in water content, suggesting increase in degradation and decreased synthesis of protein with this level of ethanol in the perfusate. Because ethanol is rapidly metabolized, we were also interested in the effects of the primary metabolite, acetaldehyde. Acetaldehyde perfusion into normal hearts was accompanied by a marked inotropic and chronotropic effect. This stimulation was associated with significant fall in incorporation of [^{14}C]lysine into protein (Table 1) whether incorporation was calculated using the ECS or ICS specific activity as that of the precursor pool. Propanolol, which blocked the inotropic and chronotropic effects, did not prevent the acetaldehyde effect on incorporation of labeled amino acids into protein [5]. There was a possibility that the acetaldehyde inotropic and chronotropic effects may deplete the high-energy stores in sufficient amounts to decrease protein synthesis. However, there were two arguments against this: First, depletion of ATP sufficient to stop protein synthesis would show up in marked impairment of contractility, which did not occur. Second, conservation of the energy by cessation of augmented contraction with propanolol still did not prevent the inhibition of synthesis (Table 1). A third argument against high-energy depletion as a cause of the acetaldehyde inhibition of synthesis was obtained by studies of subcellular systems with microsomes and polysomes synthesizing proteins (mainly peptide elongation) in excess ATP with ATP-generating systems [7]. Microsomes taken from normal hearts and incubated in ethanol solutions as high as 50 mM showed protein synthesis equal to that of controls. In contrast, acetaldehyde at levels of 0.03–0.12 mM decreased microsome synthesis to 50–60% of the controls (Table 2) [7,8] but had no inhibiting effect on polysomes freed from the sarcoplasmic reticulum [8]. Such low levels of acetaldehyde have been reported in humans after mod-

Table 1.   Ethanol and Acetaldehyde Acute Perfusion in Normal Young Guinea Pig Hearts[a]

Group	Heart rate	Amplitude	Work[b]	[14C]Lysine incorporated (μmoles/g protein N)
	Percentage of control			
Controls	100	100	100	100
Ethanol				
200 mg/100 ml	100	100	101	97
1500 mg/100 ml	85	90	91	59
				$P < 0.001$
Acetaldehyde				
0.8 mM	116	170	125	56
	$P < 0.05$	$P < 0.001$	$P < 0.02$	$P < 0.001$
Acetaldehyde				
and propanolol	100	100	100	56
				$P < 0.001$

[a] From Schreiber et al. [5].
[b] SP × R (peak systolic pressure × rate as per Opie [6]).

erate drinking [9]. The question remains as to the site of action of acetaldehyde, since it does not inhibit polysome cycling and peptide elongation in solutions freed from sarcoplasmic reticulum [8]. The presence of the latter appears to be essential for the inhibition.

The effects of chronic ethanol intake on cardiac protein synthesis have not been clear, and we were particularly interested in the effects of ethanol in the maturing animal. A model of chronic ethanol ingestion was developed in which the young guinea pig ate a normal solid diet with ethanol 5 or 10% in the drinking water [10]. This was the sole supply of fluid to the animal. The animals were paired with weight-matched controls (drinking plain water). Models of ethanol have been widely used in the past with a liquid diet containing ethanol, but the guinea pigs rejected the fluid diets and these had to be abandoned. The mean caloric intake due to ethanol in the ethanol-

Table 2.   Ethanol and Acetaldehyde in Cardiac Subcellular Systems[a]

Group	Incorporation of [14C]leucine into microsomal protein (% of control)	
Ethanol (27–54 mM)	97–108	
Acetaldehyde		
(0.03–0.12 mM)	52–65	$P < 0.001$

[a] From Schreiber et al. [7] and Oratz et al. [8].

drinking animals was 23 cal/day or 21% of the total consumed. The total calories/day ingested by ethanol-drinking animals (110–112) was approximately 10 cal/day greater than weight-matched controls, but the mean food intake by the ethanol-drinking animals was 10% lower than that of the same controls. The mean blood level of ethanol in animals 2 hr before anesthesia and operative removal of the heart was 34 ± 11 mg/100 ml. The ventricular weight/body weight ratio in ethanol-drinking animals was identical to that in weight-matched controls ($0.32 \pm 0.008\%$ compared to $0.32 \pm 0.009\%$) [10].

The protein-synthetic capacity of the heart was tested in an in vitro system after 11–15 weeks of ethanol-drinking. Hearts were removed and prepared for perfusion using a model in which the right ventricle (RV) performs work with a contractile load and the coronary perfusion is maintained at a constant level by a separate perfusion system [11]. Hearts taken from ethanol-drinking animals and weight-matched controls were perfused for 3 hr with oxygenated perfusate under standard hemodynamic conditions (RV pressure 10 mm Hg, coronary flow 6 ml/min, RV fluid load 6 ml/min). There were no significant differences in cardiac response in maintenance of RV systolic pressure, dP/dt max, and cardiac rate between hearts of ethanol-drinking animals and the matched controls. Two labeled amino acids were used simultaneously to assay protein synthesis (^{3}H- and/or ^{14}C-labeled lysine and phenylalanine). There was no difference in intracellular pool sizes or specific activities of either amino acid in both right and left ventricles of hearts from ethanol-drinking animals and controls.

In this in vitro model, the right ventricle performs work of ejecting a volume (6 ml/min) against an afterload pressure (10 mm Hg) while the left ventricle is perfused but performs work only of contraction without any volume load or work of ejection. The results of assay of incorporation of labeled amino acids into proteins are shown in Figure 1. After 3 hr of perfusion, incorporation of both labeled phenylalanine and lysine was decreased in the working right ventricle, but not in the left. That the total protein pool was the same in experimental animals and controls (Figure 2) would indicate that there was a decrease in protein synthesis in the right ventricles of hearts from ethanol-ingesting maturing guinea pigs [10]. The similarity of protein N content in perfused hearts from ethanol-drinking animals and controls would also indicate no gross change in protein degradation during perfusion because of previous ethanol exposure. These findings indicated that although chronic exposure to ethanol in the growing animal may not inhibit cardiac protein synthesis in an unstressed ventricle, the addition of a workload may result in the impairment. These data do not entirely agree with those reported by Whitman et al. [12] in the adult rat heart in vivo, in which the hypertrophy response (increased cardiac mass) to aortic banding occurred during ethanol ingestion. However, the difference may be one of degree, since the degree of response appeared to be less than that in controls after aortic banding.

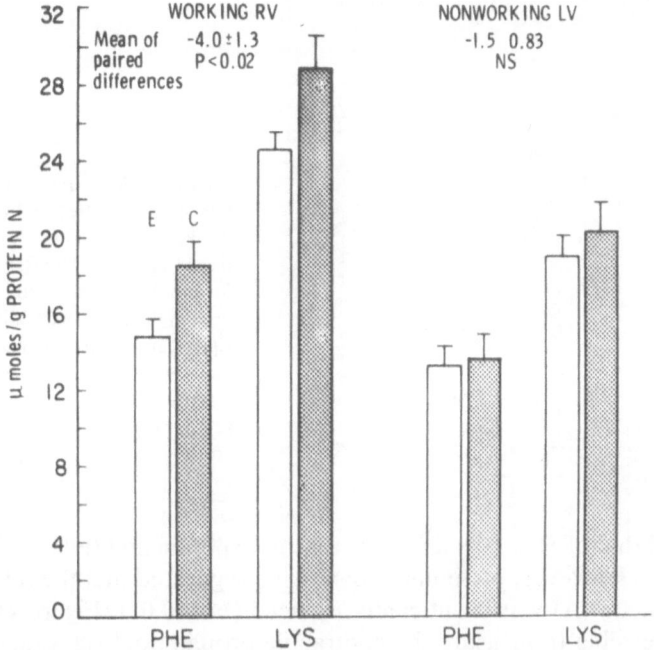

Figure 1.   Measurement of synthesis of total proteins, incorporation of labeled lysine (LYS) and phenylalanine (PHE), perfused simultaneously into hearts taken from animals ingesting ethanol for 13–15 weeks (average weight 700 g). The time of perfusion was 3 hr. The values are means ± S.E.M. The statistical differences were obtained by the method of means of paired differences (Snedecor) [10]. While there was a significant decrease in synthesis in the working right ventricles of hearts from ethanol-drinking animals (E) vs. controls (C), there was no significant difference in the nonworking left ventricles of the same animals. Originally presented at the European Section of ISHR, Bologna, Italy, 1982, and published in: C. M. Calderera and P. Harris (eds.), 1982, *Advances in Studies in Heart Metabolism*, p. 511, CLUEB, Bologna, Italy.

Assays of synthesis of some contractile proteins in hearts from ethanol-drinking animals have been attempted. Incorporation of labeled lysine and phenylalanine estimated from the specific activities of these amino acids in RV myosin heavy chains (HCs) showed no difference between hearts taken from ethanol-drinking animals and from controls (both weight-matched and controls drinking water with dextromaltose instead of ethanol) (Figure 3). The "synthesis" is expressed as the ratio of HC specific activity/perfusate specific activity, since it has been shown in earlier work that both phenylalanine and lysine in the precursor pools for synthesis of the afornamed contractile proteins equilibrate rapidly with the extracellular space or perfusate [13–15]. Since it was noted that the specific activities of labeled lysine and phenylalanine in the myosin HCs were the same in hearts from ethanol-drinking animals and controls, the HCs were used as a reference point. The relative synthesis of light chains (LC_1 and LC_2) and of tropomyosin (TM)

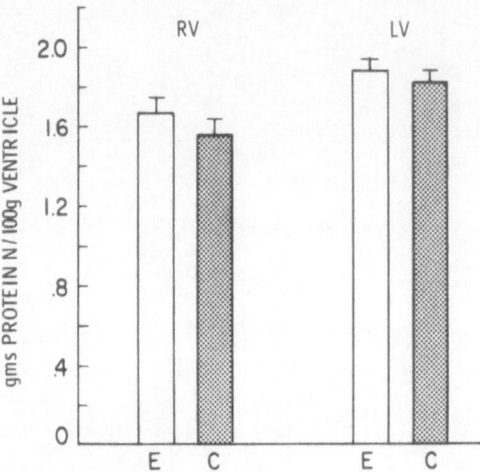

Figure 2. Measurement of total protein pools in hearts from ethanol-drinking animals (E) and matched paired controls (C) after 3 hr of perfusion. The hearts were the same as used in Figure 1. In the absence of any significant pool change, the decreased incorporation seen in Figure 1 represents a decrease in synthesis in the working RV in the ethanol group.

compared that of HCs was also the same in experimental (ethanol) and control hearts. However, preliminary data have suggested that the relative synthesis of actin (A) was significantly reduced ($P < 0.02$) (Figure 4). Since it was not feasible to measure the contractile-protein pool sizes, at this time, we cannot say whether the decreased A/HC ratio was indeed due to a decrease in synthesis of A or whether there may have been a change in the A or HC pool sizes in the hearts from ethanol-drinking animals. This difference in the relative synthesis in perfused hearts from ethanol-drinking animals remains to be explored.

The unequal protein-synthetic response in the working and nonworking ventricles following prolonged ethanol ingestion suggested additional studies with imposition of another stress on the chronically exposed ethanol heart. The stress selected was that of ischemia, induced in vitro. In this series, newly weaned (300-g) guinea pigs were raised on a standard Purina chow with 10% ethanol (weight/volume) in drinking water from 13 to 15 weeks,

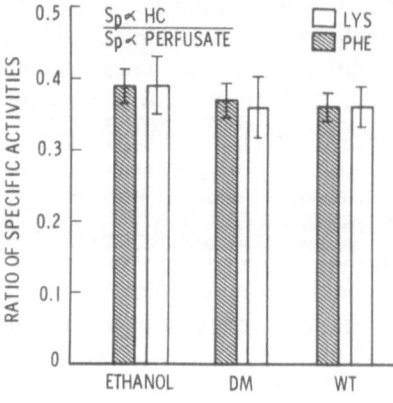

Figure 3. Specific activity of RV heavy chains (HC) expressed as a ratio of that in the perfusate with both radioactive lysine (LYS) and phenylalanine (PHE) after 3 hr of perfusion in vitro of hearts taken from ethanol-drinking, calorie-matched [(DM) dextromaltose], and weight-matched (WT) animals. The activities are expressed as a ratio of that in the perfusate, since it had been shown in earlier work that the two amino acids in the precursor pool for contractile protein synthesis equilibrated rapidly with the extracellular space [15].

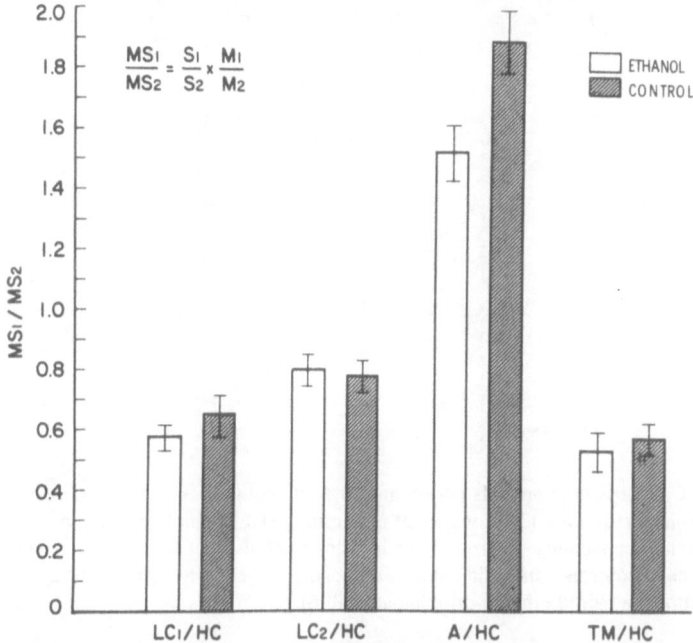

Figure 4.   Relative molar synthesis of myosin light chains 1 and 2 (LC$_1$ and LC$_2$) and of the contractile proteins actin (A) and tropomyosin (TM), with reference to the heavy chains (HC). In each individual heart, the specific activities of the proteins were determined and compared to that of the HCs. There was no significant difference in specific activity of the HCs between the hearts of ethanol-drinking animals and controls (Figure 3). Weight- and calorie-matched controls were the same and therefore pooled. Although the data would suggest that there may be a decrease in synthesis of A, one cannot exclude the possibility that a difference in pool size of A (or HC) between the ethanol-drinking and control animal hearts could explain the change in ratios. Molar synthesis (MS); rate of synthesis (S); molar proportion (M).

when they reached a weight of 700–800 g. Each ethanol-drinking animal was paired with a weight-matched and calorie-matched control (Figure 5). After 13–15 weeks, hearts were removed from anesthesized animals (Nembutal) and perfused in vitro with perfusate oxygenated with 95% O_2–5% CO_2.

The heart model [11] was adapted to allow establishment of severe ischemia with unaltered RV fluid load and pulmonary resistance [3]. There were two separate perfusion systems. The first system perfused the coronary arteries via the proximal aorta with the flow maintained at 6 ml/min (equivalent to 300–350 ml/min per 100 g ventricle). The second presented any fluid load desired to the right atrium (a closed system) via the cannulated inferior vena cava and could therefore supplement the coronary circulation, which emptied into the right atrium. The first 30 min of perfusion was called the "control period," during which the coronary flow of 6 ml/min (300 ml/100 g ventricle) emptied into the right heart; there was no additional right atrial flow, and the right ventricular output was also 6 ml/min. This was ejected

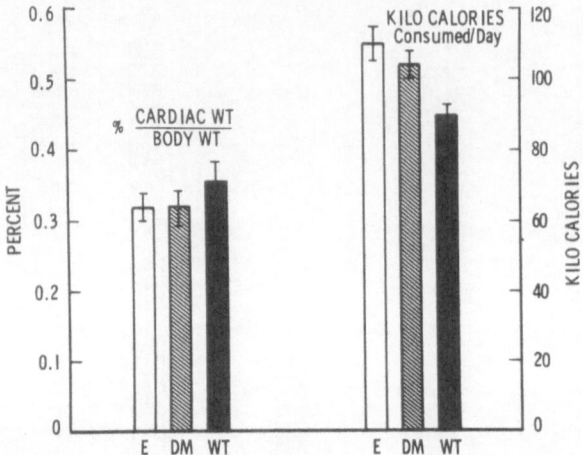

Figure 5.   Comparison of animals consuming 10% ethanol with two controls, calorie-matched and weight-matched, after 13–15 weeks of maturation. (E) Ethanol-consuming animals; (DM) calorie-matched consuming dextromaltose in calories equivalent to ethanol consumed; (WT) weight-matched controls with solid calories reduced sufficiently to maintain body weight identical to that of the paired ethanol-drinking animal [3].

by right ventricular systole against a regulated pulmonary resistance so that the right ventricular peak systolic pressure was 10–11 mm Hg, similar to that found in the right ventricles measured in vivo in this size animal. The left ventricle contracted but received no fluid load and therefore performed no work of ejection. After 30 min, the total coronary flow was reduced from 6 to 1 ml/min (Figure 6), and the right atrial perfusion was simultaneously increased from 0 to 5 ml/min via the inferior vena cava perfusion system. In this fashion, moderately severe ischemia, in both ventricles, was produced while the right atrial (and right ventricular) fluid load was maintained at preischemic levels, and the pulmonary resistance was maintained identical to that during the control period prior to the ischemia [3]. The hearts were perfused with this reduced level of coronary flow for 150 min. Thus, the right ventricle working against a fixed pulmonary resistance (afterload) with a constant preload was tested for protein-synthetic capacity with induction of severe relative ischemia. The left ventricle, which was not performing any work of ejection but was subjected to the same alterations in coronary perfusion, was also assayed for comparison. ATP and creatine phosphate levels were obtained after 30 min of normal coronary perfusion in 3 hearts of each group (ethanol-drinking animals and weight-matched and calorie-matched controls), and these values were as reported previously with normal hearts (Figure 6). In addition, at the end of the perfusion with relative ischemia, the high-energy phosphates were determined in all hearts. As expected, there was a marked decrease in the levels of ATP and creatine phosphate accompanied by a sharp increase in lactate production during the

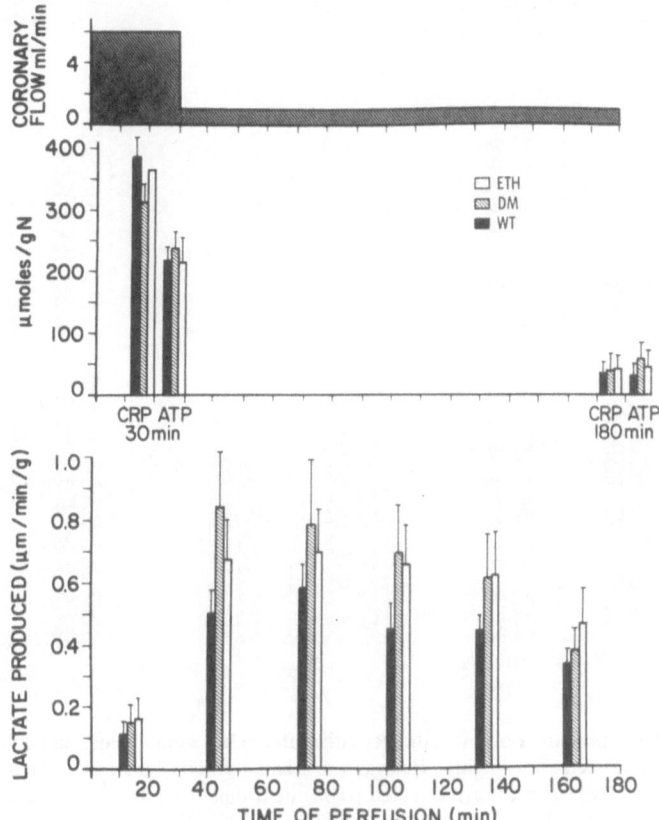

Figure 6.   Scheme of perfusion of hearts taken from ethanol-drinking animals (ETH) and the weight-matched (WT) and calorie-matched [(DM) dextromaltose] controls [3]. After 30 min of normal perfusion, the coronary flow was reduced from 6 to 1 ml/min, while the right ventricular flow was increased from 0 to 5 ml/min with maintenance of right ventricular load of 6 ml/min. The creatine phosphate (CRP) and ATP levels at 30 min were obtained from hearts perfused for only 30 min, while the levels of high-energy phosphates after 180 min were obtained in all the hearts subjected to relative ischemia. Lactate production was obtained at 30-min intervals and plotted at the midpoint of the study period. Although the lactate produced by the hearts from dextromaltose animals appeared to be higher than that in hearts from weight-controlled animals, the differences are only minimally significant. The values obtained for hearts from ethanol animals were not significantly different from controls.

ischemic perfusion (Figure 6). There was no significant difference in the levels of high-energy phosphates or in lactate production between hearts from ethanol-drinking animals and those from the matched controls.

After the ischemic perfusion, assays of total protein pools, specific activities of labeled lysine and phenylalanine in the intracellular pools, and the distribution of the labels from the ICS/ECS specific activities ratio as well as the lysine/phenylalanine ratio in the total protein were the same in hearts

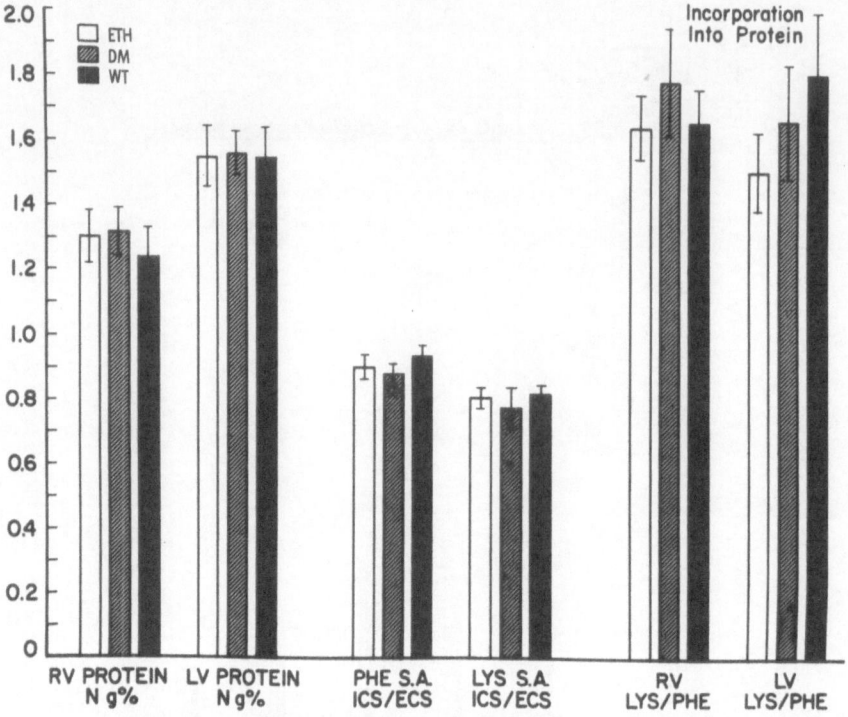

Figure 7.   Total protein pools, specific activities of labeled amino acids, and distribution of labels after 3 hr of perfusion in vitro. Hearts from ethanol-drinking growing animals (ETH) and weight-matched (WT) and calorie-matched [(DM) dextromaltose] animals were analyzed for total protein content and the specific activities of labeled lysine (LYS) and phenylalanine (PHE) in the intracellular (ICS) and extracellular (ECS) pools as well as the ratio of the two amino acid labels in the cardiac total protein. No significant differences were noted in protein nitrogen or in the distribution of the two labeled amino acids.

from ethanol-ingesting animals and those from the matched controls (Figure 7). There was a significant decline in protein synthesis (incorporation of labeled amino acids into protein) with the ischemic perfusion, but there was no greater decrease in hearts from ethanol-ingesting animals (Figure 8). Preliminary data from our laboratory suggest that there is no apparent preferential decrease in the specific activity of the labeled amino acids in the contractile proteins myosin (subunits HC and LCs) or in actin and tropomyosin.

There were, however, two significant differences in the hemodynamic reactions of the hearts from ethanol-drinking animals to the ischemic perfusion. First, as the ischemic perfusion progressed, there was a more marked diminution in the right ventricular systolic ejection pressure (Table 3). Second, there was a rise in coronary pressure in hearts from ethanol-drinking animals that was greater than that in matched controls (Table 3). There was

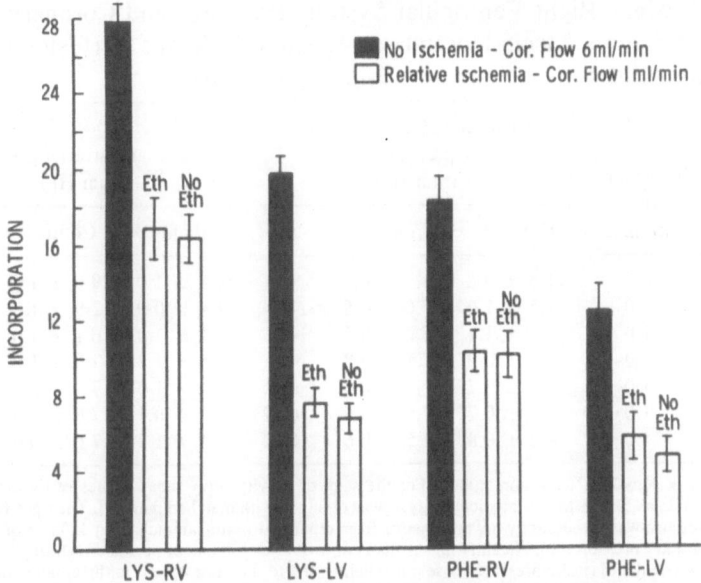

Figure 8.   Incorporation of labeled lysine (LYS) and phenylalanine (PHE) into both ventricles after 3 hr of perfusion. Hearts taken from ethanol-drinking animals and perfused with relative ischemia showed no greater decrease in protein synthesis than hearts from matched controls. These are compared to normal hearts of the same age level perfused under control conditions [3].

no decrease in the measured right ventricular output in the ethanol hearts, nor was there any visible right atrial dilatation. Furthermore, although there was a small rise in diastolic pressure after the onset of the ischemic perfusion (mean less than 1.0 mm Hg) this was not progressive and was identical in the hearts from ethanol-ingesting animals and those from the matched controls. Hence, the rise in coronary pressure was most likely due to increased coronary resistance, rather than to any backup of perfusion.

DISCUSSION

This chapter presents data to suggest that ethanol exposure may interfere with protein metabolism and contractile action, but this interference may not be uniform and may not be manifested unless an additional load or stress is placed on the heart.

In the first place, ethanol perfusion of a normal heart in vitro does not appear to change the gross parameters of contractility or protein synthesis of either the right or the left ventricle unless highly toxic concentrations are used [5]. In contrast, the primary metabolite of ethanol, acetaldehyde, inhibits protein synthesis both in acute perfusion of the normal heart and in

Table 3.   Mean Right Ventricular Systolic Pressures and Coronary Arterial Pressures during Normal and Relative Ischemic Perfusion in Hearts from Control and Ethanol-Drinking Animals[a]

Time of perfusion (min)	Coronary flow (ml/min)	Right ventricular systolic pressure (mm Hg)			Coronary arterial pressure (mm Hg)		
		Ethanol	Control	P	Ethanol	Control	P
0–30	6.0	11.8 ± 0.8	11.7 ± 0.7	NS	30.5 ± 1.0	29.0 ± 1.3	NS
30–60	1.0	4.3 ± 1.0	7.0 ± 0.6	NS	14.4 ± 0.9	12.9 ± 1.3	NS
60–100	1.0	4.6 ± 1.1	7.2 ± 0.7	NS	18.1 ± 1.0	16.1 ± 1.0	< 0.02
100–120	1.0	5.0 ± 0.9	7.1 ± 0.8	NS	22.8 ± 1.2	17.0 ± 1.0	< 0.02
120–140	1.0	4.9 ± 0.7	7.6 ± 0.6	< 0.05	23.1 ± 1.0	17.0 ± 0.9	< 0.01
140–160	1.0	4.7 ± 0.7	7.6 ± 0.6	< 0.02	23.2 ± 0.7	17.6 ± 0.8	< 0.01
160–180	1.0	4.8 ± 0.8	7.5 ± 0.6	< 0.02	23.5 ± 1.3	17.6 ± 0.9	< 0.01

[a] Recordings of pressures were continuous. For the sake of brevity, only mean values of the times listed are shown (means ± S.E.M.). Statistical analysis was obtained with matched pairs [3]. The right ventricular systolic pressure was significantly lower in hearts from ethanol-drinking animals after 120 min of perfusion and the coronary pressures significantly higher than controls after 100 min of perfusion. During this period, the right ventricular diastolic pressures rose only slightly and to the same extent in the ethanol and control groups. At 0–30, 30–60, and 150–180 min, the diastolic pressures were 3.5 ± 1.2 and 3.0 + 0.3; 4.06 + 1.3 and 4.3 + 0.7; and 4.5 + 1.5 and 4.7 + 0.8 mm Hg in ethanol and control hearts, respectively.

subcellular microsomal systems [7]. It is therefore not surprising to find that after chronic ethanol intake, there is decreased synthesis in the working right ventricle, and it has been reasoned that this may be due to repeated release of acetaldehyde by hepatic metabolism, which may exert a persistent effect as the one detected by our perfusion methods. What is surprising is that the left ventricle, not performing work of ejection in this model, shows no alteration in synthesis in in vitro testing.

This discrepancy has led to the suggestion that although ethanol reactions may not be seen in "normal" situations, the addition of another stress may produce or expose otherwise quiescent changes. This may be demonstrated by some discrepancies noted in the literature. Minimal decrease in contractility has been seen in some models in vivo [1] or in vitro [10,12]. However, with the addition of another stress such as increased arterial pressure as angiotension in vivo [1,16] or dobutamine [2], or with hypoxia [2] or ischemia [3], there is a deficiency in contractile activity. Furthermore, cardiac muscle in hearts from ethanol-exposed animals shows a decrease in response to increases in calcium in vitro [17]. The reasons for the impairments mentioned are as yet unclear, but the data would attract speculation that some protein-synthetic impairment may be a contributing cause.

ACKNOWLEDGMENTS

This research was aided in part by a grant from the Veterans Administration, The National Institute of Health HL 09562, and the Palitz Foundation.

REFERENCES

1. Bing, R. J., Tillmanns, H., Fauvel, J. M., Seeler, K., and Mao, J. C. 1974. Effect of prolonged alcohol administration on calcium transport in heart muscle in the dog. *Circ. Res.* 35:33–38.
2. Segel, L. D., Rendig, S. V., and Mason, D. T. 1979. Left ventricular dysfunction of isolated working rat hearts after chronic alcohol consumption. *Cardiovasc. Res.* 13:136–146.
3. Schreiber, S. S., Evans, C. D., Reff, F., Oratz, M., and Rothschild, M. A. 1984. Prolonged feeding of ethanol to the young growing guinea pig. II. A model to study the effects of severe ischemia on cardiac protein synthesis. *Alcoholism: Clin Exp. Res.* 8:54–61, 1984.
4. Chan, T. C. K., and Sutter, M. D. 1982. The effects of chronic ethanol consumption on cardiac function in rats. *Can. J. Physiol. Pharmacol.* 60:777–782.
5. Schreiber, S. S., Briden, K., Oratz, M., and Rothschild, M. S. 1972. Ethanol, acetaldehyde, and myocardial protein synthesis. *J. Clin. Invest.* 51:2820–2826.
6. Opie, L. H. 1965. Coronary flow rate and perfusion pressure as determinants of mechanical function and oxidative metabolism of the isolated perfused rat heart. *J. Physiol. (London)* 180:529.
7. Schreiber, S. S., Oratz, M., Rothschild, M. A., Reff, F., and Evans, C. D. 1974. Alcoholic cardiomyopathy. II. The inhibition of cardiac microsomal protein synthesis by acetaldehyde. *J. Mol. Cell. Cardiol.* 6:207–213.
8. Oratz, M., Schreiber, S. S., and Rothschild, M. A. 1977. Differing effects of acetaldehyde and ethanol on hepatic albumin synthesis and cardiac muscle protein synthesis. In: F. Seixas (ed.), *Currents in Alcoholism.* Vol. 1, pp. 47–68. Grune and Stratton, New York.
9. Korstein, M. A., Matsuzaki, S., Feinman, L., and Lieber, C. S. 1975. High blood acetaldehyde levels after ethanol administration. *N. Engl. J. Med.* 292:386–389.
10. Schreiber, S. S., Evans, C. D., Reff, F., Rothschild, M. A., and Oratz, M. 1982. Prolonged feeding of ethanol to the young growing guinea pig. 1. The effect on protein synthesis in the afterloaded right ventricle measured in vitro. *Alcoholism: Clin. Exp. Res.* 6:384–390.
11. Schreiber, S. S., Rothschild, M. A., Evans, C. D., Reff, F., and Oratz, M. 1975. The effect of pressure or flow stress on right ventricular protein synthesis in the face of constant and restricted coronary flow. *J. Clin. Invest.* 55:1–11.
12. Whitman, V., Schuler, H. G., and Musselman, J. 1980. Effects of chronic ethanol consumption on the myocardial hypertrophic response to pressure overload in the rat. *J. Mol. Cell. Cardiol.* 12:510–525.
13. McKee, E. E., Cheung, J. Y., Rannels, D. E., and Morgan, H. E. 1978. Measurement of the rate of protein synthesis and compartmentation of heart phenylalanine. *J. Biol. Chem.* 253:1030–1040.
14. Schreiber, S. S., Oratz, M., Evans, C. D., Reff, F., Klein, I., and Rothschild, M. A. 1973. Cardiac protein degradation in acute overload in vitro: Reutilization of amino acids. *Am. J. Physiol.* 224:338–345.
15. Evans, C. D., Schreiber, S. S., Oratz, M., and Rothschild, M. A. 1981. Relative synthesis of cardiac contractile proteins: Evidence for synthesis from the same precursor pool. *Biochem. J.* 194:673–678.
16. Regan, T. J., Levinson, G. E., Oldewurtel, H. A., Frank, M. J., Weisse, A. B., and Moschos, C. B. 1969. Ventricular function in non cardiacs with alcoholic fatty liver: Role of ethanol in the production of cardiomyopathy. *J. Clin. Invest.* 48:397–407.
17. Kino, M., Thorp, K. A., Bing, O. H. L., and Abelmann, W. H. 1981. Impaired myocardial performance and response to calcium in experimental alcoholic cardiomyopathy. *J. Mol. Cell. Cardiol.* 13:981–989.

The Role of Lysosomes and Microtubules in Cardiac Protein Degradation

K. Wildenthal, J. S. Crie, J. M. Ord, and J. R. Wakeland

Pauline and Adolph Weinberger Laboratory for Cardiopulmonary Research
Departments of Physiology and Internal Medicine
The University of Texas Health Science Center at Dallas
Dallas, Texas 75235

Abstract. The mechanisms and regulatory factors involved in cardiac proteolysis are incompletely understood. Agents that interfere with lysosomal function (e.g., chloroquine, leupeptin, methyladenine) cause a 25–30% reduction in the overall rate of protein degradation. In the same hearts, however, the rate of myosin breakdown remains unchanged. Disaggregation of microtubules with colchicine is accompanied by a 15% reduction in the rate of degradation of total protein and of myosin. In the same hearts, the degradation of "organellar" protein, including mitochondrial cytochromes, is reduced by over 30%. Thus, it appears that the degradation of different classes of cardiac proteins may be accomplished and regulated by different processes. Lysosomes are important in overall proteolysis, but appear not to be involved in the regulation of myosin breakdown. Microtubules are also involved in the proteolytic process, and appear to be especially important for the breakdown of proteins from mitochondria and perhaps other organelles.

INTRODUCTION

Although knowledge of the steps by which amino acids are assembled into protein is fairly complete, there is relatively little information about how proteins are degraded. The subcellular processes by which proteolysis is accomplished and the regulatory factors that are of importance remain incompletely understood. In many tissues including heart, lysosomes have been shown to play an important role, and the microtubular system seems to be involved as well.

Most studies of protein turnover have involved experimental approaches in which no distinction is made among different types of proteins within the tissue being tested. Yet there is no intrinsic reason to suppose that all proteins within a cell are degraded by exactly the same mechanisms, with the same regulatory factors being crucial. In the heart, for example, it seemed possible that the processes that are involved in the breakdown of certain classes of proteins such as myofibrillar proteins are different from the processes responsible for degradation of cytosolic proteins or mitochondrial proteins. Accordingly, our laboratory has been involved in recent

137

years in attempts not only to determine what factors may be important in overall proteolysis in the heart but also to test the hypothesis that different classes of cardiac proteins are degraded in different ways.

METHODS

As described previously [21], the rate of degradation of protein was measured in 18- to 20-day fetal mouse hearts in organ culture. This organ-culture model [17] offers the advantage of long-term stability of metabolic function combined with precise control of experimental conditions. Cultured hearts of matched littermates were labeled with L-[side chain-2,3,-^{3}H]phenylalanine and then maintained for 24 hr in control medium or medium supplemented with insulin (50 μg/ml), sucrose (100mM), leupeptin (50 μg/ml), chloroquine (0.1 mM), 3-methyladenine (10 mM), or colchicine (2.5 μM). The rate of degradation of total protein was measured from the loss of radioactive phenylalanine from trichloroacetic acid (TCA)-precipitable protein [21].

For experiments involving measurement of myosin degradation, myosin was isolated using a modification [23] of Hoh's procedure [7]. In other experiments designed to measure degradation rates in separate compartments of the cell, "myofibrillar," "organellar," and "cytosolic" fractions of the tissue homogenates were separated by differential centrifugation in various solutions as described in detail previously [4,10]. The loss of radioactive phenylalanine from the TCA-precipitable material in myosin and in each fraction of the homogenate was used as an index of the rate of protein turnover of that group of proteins. Degradation of heme proteins was measured in hearts exposed to δ-[^{14}C]aminolevulinic acid as well as [^{3}H]phenylalanine, with the rate of loss of ^{14}C radioactivity in TCA-precipitable material serving as an index of the rate of heme protein breakdown [4,11]. Because of the extensive reutilization of δ-aminolevulinic acid in heart tissue [11], cyclo-heximide was added to the media when heme protein degradation was measured.

There is some variability among fetal hearts of different litters and gestational ages, but results from within a litter are highly reproducible (S.D. < 10%). Therefore, statistical comparisons between values obtained from matched littermates under control and experimental conditions were made using Student's t test for paired samples. All results were expressed as the mean $\pm$ 1 S.E.M.

RESULTS

In keeping with previous results in this and other cardiac preparations [12,21], insulin reduced protein degradation (Figure 1, and Table 1). The degree of inhibition of total proteolysis (16–19%) was similar to the simul-

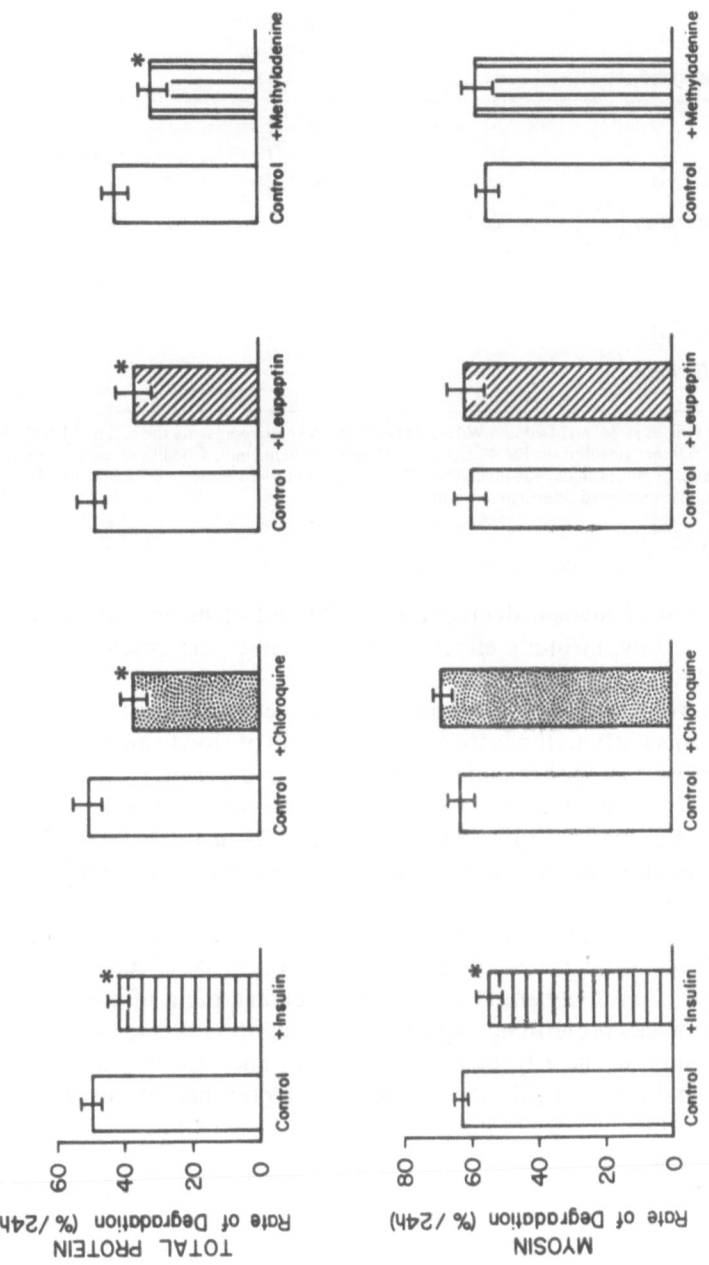

Figure 1. Effects of lysosomotropic agents and insulin on the degradation of total protein and myosin in cultured fetal mouse hearts. Each bar represents the mean ± 1 S.E.M. of at least 24 hearts from 6 litters. *$p < 0.05$ compared with matched littermate controls. Conditions of culture are described in the text. Data derived from Wildenthal et al. [23] and unpublished experiments.

Table 1.   Effects of Colchicine and Insulin on the Rate of Degradation of Total Protein and Heme Protein in Cultured Fetal Mouse Hearts[a]

Groups and results	Total protein degradation (% per day)	Heme protein degradation (% per day)
A. Control	32 ± 1	20 ± 1
B. + Insulin	26 ± 1	17 ± 2
Difference (B − A)	-6 ± 2^{b}	-3 ± 1^{b}
Percentage difference $\left(\dfrac{B - A}{A} \times 100\right)$	-19	-15
A. Control	33 ± 1	26 ± 1
B. + Colchicine	28 ± 1	18 ± 1
Difference (B − A)	-5 ± 1^{b}	-8 ± 1^{b}
Percentage difference $\left(\dfrac{B - A}{A} \times 100\right)$	-15	-31

[a] Data derived from Crie et al. [4] and Ord and Wildenthal [11]. Each value represents the mean ± 1 S.E.M. of 32 hearts from 8 litters (insulin) or 124 hearts from 31 litters (colchicine). Conditions of culture are described in the text. Cycloheximide was present in all media to inhibit reutilization of radioactive label.
[b] $P < 0.05$ compared with matched littermate controls.

taneous inhibition of myosin degradation (13%) and of heme protein degradation (15%). Thus, insulin's effect on all the classes of proteins studies was uniform [11,23].

Lysosomotropic agents also inhibited total proteolysis significantly. Sucrose, which gains entry to the lysosomal compartment slowly and produces progressive lysosomal abnormalities gradually over a period of days [20], caused a $14 \pm 7\%$ reduction in proteolysis over the first 24 hr of exposure ($p > 0.05$) and a $23 \pm 7\%$ reduction in the second 24 hr ($p < 0.01$). Thus, the inhibitory effect of sucrose on proteolysis was temporally correlated with its effect on lysosomes [22].

Chloroquine, leupeptin, and methyladenine produce rapid lysosomal dysfunction through diverse mechanisms. Chloroquine is selectively concentrated in lysosomes, where it produces major anatomic abnormalities [13], and it decreases proteolytic capacity by raising the intralysosomal pH above the optimum of most lysosomal proteinases and also by directly inhibiting lysosomal cathepsin B activity [16]. Leupeptin inhibits several important lysosomal cathepsins (e.g., cathepsins B, H, and L) as well as nonlysosomal thiol proteinases [3]. Methyladenine appears to inhibit formation of autophagosomes [14]. As reported previously [9,15,18,22], each of these agents reduced total cardiac proteolysis by 25–30% (Figure 1). Their influence on myosin was quite different, however; none of the lysosomotropic agents had any effect on the rate of myosin degradation (Figure 1). In other studies [10], the total myofibrillar protein pool was found to be unaffected by lysosomotropic agents as well. Thus, interference with lysosomal function produces uniform depression of overall proteolysis, while the degradation of myosin specifically, and of the myofibrillar pool in general, proceeds at a normal rate [23].

Disaggregation of the microtubular system produces a reduction in the rate of breakdown of endogenous and exogenous proteins in many tissues [1,6,8]. Several lines of evidence have led to suggestions that this phenomenon is somehow linked to interference with normal lysosomal function (e.g., by restricting intracellular movement of lysosomes and other organelles, limiting organellar engulfment within autophagic vacuoles, and/or preventing fusion of primary lysosomes with autophagic vacuoles). In several separate experiments [4], colchicine, the prototype of agents that disaggregate microtubules, produced a modest reduction (12–16%) in the overall rate of proteolysis in fetal mouse hearts. This inhibitory effect was minimal or absent for "cytosolic" proteins, but was major ($34 \pm 12\%$, $p < 0.05$) for "organellar" proteins [4]. Of particular interest, colchicine caused a 31% reduction in heme protein degradation in the same hearts that were simultaneously sustaining only a 15% reduction in total protein degradation (Table 1). Thus, interference with normal microtubular protein breakdown appears to exert disproportionate effects on organellar (specifically, mitochondrial) protein breakdown ($p < 0.05$).

If, as has been suggested, the effect of microtubular disruption ultimately is mediated entirely through lysosomal mechanisms, one might expect myosin degradation not to be altered by colchicine, as is the case with "lysosomotropic" agents (see above). In fact, myosin degradation was reduced by 15% in hearts in which total protein degradation was reduced simultaneously by 13% [4]. Thus, current evidence does not favor the notion that the effect of colchicine on cardiac proteolysis is mediated solely via effects on lysosomal pathways [4].

DISCUSSION AND CONCLUSIONS

Within current frameworks of our understanding of proteolytic processes, it is convenient to visualize degradation of specific proteins as occurring entirely within lysosomes, entirely outside lysosomes, or by some sort of "combination" pathway, perhaps involving initial cleavage of the protein outside the lysosomes with subsequent incorporation of large peptides within lysosomes and final hydrolysis there [2,5,18,19]. Within this context, the results described above can help put into better perspective the relative roles of lysosomal and nonlysosomal pathways in the breakdown of cardiac proteins.

Considering all cardiac proteins, a variety of agents that selectively alter lysosomal function produce a reduction of total proteolysis of 25% or more; this suggests that a sizeable fraction of cardiac proteins are degraded either solely in lysosomes or via a "combination" pathway. It is not possible to block the majority of proteolysis, however, even using large concentrations of lysosomotropic agents singly or in combination. This suggests that the purely nonlysosomal pathway is also of major importance.

In the case of myosin, interference with lysosomal proteolysis, by any of several different means, causes no reduction in breakdown. This suggests that the initial, regulatory step in myosin degradation is nonlysosomal and that the enzyme that first cleaves the myosin molecule is a nonlysosomal proteinase. This is not to say, however, that lysosomes necessarily are totally uninvolved in the breakdown of myofibrillar protein; a "combination" pathway might still be operative, since the initial cleavage products might be susceptible to further degradation in lysosomes, and this would not be detectable in the experiments described in this chapter.

In addition to normal lysosomal function, normal cardiac proteolysis is dependent on an intact microtubular system. The degradation of organellar proteins in general, and of mitochondrial cytochromes specifically, is disproportionately inhibited by microtubular disaggregation. A likely mechanism to explain this phenomenon is that microtubules are necessary for the engulfment of mitochondria (and perhaps other organelles) within autophagic vacuoles. However, since myosin breakdown is also inhibited by microtubular disaggregation (although to a lesser extent than mitochondrial protein degradation), it seems likely that microtubules are involved in nonlysosomal as well as in lysosomal proteolytic mechanisms.

In summary, lysosomes appear to have major involvement in total cardiac proteolysis, although the extent to which they play a regulatory role is not yet clear. Most probably, the degradation of different proteins involves different pathways, and the regulatory factors important for one protein may well be quite different than for another. For some of these pathways to function optimally, microtubules seem to be required. Current evidence suggests that the primary regulatory step for degradation of myosin and other contractile proteins does not involve lysosomal mechanisms.

The general conclusion that seems most likely to be true regarding the mechanisms and regulation of cardiac proteolysis is that no single proteolytic pathway is of unique importance for all cardiac proteins. Rather, different pathways are probably of importance for particular proteins and for particular conditions. Thus, there is probably no single, easy answer to the question, "What regulates cardiac proteolysis?" Finding the specific answer to this question for each of the multitude of different proteins and for each of a variety of different conditions is a fertile field for future investigation.

ACKNOWLEDGMENTS

The work described in this chapter was supported in part by the Moss Heart Fund and by the National Heart, Lung, and Blood Institute (HL 14706).

REFERENCES

1. Amenta, J. S., Sargus, M. J., and Baccino, F. M. 1977. Effect of microtubular or translational inhibitors on general cell protein degradation. *Biochem. J.* 168:223–227.
2. Ballard, F. J. 1977. Intracellular protein degradation. In: P. N. Campbell and W. N. Aldridge (eds.), *Essays in Biochemistry.* Vol. 13. pp. 1–37. Academic Press, New York.
3. Barrett, A. J. 1980. The many forms and functions of cellular proteinases. *Fed. Proc. Fed. Am. Soc. Exp. Biol.* 39:9–14.
4. Crie, J. S., Ord, J. M., Wakeland, J. R., and Wildenthal, K. 1983. Inhibition of cardiac proteolysis by colchicine. *Biochem J.* 210:63–71.
5. Dean, R. T. 1980. Regulation and mechanisms of degradation of endogenous proteins by mammalian cells: General considerations. In: K. Wildenthal (ed.), *Degradative Processes in Heart and Skeletal Muscle.* pp. 3–30. North-Holland, Amsterdam.
6. Grinde, B., and Seglen, P. O. 1981. Role of microtubuli in the lysosomal degradation of endogenous and exogenous protein in isolated rat hepatocytes. *Hoppe-Seyler's Z. Physiol. Chem.* 362:549–556.
7. Hoh, J. F. Y., McGrath, P. A., and Hale, P. T. 1978. Electrophoretic analysis of multiple forms of rat cardiac myosin: Effects of hypophysectomy and thyroxine replacement. *J. Mol. Cell. Cardiol.* 10:1053–1076.
8. Kolset, S. O., Tolleshaug, H. and Berg, T. 1979. The effects of colchicine and cytochalasin B on uptake and degradation of asialo-glycoproteins in isolated rat hepatocytes. *Exp. Cell Res.* 122:159–167.
9. Libby, P., Ingwall, J. S., and Goldberg, A. L. 1979. Reduction of protein degradation and atrophy in cultured fetal mouse hearts by leupeptin. *Am. J. Physiol.* 237:E35–E39.
10. Ord, J. M., Wakeland, J. R., Crie, J. S., and Wildenthal, K. 1983. Mechanisms of degradation of myofibrillar and nonmyofibrillar protein in heart. In: E. Chazov, V. Saks, and G. Rona (eds.), *Advances in Myocardiology.* Vol. 4, pp. 195–199. Plenum Press, New York.
11. Ord, J. M., and Wildenthal, K. 1980. Increased release of δ-aminolevulinic acid from protein during inhibition of protein synthesis in heart: Evidence for the extensive reutilization of heme in cardiac protein metabolism. *Biochem. Biophys. Res. Commun.* 93:577–582.
12. Rannels, D. R., Kao, R., and Morgan, H. E. 1975. Effect of insulin on protein turnover in heart muscle. *J. Biol. Chem.* 250:1694–1701.
13. Ridout, R. M., Decker, R. S., and Wildenthal, K. 1978. Chloroquine-induced lysosomal abnormalities in cultured foetal mouse hearts. *J. Mol. Cell. Cardiol.* 10:175–183.
14. Seglen, P. O., and Gordon, P. B. 1982. 3-Methyladenine: Specific inhibitor of autophagic/lysosomal protein degradation in isolated rat hepatocytes. *Proc. Natl. Acad. Sci. U.S.A.* 79:1889–1892.
15. Ward, W. F., Chua, B. L., Li, J. B., Morgan, H. E., and Mortimore, G. E. 1979. Inhibition of basal and deprivation-induced proteolysis by leupeptin and pepstatin in perfused rat liver and heart. *Biochem. Biophys. Res. Commun.* 87:92–98.
16. Wibo, M., and Poole, B. 1974. Protein degradation in cultured cells. II. The uptake of chloroquine by rat fibroblasts and the inhibition of cellular protein degradation and cathepsin B_1. *J. Cell Biol.* 63:430–440.
17. Wildenthal, K. 1971. Long-term maintenance of spontaneously beating mouse hearts in organ culture. *J. Appl. Physiol.* 30:153–157.
18. Wildenthal, K., and Crie, J. S. 1980. The role of lysosomes and lysosomal enzymes in cardiac protein turnover. *Fed. Proc. Fed. Am. Soc. Exp. Biol.* 39:37–41.
19. Wildenthal, K., and Crie, J. S. 1980. Lysosomes and cardiac protein catabolism. In: K. Wildenthal (ed.), *Degradative Processes in Heart and Skeletal Muscle.* pp. 113–129. North-Holland, Amsterdam.
20. Wildenthal, K., Dees, J. H., and Buja, L. M. 1977. Cardiac lysosomal derangements in mouse heart after long-term exposure to nonmetabolizable sugars. *Circ. Res.* 40:26–35.
21. Wildenthal, K., Griffin, E. E., and Ingwall, J. S. 1976. Hormonal control of cardiac protein and amino acid balance. *Circ. Res.* 38(Suppl. 1):138–144.

22. Wildenthal, K., Wakeland, J. R., Morton, P. C., and Griffin, E. E. 1978. Inhibition of protein degradation in mouse hearts by agents that cause lysosomal dysfunction. *Circ. Res.* 42:787–792.

23. Wildenthal, K., Wakeland, J. R., Ord, J. M., and Stull, J. T. 1980. Interference with lysosomal proteolysis fails to reduce cardiac myosin degradation. *Biochem. Biophys. Res. Commun.* 96:793–798.

Dependence of Protein Synthesis on Aortic Pressure and Calcium Availability

Ellen E. Gordon, Yuji Kira, and Howard E. Morgan

Department of Physiology
The Milton S. Hershey Medical Center
The Pennsylvania State University
Hershey, Pennsylvania 17033

Abstract. Increased aortic pressure accelerated protein synthesis in control–beating and arrested–drained hearts supplied with either glucose or pyruvate. Elevation of perfusion pressure from 60 to 120 mm Hg increased oxygen consumption in control–beating but not in arrested–drained preparations. Energy availability, as assessed by adenylate energy charge or creatine phosphate/creatine ratio, or both, was increased in arrested–drained hearts supplied with glucose and perfused at 60 and 120 mm Hg aortic pressure. In control–beating or arrested–drained hearts supplied with pyruvate, energy availability was not improved by elevation of aortic pressure from 60 to 120 mm Hg. An increase of perfusate calcium concentration from 0.5 to 5.0 mM in control–beating Langendorff preparations supplied with glucose and perfused at an aortic pressure of 90 mm Hg doubled oxygen consumption and decreased energy availability, but had no effect on the rate of protein synthesis. In arrested–drained hearts supplied with either glucose or pyruvate and calcium concentrations ranging from 0.5 to 5.0 mM, the rates at 120 mm Hg aortic pressure were 11–25% higher than at 60 mm Hg. These findings provide no evidence to implicate increased oxidative metabolism, energy availability, or extracellular calcium concentration as important factors in the mechanism that accounts for the effect of increased aortic pressure on protein synthesis.

INTRODUCTION

An increase in aortic pressure in vitro improved the efficiency of protein synthesis [1–4]. In these studies, incorporation of amino acids into heart protein, as well as the rate of protein synthesis, based on phenylalanyl-transfer RNA specific activities, were accelerated by higher work loads in working heart preparations or by increased aortic pressure in Langendorff preparations. In working hearts or Langendorff preparations supplied with glucose as substrate, increased protein synthesis appeared to involve prevention of the development of a block in peptide-chain initiation that occurred in Langendorff preparations that were supplied with glucose and developed low levels of ventricular pressure [3–5]. A higher pressure load, but not a higher volume load, resulted in accelerated rates of protein synthesis [2,6]. In hearts supplied with glucose and insulin, an increase in aortic pressure appeared to accelerate peptide-chain elongation [4].

The parameter that most closely relates increased pressure load to acceleration of protein synthesis has been aggressively sought. The observa-

145

tion that tetrodotoxin could stop all mechanical activity in aerobic Langendorff preparations without reducing the rate of protein synthesis suggested that protein synthesis was not dependent on contraction, per se [7]. Recent studies of Takala [8] and from our laboratory [4] showed that an increase in aortic pressure from 60 to 120 or 150 mm Hg accelerated protein synthesis in Langendorff preparations that were arrested with either high K^+ or tetrodotoxin. These findings indicated that not only the "basic" rate of protein synthesis [7,9] but also the increased rate induced by a pressure load was independent of cardiac contraction [4,8]. When higher perfusion pressures were imposed on beating Langendorff preparations, more intraventricular pressure was developed and myocardial oxygen consumption increased [10–12]. Arnold et al. [12] presented additional data showing that an elevation of perfusion pressure from 60 to 160 mm Hg in empty beating hearts increased oxygen consumption from 6.1 to 12.2 ml/min · 100 g; this result was recently confirmed in studies from our laboratory [4]. These studies were taken to indicate that the increased perfusion pressure in the coronary arteries had stretched the vessels and the ventricular wall, the so-called "erectile properties of the heart" or the "garden-hose effect" [12,13]. These results were consistent with the observation of Peterson and Lesch [14] that stretch of the right ventricular papillary muscle would increase phenylalanine incorporation. These findings appear to rule out cardiac work, intraventricular pressure development, and contraction as parameters associated with increased protein synthesis in hearts subjected to a pressure load and appear, as well, to focus attention on the relationship between wall tension and protein synthesis.

The experiments described herein were undertaken to explore the dependence on oxygen consumption, energy availability, and extracellular calcium concentration of the effects of aortic pressure on protein synthesis. The results indicated that none of these parameters was a major determinant of the faster synthetic rate that was associated with elevation of aortic pressure.

METHODS

Hearts were removed from fed male rats (Sprague–Dawley strain) and perfused as Langendorff preparations (aortic pressure, 40 mm Hg) with Krebs–Henseleit bicarbonate buffer that contained 15 mM glucose, 0.4 mM phenylalanine, normal plasma levels of all other amino acids [15], 3.0 mM Ca, and 0.1 mM EDTA (buffer A). During the first 10 min of perfusion, the buffer passed through the heart a single time and was discarded. From 10 to 70 min, 30 ml of buffer A or buffer B (10 mM pyruvate substituted for 15 mM glucose in buffer A) was recirculated through the heart at the aortic pressures noted in the tables. Concentrations of ionized Ca were varied by adding 0.6–5.1 mM total Ca to the buffers while holding the concentration of EDTA at 0.1 mM. At 70 min, [U-^{14}C]phenylalanine was added, and per-fusion was continued under the same conditions as during the first hour. After 130 min of perfusion, samples of perfusate were collected for esti-mation of phenylalanine specific activity [15], and the heart was frozen be-tween blocks of aluminum chilled to the temperature of liquid nitrogen. Perchloric acid extracts were prepared and analyzed for adenine nucleotides, creatine, and creatine phosphate, as described earlier [15]. Radioactivity in protein was determined, and rates of protein synthesis were calculated, as described earlier [15]. At the concentration of phenylalanine that was used, the specific activities of phenylalanine in the perfusate and bound to tRNA were equal and allowed for calculation of protein-synthetic rates using the specific activity of perfusate phenylalanine [16].

When oxygen consumption was measured, the pulmonary artery was cannulated, and samples of coronary effluent were collected in gas-tight syringes [11]. Arterial samples were collected from a side-arm on the tube supplying perfusate to the heart. Oxygen tension was measured with an oxygen electrode, and oxygen consumption was calculated [11].

In some experiments, cardiac contractions were arrested by addition of tetrodotoxin (9 μg/ml), and an 18-gauge Teflon catheter was inserted through the apex to prevent accumulation of fluid and pressure development [4,7].

Statistical analyses were carried out using either Student's t test (two means compared) or analysis of variance followed by the Student–Newman–Keuls multiple-range test. Differences were considered to be significant if $p < 0.05$.

RESULTS

Aortic Pressure as a Determinant of Cardiac Protein Synthesis

In our earlier work [4,17] and that of Takala [8], aortic pressure was identified as the mechanical parameter that was most closely linked to the rate of protein synthesis. Examples of experimental findings that led to this conclusion are shown in Table 1. In these experiments, rates of protein synthesis were measured during the second hour of perfusion because the effect of elevated aortic pressure became apparent only after 1h. An increase in aortic pressure from 60 to 120 mm Hg accelerated protein synthesis in either control–beating or arrested–drained hearts supplied with either glu-cose or pyruvate as oxidizable substrate. Rates of synthesis were higher in control–beating hearts provided with pyruvate than in those supplied with glucose. An elevation of perfusion pressure from 60 to 120 mm Hg increased oxygen consumption approximately 70% in control–beating hearts, but had no effect in arrested–drained preparations. Adenylate energy charge was unchanged by elevation of aortic pressure in control–beating or arrested–drained hearts provided with glucose; the higher aortic pressure decreased energy charge somewhat in hearts supplied with pyruvate. Higher aortic

Table 1. Relationship between Aortic Pressure and Rates of Protein Synthesis and Energy Metabolism in Control–Beating and Arrested–Drained Hearts[a]

Parameter	Control–beating		Arrested–drained	
	60 mm Hg	120 mm Hg	60 mm Hg	120 mm Hg
Glucose 15 mM (buffer A)				
Protein synthesis (nmoles phenylalanine/g·hr)	566 ± 11 (12)	768 ± 19 (6)[b]	630 ± 43 (9)	850 ± 27 (9)[b,c]
Oxygen consumption (mmoles/g·hr)	1.61 ± 0.10 (10)	2.74 ± 0.18 (10)[b]	0.51 ± 0.02 (7)[c]	0.58 ± 0.05 (6)[c]
Adenylate energy charge	0.899 ± 0.004 (11)	0.901 ± 0.004 (5)	0.890 ± 0.003 (5)	0.890 ± 0.004 (5)
Creatine phosphate plus creatine (μmoles/g)	70.3 ± 2.1 (11)	59.9 ± 4.4 (5)	63.0 ± 1.3 (8)[c]	52.7 ± 1.8 (8)[b]
Creatine phosphate/creatine	0.840 ± 0.039 (11)	0.789 ± 0.026 (5)	1.02 ± 0.05 (8)[c]	1.36 ± 0.10 (8)[b,c]
Pyruvate 10 mM (buffer B)				
Protein synthesis (nmoles phenylalanine/g·hr)	703 ± 32 (5)	887 ± 31 (6)[b]	657 ± 20 (6)	867 ± 24 (4)[b]
Adenylate energy charge	0.936 ± 0.002 (5)	0.915 ± 0.003 (6)[b]	0.933 ± 0.004 (6)	0.918 ± 0.001 (4)[b]
Creatine phosphate plus creatine (μmoles/g)	69.5 ± 1.3 (5)	62.5 ± 3.7 (6)[b]	65.4 ± 0.9 (6)	46.3 ± 1.9 (4)[b,c]
Creatine phosphate/creatine	2.25 ± 0.08 (5)	2.12 ± 0.14 (6)	2.29 ± 0.38 (6)	1.94 ± 0.11 (4)

[a] Adapted from Kira et al. [4]. Hearts were perfused with buffer A or buffer B as described in "Methods," except that total calcium was 3.5 mM and the EDTA concentration was 0.5 mM. Aortic pressure was adjusted to either 60 or 120 mm Hg. Values represent the means ± S.E. of the number of hearts indicated in parentheses.
[b] $p < 0.05$ vs. same conditions, 60 mm Hg aortic pressure.
[c] $p < 0.05$ vs. control–beating hearts, same conditions.

Table 2.   Relationship between Perfusate Calcium Concentration and Rates of Protein Synthesis and Oxygen Consumption and Energy Metabolism of Beating Rat Hearts Supplied with Glucose[a]

Parameter	Ionized perfusate calcium (mM)					
	0.5		2.9		5.0	
Protein synthesis (nmoles phenylalanine/g·hr)	757 ± 33	(14)	664 ± 26	(10)	700 ± 34	(10)
Oxygen consumption (mmoles/g·hr)	1.47 ± 0.08	(7)	2.24 ± 0.11	(8)[b]	2.98 ± 0.41	(5)[b]
ATP (μmoles/g)	23.5 ± 0.6	(14)	24.1 ± 0.8	(10)	22.0 ± 1.0	(10)
ADP (μmoles/g)	3.19 ± 0.46	(6)	3.83 ± 0.50	(5)	4.73 ± 0.65	(5)
AMP (μmoles/g)	0.539 ± 0.131	(6)	0.466 ± 0.090	(5)	0.629 ± 0.055	(5)
Adenylate energy charge	0.924 ± 0.013	(6)	0.918 ± 0.006	(5)	0.888 ± 0.008	(5)[b,c]
Creatine phosphate (μmoles/g)	38.1 ± 2.4	(13)	31.7 ± 1.4	(10)[b]	31.8 ± 2.1	(10)
Creatine (μmoles/g)	19.1 ± 2.4	(6)	33.5 ± 3.3	(5)[b]	35.6 ± 2.5	(5)[b]
Creatine phosphate plus creatine (μmoles/g)	54.9 ± 4.1	(6)	61.8 ± 3.8	(5)	62.3 ± 2.8	(5)
Creatine phosphate/creatine	1.97 ± 0.21	(6)	0.877 ± 0.087	(5)[b]	0.761 ± 0.058	(5)[b]

[a] Hearts were perfused as described in "Methods," using buffer A at an aortic pressure of 90 mm Hg. Values are the means ± S.E. of the number of observations shown in parentheses.
[b] $p < 0.05$ vs. 0.5 mM Ca.   [c] $p < 0.05$ vs. 29 mM Ca.

pressure decreased the total of creatine and creatine phosphate in arrested–drained hearts and forced the use of creatine phosphate/creatine ratios rather than creatine phosphate content as an index of energy availability. In control–beating hearts supplied with glucose, creatine phosphate/creatine ratios were unchanged by elevation of aortic pressure. The ratio increased in arrested–drained preparations, particularly at 120 mm Hg aortic pressure. Provision of pyruvate increased creatine phosphate/creatine ratios in control–beating and arrested–drained preparations, but this parameter of energy availability was unaffected by elevation of aortic pressure. These experiments indicated that heart rate, cardiac contraction, ventricular filling, oxygen consumption, and energy availability could be dissociated from the effects of aortic pressure on protein synthesis.

Extracellular Calcium Availability as a Determinant of Protein Synthesis, Oxygen Consumption, and Energy Availability

The next series of experiments was undertaken to determine whether variations in perfusate calcium within the experimentally feasible range would modify rates of protein synthesis (Table 2). The lower limit of calcium concentration was determined by the stability of the heart preparation. When the ionized calcium concentration was reduced below 0.5 mM, the heart lost protein and nucleotides into the perfusate and became white and markedly swollen (data not shown). Solubility of calcium in bicarbonate buffer restricted the use of calcium concentrations higher than 5 mM. An increase in extracellular ionized calcium from 0.5 to 5.0 mM had no effect on protein synthesis during the second hour of perfusion in control–beating hearts supplied with glucose and perfused at an aortic pressure of 90 mm Hg. These conditions were chosen because 90 mm Hg approximated the mean aortic pressure, in vivo, and because the combination of glucose as substrate and this perfusion pressure resulted in rates of protein synthesis that were not maximal [4,15]. Although rates of protein synthesis were unaffected by an increase in extracellular calcium from 0.5 to 5.0 mM, oxygen consumption doubled, the adenylate energy charge decreased somewhat, and the creatine phosphate/creatine ratio decreased by approximately 50%. Under these conditions, the sum of creatine phosphate and creatine was unchanged. The experiments failed to demonstrate an effect of the availability of extracellular calcium on protein synthesis even though heart rate (data not shown) and oxidative metabolism were markedly increased as extracellular calcium was raised.

Dependence on Extracellular Calcium of the Effect of Aortic Pressure on Protein Synthesis

The final series of experiments was undertaken to determine whether extracellular calcium concentration would modify the effect of aortic pressure on protein synthesis (Tables 3 and 4). The arrested–drained heart was selected for these studies to minimize the effect of calcium concentration on contractile activity and energy metabolism. An increase in aortic pressure from 60 to 120 mm Hg accelerated the rate of protein synthesis to the same extent at each perfusate calcium concentration, but had no effect on adenylate energy charge or creatine phosphate/creatine ratio at either 0.5, 2.9, or 5.0 mM calcium.

When arrested–drained hearts were supplied with pyruvate as substrate, they were less tolerant to a reduction in extracellular calcium. Under these conditions, 0.8 mM calcium represented the lower limit of calcium availability that would prevent gross protein and nucleotide loss and marked edema of the preparation. When aortic pressure was increased from 60 to 120 mm Hg, the rate of protein synthesis was faster only at a perfusate calcium concentration of 5.0 mM. The lack of an effect of aortic pressure on protein synthesis in hearts supplied with 0.8 mM calcium may have been due to the fall in ATP and creatine phosphate content at the higher perfusion pressure. When the effect of aortic pressure on protein synthesis was evaluated in hearts supplied with pyruvate and the data at 2.9 and 5.0 mM calcium were combined, the rates at 60 and 120 mm Hg were 637 ± 16 ($N = 22$) and 704 ± 17 ($N = 21$) nmoles phenylalanine/g · hr ($p < 0.01$), respectively. It should be noted that the rate of protein synthesis observed at 120 mm Hg aortic pressure (690 ± 24 nmoles phenylalanine/g · hr) in these experiments (Table

Table 3. Relationship between Perfusate Calcium Concentration and Rates of Protein Synthesis and Energy Metabolism of Arrested–Drained Hearts Supplied with Glucose[a]

Parameter	Ionized perfusate calcium (mM)					
	0.5		2.9		5.0	
	60 mm Hg	120 mm Hg	60 mm Hg	120 mm Hg	60 mm Hg	120 mm Hg
Protein synthesis (nmoles phenylalanine/g·hr)	608 ± 35	710 ± 28[b]	608 ± 59	771 ± 36[b]	517 ± 45	726 ± 39[b]
ATP (μmoles/g)	24.7 ± 0.6	21.1 ± 0.8[b]	22.8 ± 0.6	20.7 ± 0.9	22.6 ± 0.8	20.4 ± 1.2
ADP (μmoles/g)	4.23 ± 0.29	4.08 ± 0.18	4.97 ± 0.11	4.57 ± 0.09[b]	5.04 ± 0.09	4.73 ± 0.26
AMP (μmoles/g)	0.697 ± 0.13	0.687 ± 0.040	0.937 ± 0.060	0.925 ± 0.060	0.971 ± 0.050	0.880 ± 0.030
Adenylate energy charge	0.906 ± 0.008	0.895 ± 0.003	0.881 ± 0.004	0.876 ± 0.007	0.878 ± 0.004	0.874 ± 0.014
Creatine phosphate (μmoles/g)	37.7 ± 1.2	27.5 ± 1.5[b]	31.3 ± 1.1	28.4 ± 2.0	30.0 ± 1.9	30.1 ± 1.6
Creatine (μmoles/g)	17.1 ± 0.9	10.3 ± 1.0[b]	31.3 ± 1.6	29.1 ± 4.2	27.2 ± 2.8	22.8 ± 2.6
Creatine phosphate plus creatine (μmoles/g)	54.7 ± 1.5	38.1 ± 2.7[b]	62.6 ± 2.2	57.6 ± 6.0	57.1 ± 3.2	52.9 ± 3.2
Creatine phosphate/creatine	2.24 ± 0.16	2.73 ± 0.16	1.01 ± 0.05	1.03 ± 0.09	1.16 ± 0.13	1.41 ± 0.16

[a] Hearts were perfused with buffer A as described in "Methods." Aortic pressure was adjusted to either 60 or 120 mm Hg. Values are the means ± S.E. of 6 hearts.
[b] $p < 0.05$ vs. 60 mm Hg, same [Ca^{2+}].

Table 4. Relationship between Perfusate Calcium Concentration and Rates of Protein Synthesis and Energy Metabolism of Arrested–Drained Hearts Supplied with Pyruvate[a]

Parameter	Ionized perfusate calcium (mM)					
	0.8		2.9		5.0	
	60 mm Hg	120 mm Hg	60 mm Hg	120 mm Hg	60 mm Hg	120 mm Hg
Protein synthesis (nmoles phenylalanine/g·hr)	614 ± 17 (15)	666 ± 24 (11)	640 ± 20 (13)	690 ± 24 (9)	634 ± 28 (9)	714 ± 25 (12)[b]
ATP (μmoles/g)	21.5 ± 0.7 (14)	18.3 ± 0.7 (11)[b]	22.7 ± 1.0 (13)	20.1 ± 0.7 (9)	19.7 ± 1.1 (9)	18.9 ± 1.2 (12)
ADP (μmoles/g)	2.73 ± 0.15 (13)	2.74 ± 0.18 (9)	3.03 ± 0.14 (11)	3.33 ± 0.33 (8)	3.25 ± 0.56 (8)	2.81 ± 0.40 (11)
AMP (μmoles/g)	0.416 ± 0.028 (13)	0.415 ± 0.018 (9)	0.664 ± 0.053 (11)	0.588 ± 0.085 (8)	0.509 ± 0.086 (8)	0.516 ± 0.081 (11)
Adenylate energy charge	0.928 ± 0.003 (13)	0.920 ± 0.006 (9)	0.924 ± 0.006 (11)	0.905 ± 0.009 (8)	0.911 ± 0.016 (8)	0.914 ± 0.012 (11)
Creatine phosphate (μmoles/g)	35.8 ± 1.8 (14)	24.8 ± 2.1 (11)[b]	41.8 ± 3.2 (13)	33.7 ± 1.7 (9)[b]	32.9 ± 2.4 (9)	36.0 ± 2.6 (12)
Creatine (μmoles/g)	13.1 ± 1.85 (13)	12.0 ± 2.2 (9)	20.9 ± 3.2 (11)	16.4 ± 2.4 (8)	17.3 ± 3.2 (8)	17.2 ± 2.8 (11)
Creatine phosphate plus creatine (μmoles/g)	48.8 ± 3.2 (13)	38.5 ± 4.2 (9)	64.4 ± 3.7 (11)	49.6 ± 3.2 (8)[b]	50.9 ± 4.4 (8)	53.1 ± 4.3 (11)
Creatine phosphate/creatine	3.07 ± 0.28 (13)	2.52 ± 0.26 (9)	2.52 ± 0.39 (11)	2.24 ± 0.28 (8)	2.39 ± 0.40 (8)	2.62 ± 0.40 (11)

[a] Hearts were perfused with buffer B as described in "Methods." Aortic pressure was adjusted to either 60 or 120 mm Hg. Values are the means ± S.E. of the number of hearts shown in parentheses.
[b] $p < 0.05$ vs. 60 mm Hg, same $[Ca^{2+}]$.

4) was less than the value reported in Table 1 for experiments that were carried out under similar conditions (850 ± 27 nmoles phenylalanine/g · hr). The only difference in these experiments was the use of 0.1 mM EDTA (Table 4) rather than 0.5 mM EDTA (Table 1). Whether use of less chelating agent for heavy-metal contaminants accounted for this difference in rate has not been explored. Adenylate energy charge and creatine phosphate/creatine ratio were unaffected by perfusion pressure in arrested–drained hearts supplied with pyruvate.

DISCUSSION

The experiments described in this chapter were carried out in Langendorff-perfused hearts supplied with either glucose or pyruvate as substrate; rates of protein synthesis were measured during the second hour of perfusion in either control–beating or arrested–drained preparations. When aortic pressure was 60 mm Hg, a block in peptide-chain initiation was present that was more severe in hearts provided with glucose than in those provided with pyruvate [4]. Evidence for the existence of this block consisted of suboptimal rates of protein synthesis coupled with greater tissue content of ribosomal subunits. When aortic pressure was increased to 120 mm Hg, the synthetic rate increased and the content of ribosomal subunits fell, indicating that the severity of the block in peptide-chain initiation had been lessened.

As a result of Takala's studies [8] and our own [4,17], attention has been focused on aortic pressure as the parameter most closely linked to the faster rate of protein synthesis in hearts subjected to a pressure load. An increase in aortic pressure has direct effects on the ventricular wall to elevate intracoronary blood volume by as much as 60% [18], to increase sarcomere length by 10% [19], and to stretch and thicken the ventricular wall [13]. The question that next arose was the biochemical mechanism that linked stretch of the ventricular wall to more efficient peptide-chain initiation.

The biochemical parameters that were measured in an effort to determine whether they changed in a manner that would be consistent with a role in the regulatory process were oxygen consumption, energy availability, glucose-6-phosphate content, and extracellular calcium concentration. As shown in Table 1, an increase in aortic pressure from 60 to 120 mm Hg was as effective in accelerating protein synthesis in arrested–drained hearts, in which oxygen consumption did not change when aortic pressure was raised, as in control–beating hearts, in which oxygen consumption increased 70% under these conditions. These findings appeared to rule out a general increase in metabolic rate as a necessary factor for an acceleration of protein synthesis [4].

The inhibition of peptide-chain initiation in hearts supplied with glucose may have resulted from decreased formation of the eIF-2 · met-tRNA$_f^{Met}$ · GTP ternary complex due to a reduction in GTP/GDP ratio [20], a reflection of the adenylate energy charge and the ratio of creatine phosphate to creatine. However, in control–beating hearts supplied with glucose or pyruvate, the increase in protein synthesis induced by the higher aortic pressure was not accompanied by an increase in creatine phosphate/creatine ratio or adenylate energy charge (Table 1) [4]. In arrested–drained hearts supplied with glucose, however, creatine phosphate/creatine increased as aortic pressure was raised from 60 to 120 mm Hg, despite a fall in the total creatine pool (Table 1); adenylate energy charge was not affected by elevation of aortic pressure in these preparations. When arrested–drained hearts were supplied with pyruvate, creatine phosphate/creatine doubled at an aortic pressure of 60 mm Hg, but protein synthesis did not increase. These findings suggest that energy availability had not restricted protein synthesis in the preparations supplied with glucose. The finding that aortic pressure accelerated protein synthesis in arrested–drained hearts supplied with pyruvate in which energy availability remained high appears to exclude this parameter as the determinant of the effect. Similarly, glucose-6-phosphate was found to accelerate peptide-chain initiation in reticulocyte lysates, but no relationship was found between glucose-6-phosphate content in perfused rat hearts and the effect of aortic pressure on protein synthesis [4].

The effect of calcium availability on protein synthesis has been studied in only a limited manner. In guinea pig hearts, Schreiber et al. [21] reported that an increase in perfusate calcium concentration from 0.6 to 4.8 mM had no effect on the incorporation of lysine into guinea pig hearts that were perfused in vitro. Similarly, an elevation of extracellular calcium from 1 to 5 mM had no effect on the incorporation of [^{3}H]proline into collagen or noncollagen protein in fetal calvaria [22]. In this system, verapamil decreased the rate of synthesis, but this effect was not overcome by increasing the calcium concentration. Kameyama and Etlinger [23] reported that the addition of a calcium ionophore, A23187, increased tyrosine incorporation in rat soleus muscle when incubated in either a flaccid or a stretched state. This result could not be confirmed by Lewis et al. [24], who found that A23187 inhibited protein synthesis in both soleus and extensor digitorum longus under the same experimental conditions that were employed by Kameyama and Etlinger [23]. The explanation for this discrepancy is unknown. In other experiments, addition of calcium ionophore A23187 decreased ATP and creatine phosphate content and ATP/ADP ratio in rat diaphragm and epitrochlearis muscle [25]. In the experiments described herein, an increase in extracellular calcium concentration from 0.5 to 5.0 mM increased heart rate and oxygen consumption in beating hearts and decreased energy availability, but had no effect on the rate of protein synthesis. A reservation in the interpretation of these experiments is that an effect of high extracellular calcium on protein synthesis may have been obscured by the decrease in energy availability. In arrested–drained hearts supplied with glucose, rates at 120 mm Hg averaged 28% higher than at 60 mm Hg aortic pressure. In arrested–drained hearts provided with pyruvate, an increase in protein synthesis with elevation of aortic pressure occurred only at 5.0 mM calcium or when the data at 2.9 and 5 mM calcium were combined. A restriction on the rate of protein synthesis that was observed at 120 mm Hg aortic pressure in hearts supplied with 2.9 mM calcium and decreased energy availability in hearts provided with 0.8 mM calcium prevented a clear exploration of the dependence of the effect of aortic pressure on extracellular calcium in hearts supplied with pyruvate. Overall, these experiments provide no support for the possibility that calcium availability is an important controlling factor for myocardial protein synthesis.

A mechanism of regulation of peptide-chain initiation that involves a GDP exchange factor (GEF) and phosphorylation of the α-subunit of initiation factor eIF-2 has been proposed to control the rate of initiation in reticulocyte lysates (for reviews, see Safer [26], Ochoa [27], and Panniers and Henshaw [28]). GEF enhanced the exchange of GDP bound to eIF-2 for GTP. Activity of this factor was essential for catalytic activity of eIF-2 in initiation; however, phosphorylation of the α-subunit of eIF-2 inhibited this exchange function. Thus, even in the presence of normal GTP/GDP ratios, activity of eIF-2 may be inhibited by phosphorylation and subsequent failure of GTP–GDP exchange. Recently, it was shown that eIF-2 from skeletal muscle could be phosphorylated on the α-subunit by the α-subunit-specific kinase isolated from reticulocytes [29]. Whether aortic pressure affects the phosphorylation of eIF-2 or the activity of GEF is unknown.

ACKNOWLEDGMENTS

This work was supported by Grants HL-20388 and HL-07223 from the National Institutes of Health. We wish to thank Bonnie Merlino for typing the manuscript.

REFERENCES

1. Schreiber, S. S., Oratz, M., and Rothschild, M. A. 1966. Protein synthesis in the overloaded mammalian heart. *Am. J. Physiol.* 211:314–318.
2. Hjalmarson, A., and Isaksson, O. 1972. *In vitro* work load and rat heart metabolism. I. Effect on protein synthesis. *Acta Physiol. Scand.* 86:126–144.
3. Morgan, H. E., Chua, B. H. L., Fuller, E. O., and Siehl, D. 1980. Regulation of protein synthesis and degradation during *in vitro* cardiac work. *Am. J. Physiol.* 238:E431–E442.
4. Kira, Y., Kochel, P. J., Gordon, E. E., and Morgan, H. E. 1984. Aortic perfusion pressure as a determinant of cardiac protein synthesis. *Am. J. Physiol.* 246:C247–C258, 1984.
5. Hjalmarson, A., and Isaksson, O. 1972. *In Vitro* work load and rat heart metabolism. III. Effect on ribosomal aggregation. *Acta Physiol. Scand.* 86:342–352.
6. Schreiber, S. S., Rothschild, M. A., Evans, C., Reff, F., and Oratz, M. 1975. The effect of pressure or flow stress on right ventricular protein synthesis in the face of constant and restricted coronary perfusion. *J. Clin. Invest.* 55:1–11.
7. Jefferson, L. S., Wolpert, E. B., Giger, K. E., and Morgan, H. E. 1971. Regulation of protein synthesis in heart muscle. III. Effect of anoxia on protein synthesis. *J. Biol. Chem.* 246:2171–2178.

8. Takala, T. 1981. Protein synthesis in the isolated perfused rat heart: Effects of mechanical work load, diastolic ventricular pressure and coronary flow on amino acid incorporation and its transmural distribution into left ventricular protein. *Basic Res. Cardiol.* 76:44–61.

9. Schreiber, S. S., Hearse, D. J., Oratz, M., and Rothschild, M. A. 1977. Protein synthesis in prolonged cardiac arrest. *J. Mol. Cell. Cardiol.* 9:87–100.

10. Opie, L. H. 1965. Coronary flow rate and perfusion pressure as determinants of mechanical function and oxidative metabolism of isolated perfused rat heart. *J. Physiol.* 180:529–543.

11. Neely, J. R., Liebermeister, H., Battersby, E. J., and Morgan, H. E. 1967. Effect of pressure development on oxygen consumption by isolated rat heart. *Am. J. Physiol.* 212:804–814.

12. Arnold, G. F., Kosche, E., Miessner, E., Neitzert, A., and Lochner, W. 1968. The importance of the perfusion pressure in the coronary arteries for the contractility and the oxygen consumption. *Pfluegers Arch.* 299:339–356.

13. Vogel, W. M., Apstein, C. S., Briggs, L. L., Gaasch, W. H., and Ahn, J. 1982. Acute alterations in left ventricular diastolic chamber stiffness: Role of the "erectile" effect of coronary arterial pressure and flow in normal and damaged hearts. *Circ. Res.* 51:465–478.

14. Peterson, M., and Lesch, M. 1972. Protein synthesis and amino acid transport in the isolated rabbit right ventricular papillary muscle. *Circ. Res.* 31:317–327.

15. Flaim, K. E., Kochel, P. J., Kira, Y., Kobayashi, E. T., Fossel, E. T., Jefferson, L. S., and Morgan, H. E. 1983. Insulin effects on protein synthesis are independent of glucose and energy metabolism. *Am. J. Physiol.* 245(*Cell Physiol.* 14):C133–C143.

16. McKee, E. E., Cheung, J. Y., Rannels, D. E., and Morgan, H. E. 1978. Measurement of the rate of protein synthesis and compartmentation of heart phenylalanine. *J. Biol. Chem.* 253:1030–1040.

17. Kira, Y., Kochel, P., and Morgan, H. E. 1983. Aortic pressure and protein synthesis. In: J. J. Spitzer (ed.), *Myocardial Injury*. pp. 317–325, Plenum Press, New York.

18. Morgenstern, C., Höljes, U., Arnold, G., and Lochner, W. 1973. The influence of coronary pressure and coronary flow on intracoronary blood volume and geometry of the left ventricle. *Pfluegers Arch.* 340:101–111.

19. Poche, R., Arnold, G., and Gahlen, D. 1971. The influence of coronary perfusion pressure on metabolism and ultrastructure of the arrested aerobically perfused isolated guinea pig heart. *Virchows Arch. B* 8:252–266.

20. Walton, G. M., and Gill, G. N. 1976. Regulation of ternary (met-tRNA$_f$–GTP–eukaryotic initiation factor 2) protein synthesis initiation complex formation by the adenylate energy charge. *Biochem. Biophys. Acta* 418:195–203.

21. Schreiber, S. S., Oratz, M., Rothschild, M. A., and Smith, D. 1977. Increased cardiac contractility in high calcium perfusion and protein synthesis. *J. Mol. Cell. Cardiol.* 9:661–669.

22. Dietrich, J. W., and Duffield, R. 1979. Effects of the calcium antagonist verapamil on *in vitro* synthesis of skeletal collagen and noncollagen protein. *Endocrinology* 105:1168–1171.

23. Kameyama, T., and Etlinger, J. D. 1979. Calcium-dependent regulation of protein synthesis and degradation in muscle. *Nature (London)* 279:344–346.

24. Lewis, S. E. M., Anderson, P., and Goldspink, D. F. 1982. The effects of calcium on protein turnover in skeletal muscles of the rat. *Biochem J.* 204:257–264.

25. Sugden, P. H. 1980. The effects of calcium ions, ionophore A23187 and inhibition of energy metabolism on protein degradation in the rat diaphragm and epitrochlearis muscles *in vitro*. *Biochem. J.* 190:593–603.

26. Safer, B. 1983. 2B or not 2B: Regulation of the catalytic utilization of eIF-2. *Cell* 33:7–8.

27. Ochoa, S. 1983. Regulation of protein synthesis initiation in eukaryotes. *Arch. Biochem. Biophys.* 223:325–349.

28. Panniers, R., and Henshaw, E. C. 1983. A GDP/GTP exchange factor essential for eukaryotic initiation factor 2 cycling in Ehrlich ascites tumor cells and its regulation by eukaryotic initiation factor 2 phosphorylation. *J. Biol. Chem.* 258:7928–7934.

29. Proud, C. G., and Pain, V. M. 1982. Purification and phosphorylation of initiation factor eIF-2 from rabbit skeletal muscle. *FEBS Lett.* 143:55–59.

OXYGEN FREE RADICALS AND MYOCARDIAL INJURY

Identification of Hydrogen Peroxide and Hydroxyl Radical as Mediators of Leukocyte-Induced Myocardial Dysfunction
Limitation of Infarct Size with Neutrophil Inhibition and Depletion

Michael L. Hess, G. Thomas Rowe, and Martin Caplan

Department of Medicine (Cardiology)
Medical College of Virginia
Richmond, Virginia 23298

Joseph L. Romson and Benedict Lucchesi

Department of Pharmacology
University of Michigan School of Medicine
Ann Arbor, Michigan 48109

Abstract. Neutrophil infiltration of the myocardium is an important component of such diverse disease entities as myocarditis, ischemia, and ischemia–reperfusion injury. We have hypothesized that activated neutrophils are capable of disrupting myocardial function via an oxygen free-radical mechanism. Human neutrophils activated with phorbol myristate acetate disrupted calcium transport by canine cardiac sarcoplasmic reticulum, and this process was inhibited by a combination of superoxide dismutase and catalase. In addition, the activated neutrophil system was also inhibited by the combination of cyclooxygenase inhibitors (ibuprofen and indomethacin) and catalase and accelerated by MK-447. These results incriminate both hydrogen peroxide and the hydroxyl radical as mediators of neutrophil-induced myocardial dysfunction. A test of this hypothesis in vivo was performed by neutrophil-depleting dogs with anti-canine leukocyte antisera prior to coronary artery ligation. Following 6 hr of reperfusion, there was a 43% reduction in infarct size compared to non-immune-sera-injected animals. We conclude that oxygen free radicals generated by neutrophils are capable of inducing significant myocardial injury and play an important role in the pathophysiology of ischemia–reperfusion injury.

INTRODUCTION

Myocardial infarction is a dynamic disease process with several important phases in its development. Initially, an ischemic insult to the myocardium occurs due to occlusion of the coronary artery from either spasm or thrombosis. Next, since this occlusive event itself may be dynamic or intermittent, an element of reperfusion injury may be introduced. Finally, polymorphonuclear leukocytes migrate into the ischemic area within several hours of the

159

initial insult, initiating the acute inflammatory response to tissue necrosis. Whether the inflammatory response contributes to myocardial tissue injury and dysfunction is unknown. However, leukocytic infiltration in a number of cardiomyopathies is associated with myocardial dysfunction such as inflammatory myocarditis [1], Chagas's disease [2], and round cell disease of turkeys [3]. However, the mechanisms that couple leukocytic infiltration to myocardial dysfunction remain to be elucidated.

Leukocytes activated by inflammatory mediators generate cytotoxic products such as lysosomal enzymes, prostaglandins, and reduced-oxygen intermediates [4]. These reduced-oxygen intermediates [superoxide anion ($\cdot O_2^-$), hydrogen peroxide (H_2O_2), and hydroxyl radical ($\cdot OH$)] are excellent candidates for mediating leukocyte-induced cardiac dysfunction. These reduced-oxygen intermediates generated by activated leukocytes have been shown to be a mechanism of bacterial destruction by leukocytes, a mediator of the inflammatory response in synovial tissue [5], and a cytotoxic mediator in the rat model of inflammatory lung disease [6]. In addition, Kuehl et al. [7] have demonstrated that with activation of the cyclooxygenase pathway of arachidonic acid metabolism, the conversion of PGG_2 to PGH_2 is associated with the production of a reduced-oxygen intermediate that is a strong oxidizing species.

The sarcoplasmic reticulum (SR) of cardiac muscle represents a logical target organelle for reduced-oxygen intermediates. The SR has been demonstrated to serve as both a source and a sink of coupling calcium in the excitation–contraction coupling sequence [8], and numerous models of acute and chronic heart failure have been associated with SR dysfunction [9]. In addition, the acute myocarditis of cardiac allograft rejection has been associated with SR dysfunction [10], and the SR has been shown to be an antigenic site for the myocarditis of Chagas's disease [2]. In vitro studies have demonstrated that exogenous free-radical-generating systems are capable of disrupting SR calcium transport [11]. We therefore designed the following study to characterize activated leukocyte interaction with cardiac muscle and ask the following specific questions:

1. Can activated leukocytes generate reduced-oxygen intermediates that are capable of disrupting cardiac SR calcium transport?
2. Can these reduced-oxygen intermediates be identified?
3. What is the role of the arachidonic acid cascade of the leukocyte in the generation of reduced-oxygen intermediates?
4. If leukocytes disrupt cellular transport mechanisms, does inhibition of the leukocyte and/or neutrophil depletion salvage myocardium at risk from the inflammatory process?

METHODS

In Vitro Studies

Human peripheral-blood leukocytes were isolated from healthy volunteers following the method of Manson and Hess [12]. Cardiac sarcoplasmic reticulum was isolated and oxalate-dependent unidirectional calcium flux (calcium uptake rates) and calcium-stimulated, magnesium-dependent ATPase activity determined following the method of Hess et al. [9]. Inorganic phosphate was determined following the method of Penny [13].

Superoxide anion generation by phorbol myristate acetate (PMA)-activated leukocytes was measured on a dual-beam Aminco Spectrophotometer using the molar extinction coefficients of Massey [14]. Hydrogen peroxide was produced by the dismutation reaction with superoxide anion [15] and was scavenged with catalase (Sigma Chemical; 34,000 U/ml). The generation of hydroxyl radical via the Haber–Weiss reaction with superoxide anion and hydrogen peroxide was scavenged by mannitol [11].

Superoxide anion generation from the metabolism of arachidonic acid was assumed to occur during the conversion of PGG_2 to PGH_2 and feed back to deactivate cyclooxygenase [16]. This reaction can be accelerated by MK-447, an iodophenol derivative that scavenges oxygen free radicals.

In Vivo Studies: Induction of Regional Myocardial Ischemia

The effect of neutrophil depletion on the ultimate extent of irreversible myocardial injury was evaluated in male mongrel dogs anesthetized with sodium pentobarbital (30 mg/kg). A model of ischemic–reperfusion injury was established following the method of Lucchesi et al. [17]. The critical stenosis created by this model has the advantage of limiting reperfusion hyperemia, which reduces the severity of hemorrhagic infarcts and the potential for ventricular fibrillation [17,18]. Demarcation of the area at risk and the region undergoing irreversible myocardial injury was performed by the use of an ex vivo dual-perfusion technique [19]. Fishbein et al. [20] have established that this technique clearly differentiates irreversibly injured myocardium from viable tissue as early as 6 hr after the ischemic insult. Antiserum to canine polymorphonuclear leukocytes was prepared following the method of English and Abrams [21]. The experimental design and tissue techniques have previously been reported [22].

In a separate group of animals, leukocyte accumulation in the region of infarcted myocardium was assessed by the use of [111] In-labeled leukocytes. The [111] In autologous labeled leukocytes were prepared by drawing 50 ml venous blood into 330 IU heparin. To this blood sample, 3.0 ml hydroxyethyl starch and 3.0 ml normal saline were added. The blood sample was allowed to incubate at room temperature for 60 min to allow the separation of the leukocyte-rich plasma. The leukocytes were pelleted by centrifugation of the leukocyte-rich plasma for 5 min at 450g. The leukocyte pellet was washed twice by centrifugation and resuspended in normal saline. The washed leukocytes were then incubated with 500 μCi [^{111}In]oxine for 15 min at room temperature. Labeled leukocytes were then pelleted and resuspended in autologous leukocyte-free plasma. Leukocyte labeling efficiency was 86 ± 2% (range 64–97%). Leukocyte viability after ^{111}In labeling was assessed by in vivo recovery of radioactivity 30 min after administration.

Table 1.   Effects of Activated Leukocytes, SOD, Catalase, and SOD + Catalase on Calcium Uptake Rates and Ca^{2+}-Stimulated, Mg^{2+}-Dependent ATPase Activity on Cardiac Sarcoplasmic Reticulum

Group[a]	Ca^{2+} uptake rates (μmoles Ca^{2+}/mg-min)	ATPase activity (μmoles Ca^{2+}/mg-min)
Control	1.16 ± 0.03	1.64 ± 0.03
PMA	0.52 ± 0.02[b]	0.74 ± 0.04[b]
SOD	0.44 ± 0.02[b]	1.02 ± 0.02[b]
CAT	1.0 ± 0.02[b]	1.10 ± 0.04[b]
SOD + CAT	1.18 ± 0.04	1.66 ± 0.03

[a] (PMA) Phorbol myristate acetate; (SOD) superoxide dismutase (10 μg/ml); (CAT) catalase (10 μg/ml).
[b] Significantly different from control.

Ibuprofen was prepared for intravenous administration by dissolving the crystalline material in 0.2 mole Na_2CO_3. The pH was adjusted to 7.5–8.0 with 1.0 N hydrochloric acid. Ibuprofen was administered intravenously at a dose of 12.5 mg/kg, 30 min before occlusion of the circumflex coronary artery. Subsequent doses of 12.5 mg/kg were given every 4 hr so that total dose of 75 mg/kg was administered over 24 hr. Control dogs received drug vehicle in equal volume to that given to ibuprofen treated dogs. Dogs were sacrificed at the end of 24 hr, and infarct size was assessed as described above.

RESULTS

Our method for isolating leukocytes resulted in a cell population of 69% polymorphonuclear leukocytes, 20% monocytes, and 11% lymphocytes. Using superoxide dismutase [(SOD) 10 μg/ml]-inhibitable reduction of ferricytochrome C at 37°C, pH 7.0, this leukocyte system resulted in an initial rate of 82.3 nmoles $\cdot O_2^-$/liter $\cdot$ sec. All leukocyte preparations were isolated on the day of the study, and viability was confirmed by trypan blue exclusion.

Table 1 presents the results of PMA activation of our leukocyte population (4 × 10⁶ cells/ml) on cardiac sarcoplasmic reticulum (SR) calcium uptake and ATPase activity. Control calcium uptake rate after 10 min of preincubation at 37°C was 1.16 ± 0.03 μmoles Ca^{2+}/mg-min, a value in good agreement with previous reported uptake rates at 37°C with no incubation [9,10]. PMA-activated leukocytes resulted in a 60% depression of calcium uptake rates. PMA alone and nonactivated leukocytes had no effect on calcium uptake rates. Sodium azide (0.1 mM) completely inhibited the effects of PMA-activated leukocytes (C = 1.16 ± 0.03; PMA + leukocytes + azide

Table 2.   Effects of Hydrogen Peroxide and Catalase on
Calcium Uptake Rates and Ca^{2+}-Stimulated, Mg^{2+}-
Dependent ATPase Activity on Cardiac Sarcoplasmic
Reticulum

Group[a]	Ca^{2+} uptake rate (μmoles Ca^{2+}/mg-min)	ATPase activity (μmoles P_i/mg-min)
Control	1.16 ± 0.03	1.643 ± 0.03
+ H_2O_2 (0.441 mM)	1.08 ± 0.03	1.664 ± 0.03
+ CAT (10 μg/ml)	1.20 ± 0.03	1.681 ± 0.02
+ H_2O_2 (4.41 mM)	0.631 ± 0.02[b]	1.651 ± 0.03
+ CAT (10 μg/ml)	1.19 ± 0.03	1.703 ± 0.02
+ H_2O_2 (44.1 mM)	0.194 ± 0.02[b]	1.639 ± 0.03
+ CAT (10 μg/ml)	1.19 ± 0.02	1.676 ± 0.02

[a] (H_2O_2) Hydrogen peroxide; (CAT) catalase.
[b] Significantly different from control.

= 1.23 ± 0.02 μmoles CA^{2+}/mg-min; N = 4). In the presence of SOD, there was a small but statistically significant additional depression of calcium uptake rates. In the presence of catalase, there was significant inhibition of the effects of PMA-activated leukocytes, but this was still significantly depressed from control. Neither boiled catalase nor boiled SOD had any effects on PMA-activated leukocyte depression of cardiac SR. The presence of SOD and catalase completely inhibited the effects of PMA-activated leukocyte depression of cardiac SR. PMA-activated leukocytes resulted in a 55% depression of ATPase activity. The addition of SOD alone or catalase alone resulted in a small but significant inhibition of the PMA-activated leukocytes. In the presence of SOD + catalase, the PMA-activated-leukocyte system was completely inhibited.

The preceding data would appear to incriminate either hydrogen peroxide or the hydroxyl radical as the disruptive species of leukocyte-derived oxygen free radicals that interact with cardiac SR. To test this possibility, an exogenous hydrogen peroxide concentration–response study with and without catalase (10 μg/ml) was performed. Table 2 presents the results of this study. Exogenous hydrogen peroxide significantly depressed calcium uptake by cardiac SR in a dose–response fashion in a concentration range between 0.441 and 44.1 mM that was catalase-inhibitable. In contrast to the activated-leukocyte system, exogenous hydrogen peroxide had no effect on the calcium-stimulated, magnesium-dependent ATPase activity. The effects of mannitol, a known scavenger of the hydroxyl radical, in concentrations between 20 and 100 mM are presented in Table 3.Mannitol alone had no effect on calcium uptake rates, but resulted in a small, statistically significant inhibition of the PMA-activated-leukocyte effect on SR ATPase activity. In combination with SOD, there again was no effect on calcium uptake activity,

Table 3.   Effects of Mannitol and SOD + Mannitol on Calcium Uptake Rates and Ca^{2+}-Stimulated, Mg^{2+}-Dependent ATPase Activity on Cardiac Sarcoplasmic Reticulum in the Presence of PMA-Activated Leukocytes

Group[a]	Ca^{2+} uptake rate (μmoles Ca^{2+}/mg-min)	ATPase activity (μmoles P_i/mg-min)
Control	1.18 ± 0.035	1.516 ± 0.02
PMA	0.571 ± 0.02[b]	0.706 ± 0.069[b]
+MAN (20 mM)	0.608 ± 0.017[b]	0.912 ± 0.031[b]
+MAN (50 mM)	0.609 ± 0.014[b]	0.919 ± 0.034[b]
+MAN (100 mM)	0.606 ± 0.021[b]	1.046 ± 0.041[b]
+SOD-MAN (20 mM)	0.515 ± 0.011[b]	1.293 ± 0.028[b]
+SOD-MAN (50 mM)	0.509 ± 0.038[b]	1.464 ± 0.045[b]
+SOD-MAN (100 mM)	0.516 ± 0.030[b]	1.595 ± 0.026

[a] (PMA) Phorbol-myristate-acetate-activated leukocytes; (MAN) mannitol; (SOD) superoxide dismutase.
[b] Significantly different from control.

but there was a significant dose–response inhibition of the effect of PMA-activated leukocytes on the ATPase activity of cardiac SR.

With the demonstration that leukocyte reduced-oxygen intermediates can cause SR dysfunction, the possible participation of the cyclooxygenase system in the production of reduced-oxygen intermediates was then investigated. Table 4 presents the results of PMA-activated leukocytes incubated with the cyclooxygenase inhibitors indomethacin and ibuprofen. Neither indomethacin nor ibuprofen alone had any effect on calcium uptake rates or ATPase activity. Both cyclooxygenase inhibitors resulted in a slight inhibition in the depression of SR calcium uptake activity caused by PMA-activated leukocytes. In contrast, the ATPase activity was normalized in the presence of the cyclooxygenase inhibitors.

Table 4.   Effects of Indomethacin and Ibuprofen on Calcium Uptake Rates and Ca^{2+}-Stimulated Mg^{-2+}-Dependent ATPase Activity on Cardiac Sarcoplasmic Reticulum in the Presence of PMA-Activated Leukocytes

Group	Calcium uptake rate (μmoles Ca^{2+}/mg-min)	ATPase activity (μmoles P_i/mg-min)
Control	1.16 ± 0.03	1.64 ± 0.03
PMA	0.52 ± 0.02[a]	0.74 ± 0.04[a]
Indomethacin (10 μg/ml)	0.61 ± 0.03[a]	1.66 ± 0.04
Ibuprofen (10 μg/ml)	0.59 ± 0.03[a]	1.58 ± 0.02

[a] Significantly different from control.

Table 5.   Effects of MK-447, Indomethacin, and Indomethacin and Calcium Uptake Rates and Ca^{2+}-Stimulated, Mg^{2+}-Dependent ATPase Activity and Superoxide Anion Production

Group	Calcium uptake rate (μmoles Ca^{2+}/mg-min)	ATPase Activity (μmoles P_i/mg-min)	Superoxide anion production (nmoles·O_2^-/liter·sec)
Control	1.16 ± 0.03	1.64 ± 0.03	<5
PMA-WBC	0.52 ± 0.02	0.74 ± 0.04[a]	82.3 ± 10
+MK-447	0.31 ± 0.02[a]	1.15 ± 0.04[a]	140.7 ± 12
+MK-447-INDO	0.50 ± 0.01[a]	1.59 ± 0.04	76.2 ± 7
+INDO	0.61 ± 0.03[a]	1.66 ± 0.04	78.1 ± 5
+INDO-CAT	1.18 ± 0.02	1.59 ± 0.02	77.3 ± 8

[a] Significantly different from control.

Having incriminated the leukocyte–cyclooxygenase system in the production of reduced-oxygen intermediates, we attempted a more precise localization of this process with the compound 2-aminomethyl-4-t-butyl-6-iodophenol (MK-447), which accelerates the conversion of PGG_2 to PGH_2 with the production of reduced-oxygen intermediates. Table 5 presents the results of this study. In the presence of PMA-activated leukocytes, MK-447 produced a further significant depression in calcium uptake rates and resulted in a significant inhibition of activated-leukocyte depression of SR ATPase activity. Indomethacin inhibited the additional depression of SR calcium uptake induced by MK-447 and completely inhibited the effects of PMA-activated leukocytes, in the presence of MK-447, on ATPase activity.

The preceding study was repeated using SOD-inhibitable ferricytochrome C as a measure of superoxide anion production. PMA-activated leukocytes produced 82.3 nmoles ·O_2^-/liter · sec, which significantly increased (140 ± 12.0 nmoles ·O_2^-/liter · sec) in the presence of MK-447. Indomethacin completely inhibited the stimulatory effects of MK-447. The amount of superoxide anion production in the presence of PMA-activated leukocytes and indomethacin (INDO), or of PMA-activated leukocytes, indomethacin, and catalase (INDO-CAT), did not significantly differ from the amount of superoxide anion production from PMA-activated leukocytes alone. Our data would appear to incriminate two species of destructive reduced-oxygen intermediates generated from PMA-activated leukocytes: hydrogen peroxide (Tables 1 and 2) and a species produced from the cyclooxygenase pathway that is most likely a superoxide anion that via a Fenton reaction results in the production of hydroxyl radical (Tables 3–5). Therefore, we hypothesized that a combination of catalase and a cyclooxygenase inhibitor would completely normalize the effects of PMA-activated leukocytes on calcium transport by cardiac SR. In this study (Table 5), the combination of catalase and indomethacin completely normalized the effects of

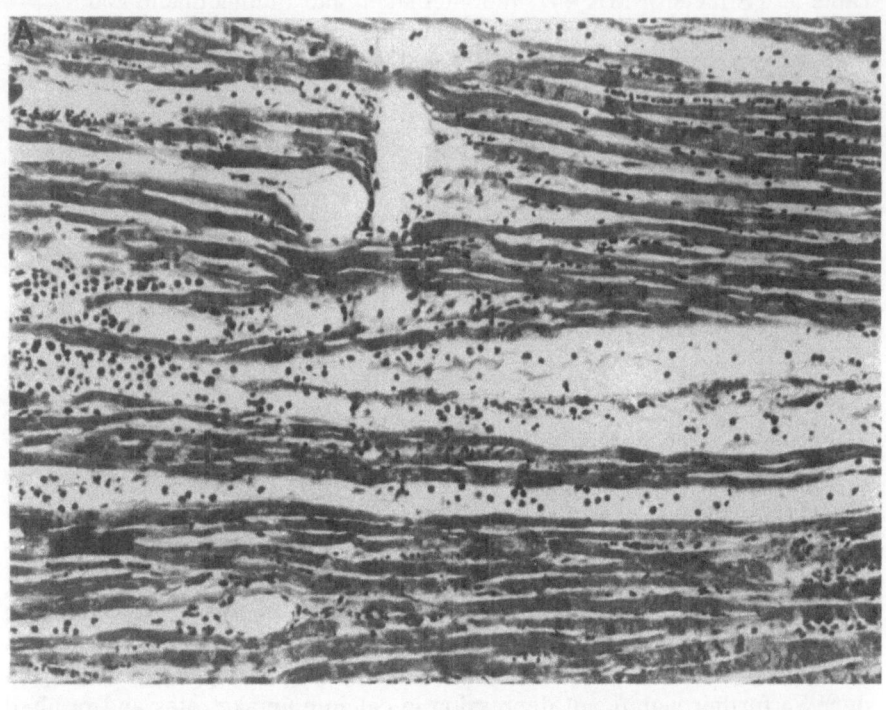

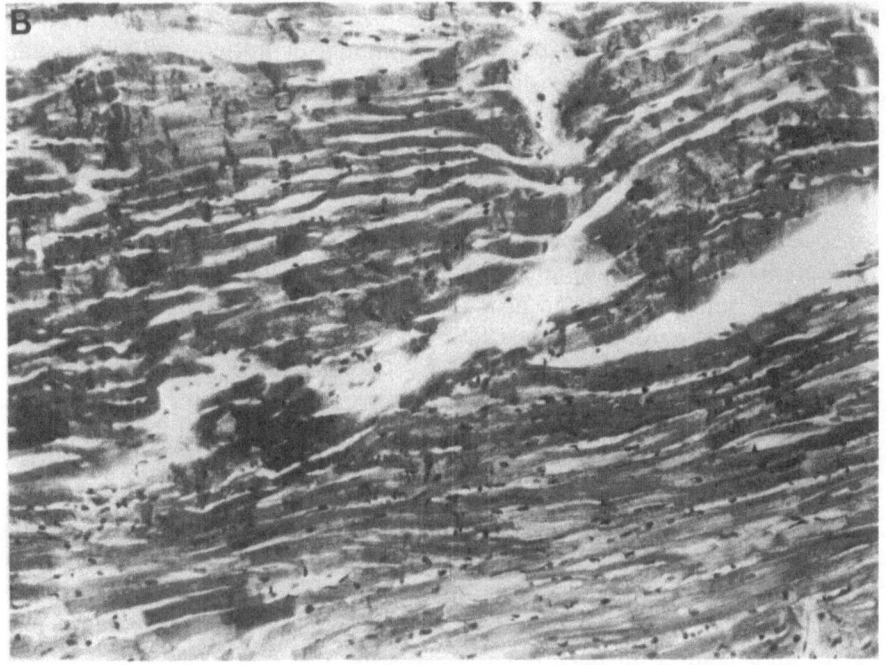

PMA-activated leukocytes on cardiac SR calcium uptake and ATPase activity.

Since activated leukocytes are capable of disrupting in vitro SR calcium transport by the production of reduced-oxygen intermediates, this observation was compared to an in vivo model of regional myocardial ischemia with a well-documented acute inflammatory response in the periinfarction zone. The hypothesis was established that prior neutrophil depletion would limit infarct size. To test this hypothesis, anti-canine leukocyte antiserum was administered to dogs, which resulted in a 77 ± 2% reduction in circulating neutrophils. Acute myocardial infarction was then induced, and following 6 hr of reperfusion, myocardial infarction in the antibody-treated group demonstrated a 43% reduction in infarct size compared to non-immune-sera-injected animals. As demonstrated by Figure 1, histopathological examination revealed that infarcted myocardium from the sham-injected group demonstrated a substantial neutrophilic infiltration that was virtually absent in the group that received neutrophil antiserum [22].

The time–course of infiltration of leukocytes into infarcted myocardium has been well characterized. In animal models of permanent coronary artery occlusion, leukocytes migrate to regions of myocardial injury within 24 hr reaching a peak within 4–5 days [23]. However, Sommers and Jennings [24] reported that reinstituting myocardial blood flow after temporary coronary occlusion accelerated the infiltration of inflammatory cells into injured myocardium. The experimental model employed in our study [22,25] made use of a model of myocardial ischemic injury resulting from a temporary occlusion (60 min) of the circumflex coronary artery followed by reperfusion, after which the accumulation of leukocytes in infarcted myocardium was assessed 24 hr after the ischemic insult.

Since neutrophil depletion limits infarct size in the canine model of ischemic–reperfusion injury and ibuprofen can inhibit the lethal hydroxyl radical generation from the leukocyte, the effects of ibuprofen pretreatment on inhibition of infarct size were studied. In this study, myocardial infarct size, as a percentage of area at risk, was reduced in the ibuprofen-pretreated group by 40%, from 48 ± 4% in control animals to 29 ± 4% ($p = 0.005$) [25]. Figure 2 presents a summary of the effects of ibuprofen on leukocyte

←——————————————————————————————————

Figure 1.   (A) Myocardium from a control dog treated with nonimmune serum. None of the myocardium in this field appears viable. Many fibers, particularly in the upper right quadrant, appear dark because of increased cytoplasmic eosinophilia. Contraction bands are evident in the lower right and upper midportions of the field. Karyolysis and pyknosis, although present, are difficult to discern at this magnification. An interstitial leukocytic infiltrate is obvious. Hematoxylin–eosin stain; original magnification: × 141. (B) Myocardium from a neutrophil-depleted dog. Some viable myocardium remains in the upper left quadrant of the field. The necrotic fibers, particularly at the extreme right, appear dark because of increased eosinophilia and homogenization of cytoplasm. Contraction bands are also prominent, especially in the lower right quadrant. In contrast to (A), there is virtually no leukocytic infiltrate. Hematoxylin–eosin stain; original magnification: × 141.

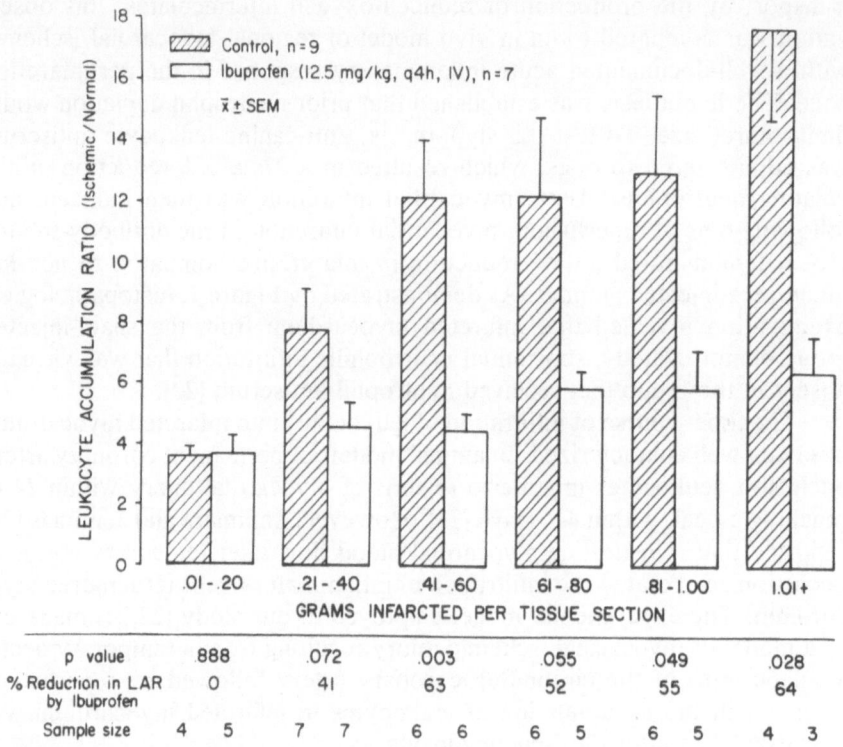

p value	888		.072		.003		.055		.049		.028	
% Reduction in LAR by Ibuprofen	0		41		63		52		55		64	
Sample size	4	5	7	7	6	6	6	5	6	5	4	3

Figure 2. Effect of ibuprofen on the accumulation of ^{111}In-labeled leukocytes in infarcted myocardium. Quantitative assessment of the accumulation of ^{111}In-labeled leukocytes was accomplished by calculating the leukocyte accumulation ratio (LAR), defined as the increase in radioactivity present in infarcted myocardium compared with the ^{111}In activity present in nonischemic tissue. The LAR was calculated for each transmural myocardial tissue section taken from the area at risk. These values were then grouped according to the number of grams of infarcted tissue in each transmural section. In control dogs, LAR increased substantially with greater amounts of infarcted tissue in each section. Treating the dogs with ibuprofen markedly suppressed leukocyte accumulation in infarcted myocardium. Statistical comparison of the LAR between control and ibuprofen-treated dogs for each of the gram-infarct intervals yielded the p values listed at the bottom of the figure. The percentage reduction in LAR by ibuprofen treatment, within each gram-infarct interval, is also presented. Thus, ibuprofen treatment markedly suppresses leukocyte accumulation in irreversibly injured myocardium. The number of dogs presented in each 0.2-g division for control and ibuprofen-treated dogs is shown at the bottom of the figure. Each animal is not represented in each infarct interval due to the random distribution of tissue sections with varying degrees of injury. The 1.01 + gram-infarct division includes tissue samples with more than 1.0 g but less than 1.4 g of infarcted tissue (Romson et al. [25]).

accumulation in the canine heart subjected to temporary coronary artery occlusion followed by 24 hr of reperfusion. The leukocyte accumulation ratio is defined as the increase in ^{111}In radioactivity of tissue sections from the area at risk compared with the radioactivity present in nonischemic tissue samples. Heart muscle sections from nontreated control animals revealed a marked increase in the leukocyte accumulation ratio that was related directly to the use of infarcted myocardium in any segment. Treatment with ibuprofen (12.5 mg/kg i.v. every 4 hr) markedly reduced the leukocyte accumulation ratio, so that only a 76% increase was noted as compared to a 397% increase in the ratio from myocardial sections obtained from nontreated control animals.

DISCUSSION

Our study makes the following significant points: (1) Phorbol myristate acetate (PMA)-activated leukocytes disrupt cardiac muscle cell calcium transport mechanisms via a reduced-oxygen-intermediate mechanism. (2) The destructive species of reduced-oxygen intermediates would appear to be hydrogen peroxide generated from the NADPH system and hydroxyl radical generated from the metabolism of arachidonic acid. (3) Pharmacological inhibition of the leukocyte reduced-oxygen-intermediate system results in a decrease in the inflammatory response and a decrease in the consequences of the acute inflammatory response of ischemic reperfusion injury, and complete inhibition of the neutrophil system results in a similar histological picture. This study also further characterizes the interaction of the activated-leukocyte system in the generation of reduced-oxygen intermediates and its potential interaction with cardiac muscle. Our activated-leukocyte system produces similar quantities of superoxide anion compared to other studies as measured by ferricytochrome C. The generation of these reduced-oxygen intermediates is capable of interacting with cardiac sarcoplasmic reticulum (SR) and depresses both calcium uptake rates and ATPase activity. The depression of calcium uptake in the presence of increasing doses of superoxide dismutase (SOD) and the demonstration that exogenous hydrogen peroxide uncouples calcium transport from ATP hydrolysis incriminates hydrogen peroxide as a mediator of calcium-uptake depression in the SR. In our in vitro system, activated leukocytes were not inhibited by either SOD or catalase alone, but required both SOD and catalase. This would strongly incriminate the generation of the hydroxyl radical. The complete inhibition of leukocyte-induced depression of the SR ATPase with SOD plus mannitol strongly suggests that the hydroxyl radical is the destructive species responsible for the depression of the enzyme system. This production of hydroxyl radical by peripheral-blood neutrophils has been previously demonstrated by Tauber and Babior [26]. Thus, one could postulate that the superoxide anion per se is not a destructive species in our system, but the dismutation of the superoxide anion to hydrogen peroxide and then by either a Fenton reaction or a Haber–Weiss reaction results in the production of the hydroxyl radical. This concept would fit with the suggestion of Fee and Valentine [27], who claim that the toxicity of the superoxide anion may be quite low.

Insight into the production of these reduced-oxygen intermediates is also extended by the study discussed above. PMA activates the membrane-bound NADPH oxidase system, resulting in the generation of both super-oxide anion and hydrogen peroxide [28]. However, in the presence of cy-clooxygenase inhibitors, the depression of SR ATPase activity is inhibited, whereas the SR calcium uptake remains uncoupled from ATP hydrolysis identical to that observed in the exogenous-hydrogen-peroxide study. In addition, MK-447, a compound known to accelerate the conversion of PGG_2 to PGH_2, increased the production of superoxide anion, and this increased production was inhibited by indomethacin. These data suggest that the cy-clooxygenase system of the leukocyte is an active participant in the gen-eration of oxygen free radicals. This is in agreement with the findings of Kuehl et al. [7], who describe an oxidizing species (OX) resulting from the conversion of PGG_2 to PGH_2. Our results demonstrating a decrease in SR calcium uptake and partial protection of the SR and calcium ATPase with MK-447 also adds credibility to the participation of cyclooxygenase in the generation of free radicals. With the increase in superoxide anion generated from the conversion of PGG_2 to PGH_2, hydrogen peroxide production is increased. The partial protection of the calcium ATPase agrees with the concept that generation of an oxygen radical by the cyclooxygenase system acts as a negative-feedback mechanism on cyclooxygenase and suggests that MK-447 scavenges this oxidizing species, probably hydroxyl radical. Fur-ther, our data would agree with the work of Kontos et al. [29], who incrim-inate superoxide anion and hydroxyl radical in the cerebral vascular injury induced by PGG_2 but not by PGH_2, and with the work of Okabe et al. [30], who, in an in vitro free-radical-generating system, also found that PGG_2 disrupted skeletal muscle SR in calcium transport, this effect being inhib-itable by scavengers of oxygen free radicals. Thus, we would suggest that in PMA-activated leukocytes, activation of the NADPH system results in-itially in the generation of the superoxide anion that then dismutates to hy-drogen peroxide, which is a destructive species in our system and is re-sponsible for the uncoupling of calcium transport from ATP hydrolysis. Further, PMA would appear to activate the arachidonic acid system with the initial generation of the superoxide anion and hydrogen peroxide, but then by a Fenton reaction, the increase in superoxide anion and hydrogen peroxide production could result in the production of the hydroxyl radical. Our study, using catalase and indomethacin to completely inhibit the effects of PMA-activated leukocytes, would appear to support this hypothesis.

The SR of cardiac muscle represents a logical target organelle for leu-kocyte-generated oxygen free radicals. There is an abundant subsarcolemmal network of SR in cardiac muscle, and the SR has been shown to be capable of serving as both the source of and a sink for calcium in the excitation–contraction coupling system. In addition, the SR ATPase of cardiac muscle has been shown by Sadigursky et al. [2] to share antigenic recognition with *Trypanosoma cruzi* in the myocarditis of Chagas's disease. In the myocarditis of acute cardiac allograft rejection, Hess et al. [10] have identified significant depression of SR calcium transport and ATPase activity. In the acute myocarditis of congenital round cell disease in turkeys, Staley et al. [3] have correlated leukocytic infiltration with a depressed SR calcium transport system. In addition, they were able to show a protective effect of broad-spectrum immunosuppression using cyclophosphamide. The importance of the inflammatory response to the field of ischemic cardiac disease is also highlighted by this study. The studies on ischemia–reperfusion injury presented herein clearly incriminate the acute inflammatory response as a potential mediator of the loss of viability of the periinfarction zone. The use of the nonsteroidal antiinflammatory agent to modify infarct size clearly suggests that the neutrophil plays an important role in ischemic reperfusion injury. In this study, the use of ibuprofen could have two potential mechanisms: One, as demonstrated by the in vitro studies, is the inhibition of the cyclooxygenase system and thereby the inhibition of the generation of the hydroxyl radical. The second major mechanism by which ibuprofen may be working is the inhibition of the lipoxygenase [26,31] system, which would decrease the production of chemotactic leukotrienes. The leukotrienes produced from the metabolism of arachidonic acid are strong chemotactic agents, and by inhibition of this system, there would be a decrease in migration of neutrophils to the periinfarction zone and therefore a reduction in the generation of reduced-oxygen intermediates. This pathway would then preserve still-viable myocardial tissue. This hypothesis is quite compatible with the data of McCluskey et al. [32], who demonstrated that at 72 hr postinfarction, the acute inflammatory reaction in the area of the infarction correlated with an increase in arachidonic acid metabolites. These investigators suggest that the enhanced ability of the postinfarction region to metabolize arachidonic acid may truly result from the inflammatory-cell invasion or fibroblast activation that accompanies the healing myocardial infarction. Our findings are also compatible with the work of Judgett et al. [33], who found that ibuprofen afforded protection 2 days post myocardial infarction, protection that was not due to changes in myocardial flow or myocardial oxygen demands, and suggested that cellular and metabolic effects may be important. A similar conclusion has been found by Romson et al. [34] following ischemia–reperfusion injury and global ischemic injury in the isolated blood-perfused feline heart. These authors have demonstrated that the reduction in myocardial oxygen consumption or a redistribution of blood flow is not an important mechanism underlying the protective effects of ibuprofen in experimental myocardial ischemia. Thus, it would appear that the role of the leukocyte–cyclooxygenase system and the oxygen free-radical system is an important component of both ischemic reperfusion injury and leukocytic infiltration of the myocardium, that the mechanism underlying the destruction of cardiac tissue is based on the production of reduced-oxygen intermediates. This pathophysiological cascade should open up new avenues for the potential application of scavengers and/or inhibitors of reduced-oxygen-intermediate systems as another potential mechanism in the protection of the myocardium during ischemic reperfusion injury. Mullane and Moncada [35] have reported that BW-755C, a dual inhibitor of the lipoxygenase and cyclooxygenase pathway of arachidonic acid metabolism, reduces the size of an infarct produced by 60 min of coronary occlusion followed by 5 hr of reperfusion in anesthetized dogs. The authors concluded that the efficacy of BW-755C is due to the inhibition of lipoxygenase product formation by migrating cells that invade the damaged myocardium to produce an inflammatory response.

Most recently, it has been reported [36] that the combined intracoronary administration of superoxide dismutase (SOD) and catalase (CAT) resulted in a significant reduction in ultimate infarct size in the canine heart subjected to temporary coronary occlusion followed by 24 hr of reperfusion. Thus, nontreated control hearts had significantly larger infarcts, expressed as a percentage of the area at risk, as compared to hearts that received both SOD and CAT (45.54% vs. 23.0 + 6.9%). These results suggest that the SOD + CAT combination reduced irreversible ischemic injury by removing free radicals generated in ischemic tissue.

The observations presented in this review may be deserving of careful extrapolation to clinical situations in which myocardial ischemia is followed by reperfusion. During cardiac surgery, the heart is subjected to varying periods of global ischemic arrest. Despite the use of hypothermia and cardioplegic solution, there is the potential to develop reperfusion-related injury that may be attributed to the mechanisms discussed and may be preventable by pharmacological maneuvers directed at the leukocyte or toxic oxygen species or both. Other areas that warrant consideration are those in which patients with evolving myocardial infarction are candidates for emergency reperfusion by any or a combination of thrombolytic therapy, angioplasty, and coronary bypass surgery.

The studies reported by us as well as those of others cited above should provide basic evidence that toxic oxygen species derived in part from myocardial tissue as well as from invading inflammatory cells constitute a major mechanism whereby myocardial tissue that is reperfused, but otherwise viable and salvageable, becomes irreversibly injured. We have been able to identify protective effects of several interventions, each of which, in some way, reduces the generation of toxic oxygen species in a region of myocardial tissue that has been made ischemic and is subsequently reperfused. A potential clinical application of these observations would be the use of appropriate scavengers of oxygen radicals in patients with an acute coronary artery occlusion who are to undergo emergency reperfusion. Such interventions should enhance the amount of myocardium that is salvageable by the restoration of blood flow.

ACKNOWLEDGMENTS

This research was supported by Grants HL 30716 and HL 24517 (Medical College of Virginia) and Grants HL 19784 and HL 27817 and a grant from the Michigan Heart Association (University of Michigan).

REFERENCES

1. Hastillo, A., Willis, M. E., and Hess, M. L. 1982. The heart as a target organ of immune injury. In: P. Harvey (ed), *Current Problems in Cardiology* Vol. 6, pp. 1–51. Year Book Medical Publishers, Chicago.
2. Sadigursky, M., Acosta, A. M., and Santos-Buch, C. A. 1982. Muscle sarcoplasmic reticulum antigen shared by a *Trypanosoma cruzi* clone. *Am. J. Trop. Med. Hyg.* 31(5):934–941.
3. Staley, N. A., Noren, G. R., and Enzig, S. 1981. Early alterations in the functional SR in a naturally occurring model of congestive cardiomyopathy. *Cardiovasc. Res.* 15:276–281.
4. Babior B. M. 1982. The enzymatic basis for $\cdot O_2^-$ production by human neutrophils. *Can. J. Physiol. Pharmacol.* 60:1353–1358.
5. Del Maestro, R. 1980. An approach to free radicals in medicine and biology. *Acta Physiol. Scand. Suppl.* 492:153–168.
6. Fantone, J. C., and Ward, P. A. 1982. Roles of oxygen derived free radicals and metabolites in leukocyte-dependent inflammatory reactions. *Am. J. Pathol.* 107:397–418.
7. Kuehl, F. A., Humes, J. L., Torchiana, M. L., Ham, E. A., and Egan, R. W. 1979. Oxygen centered radicals in the inflammatory process. In: G. Weissman (ed.), *Advances in Inflammation Research*. Vol. I, pp. 419–430. Raven Press, New York.
8. Fabiato, I., and Fabiato, F. 1977. Calcium release from the sarcoplasmic reticulum. *Circ. Res.* 40:119–129.
9. Hess, M. L., Warner, M., Robbins, A. D., Crute, S., and Greenfield, L. J. 1981. Characterization of the E–C coupling system of the hypothermic myocardium following ischemia and reperfusion. *Cardiovasc. Res.* 15:380–389.
10. Hess, M. L., Manson, N. H., Warner, M. F., and Lower, R. R. 1981. Mechanical and subcellular function of the canine heterotopic transplanted myocardium during active transplant injury. *Transplantation* 32:194–202.
11. Hess, M. L., Okabe, E. and Kontos, H. A. 1981. Proton and free oxygen radical interaction with the calcium transport system of cardiac SR. *J. Mol. Cell. Cardiol.* 13:767–772.
12. Manson, N. H., and Hess, M. L. 1983. Interaction of oxygen free radicals and cardiac sarcoplasmic reticulum: Proposed role in the pathogenesis of endotoxin shock. *Circ. Shock* 10:205–213.
13. Penny C. L. 1976. A simple microassay for inorganic phosphate. *Ann. Biochem.* 75:201–210.
14. Massey, V. 1959. The microestimation of succinate and the extinction coefficient of cytochrome C. *Biochim. Biophys. Acta* 34:255–256.
15. Beauchamp, C. and Fridovich, I. 1970. A mechanism for the production of ethylene from methional: The generation of the hydroxyl radical by xanthine oxidase. *J. Biol. Chem.* 245:4641–4646.
16. Blackwell, G. J., Duncombe, W. G., Flower, R. J., Parsons, M. F., and Vane, J. R. 1977. The distribution and metabolism of arachidonic acid in rabbit platelets during aggregation and its modification by drugs. *Br. J. Pharmacol.* 59:353.

17. Lucchesi, B., Burmeister, W., Lomas, T., and Abrams G. 1976. Ischemic changes in the canine heart as affected by the dimethyl quaternary analog of propranolol, UM-272 (SC-27761). *J. Pharmacol. Exp. Ther.* 199:310–328.
18. Sheehan, F., and Epstein, S. 1982. Determinants of arrhythmic death due to coronary spasm: Effect of preexisting coronary artery stenosis on the incidence of reperfusion arrhythmias. *Circulation* 65:259–264.
19. Romson, J., Bush, L., Jolly, S., and Lucchesi, B. 1982. Cardioprotective effects of ibuprofen in experimental regional and global myocardial ischemia. *J. Cardiovasc. Pharmacol.* 4:187–196.
20. Fishbein, M., Meerbaum, S., Rit, J., Lando, U., Kanmatsuse, K., Mercier, J., Corday, E., and Ganz, W. 1981. Early phase acute myocardial infarct size quantification: Validation of the triphenyl tetrazolium chloride tissue enzyme staining technique. *Am. Heart J.* 101:593–600.
21. English, D., and Abrams, B. 1974. Single-step separation of red blood cells, granulocytes and mononuclear cells on discontinuous density gradients of Ficoll–Hypaque. *J. Immunol. Methods* 5:249–258.
22. Romson, J. L., Hook, B. G., Kunkel, S. L., Abrams, G. D., Schork, A., and Lucchesi, B. R. 1983. Reduction of the extent of ischemic myocardial injury by neutrophil depletion in the dog. *Circulation* 67:1016–1023.
23. Mallory, G., White, P., and Salcedo-Salgar, J. 1939. The speed of healing of myocardial infarction. *Am. Heart J.* 18:647–671.
24. Sommers, H., and Jennings, R. 1964. Experimental acute myocardial infarction: Histologic and histochemical studies of early myocardial infarcts by temporary or permanent occlusion of a coronary artery. *Lab. Invest.* 13:1491–1503.
25. Romson, J. L., Hook, B. G., Rigot, V. H., Schork, M. A., Swanson, P. P., and Lucchesi, B. R. 1982. The effect of ibuprofen on accumulation of indium-111-labeled platelets and leukocytes in experimental myocardial infarction. *Circulation* 66:1002–1011.
26. Tauber, A. I., and Babior, B. M. 1977. Evidence for hydroxyl radical production by human neutrophils. *J. Clin. Invest.* 60:374–399.
27. Fee, J. A., and Valentine, J. S. 1977. Chemical and physical properties of superoxide. In: A. M. Michelson, J. M. McCord, and I. Fridovich (eds.), *Superoxide and Superoxide Dismutase.* pp. 19–60. Academic Press, New York.
28. DeChatelet, R., Shirley, P. S., and Johnson, R. B., Jr. 1976. Effect of phorbol myristate acetate on the oxidative metabolism of human polymorphonuclear leukocytes. *Blood* 47:545–554.
29. Kontos, H. A., Wei, E. P., Povlishock, J. T., Dietrich, W. D., Magiera, C. J., and Ellis, E. F. 1980. Cerebral arteriolar damage by arachidonic acid and prostaglandin G_2. *Science* 209:1242–1245.
30. Okabe, E., Hiyama, E., Oyama, M., Odajima, C., Ito, H., and Cho, Y. 1982. Free radical damage to sarcoplasmic reticulum of masseter muscle by arachidonic acid and prostaglandin G_2. *Pharmacology* 25:138–148.
31. Sircar, J. C., Schwender, C. F., and Johnson, E. A. 1983. Soybean lipoxygenase inhibition by non-steroidal anti-inflammatory drugs. *Prostaglandins* 25:393–396.
32. McCluskey, E. R., Corr, P. B., Lee, B. I., Saffitz, J. E., and Needleman, P. 1982. The arachidonic acid metabolic capacity of canine myocardium is increased during healing of acute myocardial infarction. *Circ. Res.* 51:743–750.
33. Judgett, B. I., Hutchins, G. M., Bulkley, B. H., and Becker, L. C. 1980. Salvage of ischemic myocardium by ibuprofen during infarction in the conscious dog. *Am. J. Cardiol.* 46:74–82.
34. Romson, J. L., Brush, L. R., Jolly, S. R., and Lucchesi, B. R. 1982. Cardioprotective effects of ibuprofen in experimental regional and global myocardial ischemia. *J. Cardiovasc. Pharmacol.* 4:187–196.

35. Mullane, K. M., and Moncada, S. 1982. The salvage of ischemic myocardium by BW-755C in anesthetized dogs. *Prostaglandins* 24:255–266.
36. Jolly S. R., Kane W. J., Bailie M. B., Abrams, G. D., Lucchesi B. R. 1984. Canine myocardial reperfusion injury: Its reduction by the combined administration of superoxide dismutase and catalase. *Circ. Res.* 54:277–285.

The Oxygen Free Radical System and Myocardial Dysfunction

Michael L. Hess and Nancy H. Manson

Department of Medicine (Cardiology)
Medical College of Virginia
Richmond, Virginia 23298

Abstract. The pathways for the metabolism of molecular oxygen involve one electron-transfer reaction with the subsequent production of reduced-oxygen intermediates. These reduced-oxygen intermediates include the superoxide anion ($\cdot O_2^-$), hydrogen peroxide (H_2O_2), and the hydroxyl radical ($\cdot OH$), which are highly reactive, short-lived species. Normally, intracellular enzyme systems that include superoxide dismutase, catalase, and glutathione peroxidase are responsible for "scavenging" these products of oxygen metabolism. However, in many pathological states such as inflammation, ischemia, and reperfusion, there is an increased production of these reduced-oxygen intermediates, which are capable of extensive tissue damage. It is the purpose of this symposium to examine, in depth, the role of oxygen free radical systems as mediators of myocardial dysfunction and expand our knowledge of myocardial ischemia, ischemia–reperfusion injury, and the inflammatory response of the myocardium.

Molecular oxygen has an unusual structure in that it contains two unpaired electrons with parallel electron spins. Most organic compounds that might react with oxygen contain paired electrons. The simultaneous insertion of two paired electrons into a molecule of oxygen would violate the rules of quantum mechanics. The result of this restriction is that ordinary molecular oxygen is relatively nonreactive. The reduction of oxygen to water in living tissues can proceed by one of two pathways. Mitochondrial enzymes have the capability of overcoming quantum mechanical restrictions to reduce oxygen to water by tetravalent reduction without the production of any intermediates. This pathway ordinarily accounts for 95% of the oxygen consumption of itssues [1]. The remaining 5% proceeds by a univalent pathway in which several intermediates are produced:

$$O_2 \xrightarrow{e^-} \cdot O_2^- \xrightarrow{e^- + 2H^+} H_2O_2 \xrightarrow{e^- + H^+} \cdot OH \xrightarrow{e^- + H^+} \qquad (1)$$
$$\searrow \qquad\qquad \searrow$$
$$H_2O \qquad\qquad H_2O$$

in which $\cdot O_2^-$ is the superoxide anion, H_2O_2 is hydrogen peroxide, and $\cdot OH$ is the hydroxyl radical.

Superoxide anion ($\cdot O_2^-$) is the best-studied free-radical species. This free radical may act as a reducing agent, donating its electrons, or as an oxidizing agent, in which case it is reduced to H_2O_2. Thomas et al. [2,3] have demonstrated that $\cdot O_2^-$ may react with lipid hydroperoxides to form alkoxy radicals ($RO\cdot$) in phospholipid membranes. Formation of the alkoxy radical is prevented in normal biological tissue by the dismutation reaction:

$$\cdot O_2^- + \cdot O_2^- + 2H^+ \longrightarrow H_2O_2 + O_2$$

This reaction can proceed spontaneously or it can be catalyzed by superoxide dismutase (SOD), which increases the rate of intracellular dismutation by a factor of 10^9. SOD is a ubiquitous mammalian enzyme, and in the presence of normal intracellular levels of catalase and peroxidase is responsible for the reduction of H_2O_2 to H_2O, thus serving as a normal biological defense against the formation and accumulation of the reactive free radicals.

Additionally, NADPH oxidase on the surface of polymorphonuclear leukocytes, monocytes, and macrophages reduces molecular oxygen to superoxide anion [14]. The ability of leukocytes to reduce oxygen to superoxide anion is important for bacteriological phagocytosis and killing. The generation of free oxygen radicals is an established and important mechanism by which leukocytes phagocytize and kill [5].

Hydrogen peroxide (H_2O_2) produced by the univalent reduction of oxygen is catalytically reduced in the cell to H_2O by catalase [equation (3b)] or glutathione peroxidase [equation (3c)]:

$$\cdot O_2^- + \cdot O_2^- + 2H^+ \longrightarrow H_2O_2 + O_2 \qquad (3a)$$

$$2H_2O_2 \xrightarrow{\text{catalase}} O_2 + 2H_2O \qquad (3b)$$

$$2\,GSH + H_2O_2 \longrightarrow GSSG + 2H_2O \qquad (3c)$$

$$GSSH + \text{glutathione reductase} \longrightarrow GSH$$

This system constitutes the major intracellular hydrogen peroxide decomposition system. Although H_2O_2 may be toxic at high concentrations, these concentrations are orders of magnitude higher than the intracellular flux. The major danger of H_2O_2 accumulation is the production of hydroxyl radical ($\cdot OH$) by the Fenton-type reaction with a metal chelate [equation (4a)] or the Haber–Weiss reaction [equation (4b)] [6]:

$$Me^{n+} + chelate + \cdot O_2^- \rightarrow Me^{(n-1)+} chelate + O_2 \qquad (4a)$$

$$Me^{(n-1)+} + chelate + H_2O_2 \rightarrow Me^{n+} chelate + OH + \cdot OH$$

$$Fe^{2+} + H_2O_2 \rightarrow Fe^{3+} + \cdot OH + OH^- \qquad (4b)$$

$$\cdot OH + H_2O_2 \rightarrow H_2O + \cdot O_2^- + H^+$$

$$\cdot O_2^- + H_2O_2 \rightarrow O_2 + OH^- + \cdot OH$$

$$Fe^{2+} + \cdot OH^- \rightarrow Fe^{3+} + OH^-$$

The hydroxyl radical ($\cdot OH$) is a very reactive and an unstable oxidizing species that reacts with a large variety of organic compounds and bio-membranes. The potential for generating hydroxyl radicals [equations (4a) and(4b)] is very real, but under normal physiological conditions, hydroxyl radicals would not be formed. This can be seen from equation (1). Since $\cdot OH$ is a trivalent reduction product of O_2, it requires both $\cdot O_2^-$, which is normally scavenged by SOD, and H_2O_2, which is scavenged by the catalase–peroxidase system. Hydroxyl radicals, therefore, do not exist under physiological conditions. It must also be pointed out that there are no physiological defense or enzyme systems that can scavenge hydroxyl radicals. In pathological conditions known to generate hydroxyl radicals, tissue destruction is extensive. Therapeutic use of this concept is observed in radiation therapy, which induces hydroxyl radicals and destroys tumor tissue [7]. Two important pathophysiological states involving the generation of free radicals with subsequent tissue destruction have been fairly well studied and have application to the myocardium: central nervous system (CNS) ischemia and the acute inflammatory response.

There is a growing body of evidence that free-radical production is an important mediator of CNS ischemia. Demopolous et al. have reviewed this subject [8] and have recently demonstrated [9] in the cat model of CNS ischemia and spinal cord trauma distinct free-radical pathology that affects predominantly membrane lipids in the ischemic or traumatized tissue. Wei et al. [11] were able to extend the results of Demopolous in a cat model of experimental brain injury. Kontos et al. [10] have demonstrated the potential role of free-radical-mediated cerebral vascular damage during acute hypertension. In each of these studies, agents postulated to inhibit CNS ischemia damage were found to also inhibit the production and/or effects of free radicals, e.g., nonsteroidal antiinflammatory agents and mannitol. Nonsteroidal antiinflammatory agents inhibit the synthesis of prostaglandins primarily by inhibiting the activity of cyclooxygenase. Intermediate steps in the synthesis of prostaglandins involve the generation of free oxygen radicals. One possible mechanism for the beneficial effects of nonsteroidal antiinflammatory

agents in CNS ischemia may be a decreased production of free oxygen radicals. Mannitol is a scavenger of the hydroxyl radical [12]. It is now postulated that the beneficial effects of mannitol on ischemic CNS damage may
be related not entirely to its osmotic effect, but also to its ability to scavenge
the highly destructive hydroxyl radical.

The acute inflammatory reaction presents a second example of extracellular free-radical generation with subsequent tissue destruction [13,14].
This exciting field evolved when a physiological function of the oxygen free-
radical system was demonstrated by Babior and co-workers. They found
that normal human leukocytes (subsequently found to be neutrophils and
monocytes) generate superoxide anion and hydrogen peroxide during phagocytosis [4]. The physiological importance of this free-radical system was
shown by Johnston et al. [15], who demonstrated that the oxygen free-radical
system is a mechanism of leukocyte-mediated phagocytic bactericidal activity. These two observations are important for our developing hypothesis,
for they demonstrate that leukocytes are capable of generating cytotoxic
free-radical species to the extracellular space and that these radicals are
capable of crossing cell-membrane barriers and exerting a cytotoxic effect.

On the basis of this sort of background information, investigators in
Europe, Canada, and the United States have studied the potential role for
free-radical mechanisms in the pathophysiology of cardiac disease. There
are three major areas in which a free-radical mechanism should play an
important role as mediator of cardiac tissue destruction: ischemia, reperfusion, and inflammation. During the course of myocardial ischemia with
the decrease in supply of molecular oxygen, there is an abrupt increase in
reducing equivalents, decrease in intracellular pH, and loss of physiological
scavengers of superoxide anion and hydrogen peroxide. This ischemic intracellular milieu is very conducive to the generation of reduced-oxygen
intermediates, which in turn are capable of lipid peroxidation and contributing to the negative inotropic process of ischemia. Reperfusion injury presents an ideal free-radical-mediated process. With the reintroduction of molecular oxygen to an ischemic vascular bed, there could be a burst of free-
radical generation and, with little or no scavenging ability available, significant myocardial injury. Inflammation represents a third important free-radical-mediated process. Although not as well studied as ischemia–reperfusion
injury, acute inflammation occurs within 24 hr of myocardial infarction and
in several significant myopathic processes such as Chagas's disease, viral
and nonviral myocarditis, acute rheumatic fever, and acute cardiac allograft
rejection. In all these processes, leukocyte-derived free radicals may contribute to the development of myocardial failure.

This symposium has brought together a distinguished panel of experts
in the field of free-radical mediation of myocardial dysfunction. The three
major areas of ischemia, reperfusion, and inflammation have been discussed,
and new and exciting information has been presented. With the elucidation
of free-radical mechanisms in cardiac pathophysiology, a new avenue of

approach should emerge for protection of the myocardium during the course of ischemia, reperfusion, and inflammation.

ACKNOWLEDGMENTS

This research was supported by Grants HL 30716 and HL 24517.

REFERENCES

1. Fridovich, I. 1978. The biology of oxygen radicals. *Science* 201:875–888.
2. Pryor, W. A. 1976. The role of free radical reactions in biological systems. In: W. Pryor (ed.), *Free Radicals in Biology*. pp. 1–49. Academic Press, New York.
3. Thomas, M. J., Mehl, K. S., and Pryor, W. A. 1978. The role of superoxide anion in the xanthine-oxidase induced autoxidation of linoleic acid. *Biochem. Biophys. Res. Commun.* 83:927–932.
4. Babior, B. M. 1978. Oxygen-dependent microbial killing by phagocytes. Parts I and II. *N. Engl. J. Med.* 298:659–668 and 732–725.
5. Klebanoff, J. J. 1980. Oxygen metabolism and the toxic properties of phagocytes. *Ann. Intern. Med.* 93:480–489.
6. Haber, F., and Weiss, J. 1934. The catalytic decomposition of hydrogen peroxide by ion salts. *Proc. R. Soc.* 147:332–351.
7. Benon, H., Bielski, J., and Gebicki, J. M. 1977. Application of radiation chemistry to biology. In: W. Pryor (ed.), *Free Radicals in Biology*. Vol. 3, pp. 1–51. Academic Press, New York.
8. Demopoulos, H. G., Glamm, E. S., Seligman, M. L., Mitamura, J. A., and Ransohoff, J. 1979. Membrane perturbations in central nervous system injury: Theoretical basis for free radical damage. In: A. J. Popp, R. S. Bourke, L. R. Nelson, and H. K. Kimelberg (eds.), *Neural Trauma*. pp. 63–78. Raven Press, New York.
9. Demopoulos, H. B., Flamm, E. S., Pietronigro, D. D., and Seligman, M. L. 1980. The free radical pathology and the microcirculation in the major central nervous system disorders. *Acta Physiol. Scand. Suppl.* 492:91–119.
10. Kontos, H. A., Wei, E. P., Dietrich, W. D., Navari, R. M., Povlishock, J. T., Ghatak, N. R., Ellis, E. F., Patterson, J. L. Mechanism of cerebral arteriolar abnormalities after acute hypertension. *Am. J. Physiol.* 240:H511–H527.
11. Wei, E. P., Kontos, H. A., Dietrich, W. D., Povlishock, J. T., and Ellis, E. F. 1981. Inhibition by free radical scavengers and by cyclooxygenase inhibitors of pial arteriolar abnormalities. *Circ. Res.* 48:95–103.
12. Dorfman, L. M., and Adams, G. E. 1973. Reactivity of hydroxyl free radicals in aqueous solutions. NSRDS NL35, No 46, United States Department of Commerce, National Bureau of Standards.
13. Kuehl, F. A., Humes, J. L., Ham, E. A., Egan, R. W., Dougherty, H. W. 1980. Inflammation: The role of peroxidase-derived products. *Adv. Prostaglandin Thromb. Res.* 6:77–86.
14. McCord, J. M. 1974 Free radicals and inflammation: Protection of synovial fluid by superoxide dismutase. *Science* 185:529–531.
15. Johnson, R. B., Keele, B. B., Misra, H. P., Lehmeyer, J. P., Webb, L. S., Baehner, R. L., Rajagopalan, K. V. 1975. The role of superoxide anion generation in phagocytic bacterial activity: Studies with normal and chronic granulomatous disease leukocytes. *J. Clin. Invest.* 55:1357–1372.

Free Radicals and Myocardial Ischemia
The Role of Xanthine Oxidase

Joe M. McCord and Ranjan S. Roy

Department of Biochemistry
College of Medicine
University of South Alabama
Mobile, Alabama 36688

Stephen W. Schaffer

Department of Pharmacology
College of Medicine
University of South Alabama
Mobile, Alabama 36688

Abstract.   Recent studies have established a major role for oxygen-derived free radicals in post ischemic tissue injury to the intestine. During ischemia, there appears to be a calcium-triggered, protease-dependent conversion of the native xanthine dehydrogenase to a superoxide-producing xanthine oxidase. The catabolic degradation of ATP during ischemia provides an oxidizable substrate, hypoxanthine. On reperfusion, molecular oxygen is resupplied and a burst of superoxide production ensues, resulting in extensive tissue damage. The same mechanism appears to occur in myocardial ischemia. Xanthine dehydrogenase rapidly converts to the oxidase during nonperfusion in the rat heart. In the isolated perfused working rat heart model, 40 min of anoxia followed by reoxygenation results in substantial release of creatine kinase. The release of creatine kinase is blocked almost completely by pretreatment of the rats with allopurinol, a specific inhibitor of xanthine oxidase.

INTRODUCTION

The superoxide free radical ($\cdot O_2^-$) was recognized in 1968 to be a product of the enzyme xanthine oxidase, resulting from a one-electron reduction of molecular oxygen [1]. Since that time, much interest has centered on the various biological sources of the radical, as well as its involvement as a cytotoxic agent in a number of pathophysiological circumstances including oxygen toxicity, radiation injury, phagocyte-mediated inflammation, and, most recently, postischemic tissue injury [2–5]. A number of different sources of superoxide have been identified and studied, such as the NADPH oxidase of phagocytes and the nonenzymatic leakage of electrons to oxygen from certain carriers in the electron-transport system of the mitochondria [2]. Ironically, not much attention has been given to the first-described biological source of the radical: the enzyme xanthine oxidase. The reason for this is clear. In vivo, the enzyme has been shown to exist as an NAD^+-reducing dehydrogenase, not as the superoxide-producing oxidase [6]. During the course of purification of xanthine dehydrogenases from a variety of sources, the enzymes are typically observed to convert spontaneously to xanthine oxidases. This has been shown to be the result of attack by proteases released during the homogenization of tissue or by the oxidation of sulfhydryl groups within the enzyme. Thus, while the phenomenon of protease-catalyzed dehydrogenase-to-oxidase conversion has been known for some time [7], there had been no evidence that the conversion could occur in intact cells under physiological or pathological conditions.

In recent studies of intestinal ischemia, however, we have found that xanthine dehydrogenase rapidly converts in the non-perfused ileum to the radical-producing xanthine oxidase [8,9]. The conversion appears to be the result of limited proteolysis, perhaps triggered by an influx of calcium into the energy-starved cell. Furthermore, we found that essentially all the postischemic tissue injury resulting from 30 min [4] or 3 hr [5] of partial ischemia in the feline ileum could be attributed to superoxide production in the reoxygenated tissue. This conclusion was based on the observations that dramatic protection was provided by pretreatment of the animals with either superoxide dismutase, to enzymatically scavenge superoxide free radicals, or allopurinol [4-hydroxypyrazolo (3,4-d)pyrimidine], a specific inhibitor of xanthine oxidase that would prevent the formation of the free radicals in the reperfused tissues.

It has been known for some time that ischemic tissues accumulate hypoxanthine, a substrate for xanthine oxidase, from the catabolic breakdown of ATP due to oxygen starvation [10]. We have now shown that xanthine dehydrogenase is likewise converted to the oxygen-reducing xanthine oxidase during ischemia [8,9]. That is, during the period of low blood flow, a new enzyme activity, xanthine oxidase, appears. Concomitantly, and for altogether independent reasons, one of the two necessary substrates for that enzyme appears. The second substrate, molecular oxygen, is supplied when the tissue is reperfused. At that point, all the ingredients necessary for the reaction to proceed are present, and a burst of tissue-damaging superoxide production ensues. This scheme of events is diagrammed in Figure 1.

Xanthine dehydrogenase activity is widely distributed among species and among tissues [11]. We have found that the intestinal mucosa not only contains the highest concentration of the enzyme, but also displays the most rapid rate of conversion of the dehydrogenase to oxidase when subjected to nonperfusion [9]. These facts correlate well with the clinically observable extreme sensitivity of the intestinal mucosa to reperfusion injury.

It is of obvious interest to determine whether this free-radical-based mechanism of ischemic injury is peculiar to the intestine or rather represents a general mechanism applicable to many, if not all, tissues. We now report that the conversion of xanthine dehydrogenase to oxidase occurs in the nonperfused rat heart, as well as in the anoxic isolated perfused working rat

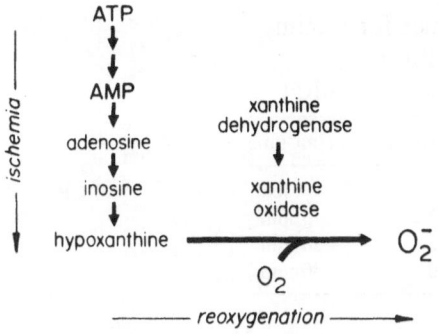

Figure 1. Proposed mechanism for super-oxide production during reperfusion of ischemic tissues.

heart, and that the superoxide produced on reoxygenation appears to be responsible for the tissue damage leading to release of creatine kinase into the perfusate.

METHODS

Xanthine Dehydrogenase-to-Oxidase Conversion

Male Lewis rats were anesthetized with sodium pentobarbital (30 mg/kg, intraperitoneally). The desired tissue was surgically exposed and excised. The tissue was dropped immediately into liquid nitrogen, then homogenized while frozen in ice-cold buffer containing 1 mM phenylmethylsulfonylfluoride (PMSF) (a potent serine protease inhibitor). To determine whether a period of nonperfusion might trigger dehydrogenase-to-oxidase conversion, identical procedures were performed except for the introduction of periods of time varying from 5 sec to 1 hr between the surgical excision of the tissue and freezing it in liquid nitrogen. During these periods, the tissue was completely ischemic. Tissue homogenates were centrifuged at 27,000g for 120 min at 4°C. The supernates were passed through a Sephadex G-25 column prior to assay to remove metabolites that interfere optically with the enzymatic assays. Xanthine oxidase and dehydrogenase activities were determined spectrophotometrically at 37°C by following urate production without added NAD^+ (oxidase activity) and in the presence of NAD^+ (oxidase plus dehydrogenase activity) as described by Stirpe and Della Corte [7]. Formation of uric acid was followed at 295 nm; formation of NADH, at 340 nm.

Isolated Perfused Working Rat Heart Model

Male Wistar rats (220–260 g) were decapitated and hearts were cannulated on a standard working-heart apparatus within 1 min after excision [12]. All hearts were perfused from a reservoir placed 100 cm above the

Table 1.   Half-Times for Decline
of D/O Ratios in Situ in
Nonperfused Tissues of the Rat

Tissue	Units/g protein	Half-time
Intestine	10	4 sec
Heart	0.82	5 min
Liver	0.78	30 min
Kidney	0.40	30 min

aortic cannula, while the left atrium received fluid from an atrial filling vessel maintained at a filling pressure of 13 cm H_2O. When the left atrial cannula was open, there was a net ejection of fluid against the 100-cm aortic pressure head. Coronary flow and aortic pressure under these conditions were 15 ± 1 ml/min and 150 ± 5 cm H_2O, respectively. The standard perfusate was 37°C Krebs–Henseleit buffer gassed with either 95% O_2–5% CO_2 or 95% N_2–5% CO_2 to yield a final pH of 7.4. When appropriate, the buffer was supplemented with 11 mM glucose or 50 μM allopurinol or both. All hearts were paced at 300 beats/min.

To examine the effects of allopurinol on cellular damage resulting from an anoxic insult, hearts obtained from animals pretreated intraperitoneally with 30 mg/kg allopurinol for 4 days were subjected to the following protocol: After being initially perfused for a 15-min stabilization period with buffer containing 11 mM glucose and 50 μM allopurinol, they were abruptly exposed to deoxygenated buffer containing allopurinol, but no substrate. The anoxic, substrate-free perfusion period was maintained for 40 min, at which time the hearts were reoxygenated with the original stabilizing buffer. Perfusate samples were collected at 1-min intervals following reoxygenation and assayed for creatine kinase using a standard procedure [13]. Hearts from untreated control animals underwent the same protocol except that allopurinol was excluded from all buffers.

RESULTS

The conversion of xanthine dehydrogenase to xanthine oxidase in situ in nonperfused tissues of the rat was observed in all tissues except skeletal muscle. The rates of conversion varied dramatically, as shown in Table 1. The data are presented as ratios of dehydrogenase to oxidase activities (D/O) and the half-times reported are the times required for the D/O ratio to decline to a value one half of its original value.

The effects of 40 min of anoxia on the isolated perfused working rat heart are shown in Figure 2. Note that the release of creatine kinase into the perfusate did not commence until the heart was reoxygenated. In sharp

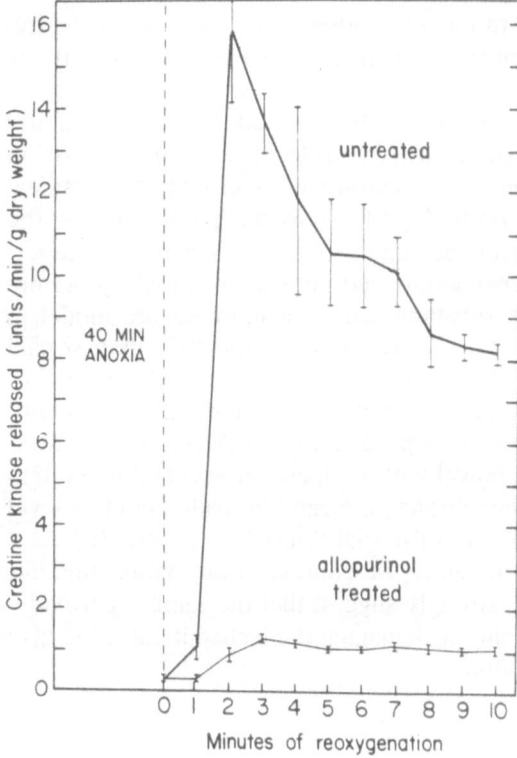

Figure 2. Prevention of creatine kinase release from the reoxygenated myocardium by allopurinol. Hearts were prepared and stabilized as described under "Methods," then perfused for 40 min with a deoxygenated, glucose-free buffer. When oxygen and glucose were reintroduced, perfusate was collected in 1-min fractions and assayed for creatine kinase. Points represent means ± S.E.M. For the control group, $N = 3$; for the allopurinol-treated group, $N = 5$.

contrast, hearts from rats that had been pretreated with the xanthine oxidase inhibitor allopurinol showed almost no release of creatine kinase when subjected to the same regimen of anoxia followed by reperfusion.

DISCUSSION

In 1969, Crowell et al. [14] reported that the drug allopurinol protected against hemorrhagic shock. In 1971, DeWall and co-workers reported that the drug protected against the damage produced by myocardial ischemia [15]. The relative specificity of allopurinol as an inhibitor of xanthine oxidase strongly implicated that enzyme as being somehow responsible for the tissue damage. Further, it was shown that in ischemic tissues, ATP is catabolically but reversibly converted to hypoxanthine, which accumulates in the tissues (see Figure 1) [10]. The conversion of hypoxanthine to xanthine and finally to uric acid by the action of xanthine dehydrogenase or xanthine oxidase is the first irreversible step in this catabolic pathway. Accordingly, these investigators hypothesized that the action of allopurinol might be to block the irreversible loss of the purine pool of the cell, such that when reoxygenation occurred, ATP might be quickly resynthesized from the hypoxanthine. An experiment predicted from this rational hypothesis, however—i.e., the hypothesis that the infusion of hypoxanthine might also ameliorate the effects of hemorrhagic shock—failed to support the hypothesis [14].

Based initially on studies of feline intestinal ischemia, we have offered an alternative hypothesis for the destructive role of xanthine oxidase in ischemic shock: the production of the cytotoxic superoxide free radical [4,5,8,9]. The primary observation that gave rise to our hypothesis was the protection afforded by the intravenous administration of the enzyme superoxide dismutase against the ischemia-induced increase in capillary permeability [4]. The hypothesis was substantiated by a more severe model in which the tissue damage was histologically and morphometrically assessed [5]. In this case, a high degree of protection was obtained with either allopurinol (which prevents superoxide production) or superoxide dismutase (which scavenges the radical after it is produced). Furthermore, the intraluminal perfusion of the normal bowel with a superoxide-generating system was found to increase mucosal membrane permeability to albumin to a level comparable to that produced by 2 hr of partial arterial occlusion [16].

The data presented herein, taken in the context of our earlier findings in studies of intestinal ischemia, strongly suggest that the same superoxide-dependent mechanism responsible for damaging the ischemic intestine also occurs in the ischemic myocardium.

ACKNOWLEDGMENTS

This work was supported in part by Grants 20527 and 00595 from the National Institute of Arthritis, Metabolism and Digestive Diseases.

REFERENCES

1. McCord, J. M., and Fridovich, I. 1968. The reduction of cytochrome c by milk xanthine oxidase. *J. Biol. Chem.* 243:5753–5760.
2. McCord, J. M., and Fridovich, I. 1978. The biology and pathology of oxygen radicals. *Ann. Intern. Med.* 89:122–127.
3. Petrone, W. F., English, D. K., Wong, K., and McCord, J. M. 1980. Free radicals and inflammation: Superoxide-dependent activation of a neutrophil chemotactic factor in plasma. *Proc. Natl. Acad. Sci. U.S.A.* 77:1159–1163.
4. Granger, D. N., Rutili, G., and McCord, J. M. 1981. Superoxide radicals in feline intestinal ischemia. *Gastroenterology* 81:22–29.
5. Parks, D. A., Bulkley, G. B., Granger, D. N., Hamilton, S. R., and McCord, J. M. 1982. Ischemic injury in the cat small intestine: Role of superoxide radicals. *Gastroenterology* 82:9–15.
6. Battelli, M. G., Della Corte, E., and Stirpe, F. 1972. Xanthine oxidase type D (dehydrogenase) in the intestine and other organs of the rat. *Biochem. J.* 126:747–749.
7. Stirpe, F., and Della Corte, E. 1969. The regulation of rat liver xanthine oxidase: Conversion in vitro of the enzyme activity from dehydrogenase (type D) to oxidase (Type O). *J. Biol. Chem.* 244:3855–3863.

8. McCord, J. M., and Roy, R. S. 1982. The pathophysiology of superoxide: Roles in inflammation and ischemia. *Can. J. Physiol. Pharmacol.* 60:1346–1352.

9. Roy, R. S., and McCord, J. M. 1983. Superoxide and ischemia: Conversion of xanthine dehydrogenase to xanthine oxidase. In: R. A. Greenwald and G. Cohen (eds.), *Oxy Radicals and Their Scavenger Systems. Volume II. Cellular and Medical Aspects.* pp. 145–153. Elsevier Science, New York.

10. Jones, C. E., Crowell, J. W., and Smith, E. E. 1968. Significance of increased blood uric acid following extensive hemorrhage. *Am. J. Physiol.* 214:1374–1377.

11. Krenitsky, T. A., Tuttle, J. V., Cattau, E. L., Jr., and Wang, P. 1974. A comparison of the distribution and electron acceptor specificities of xanthine oxidase and aldehyde oxidase. *Comp. Biochem. Physiol.* 49B:687–703.

12. Neely, J. R., Liebermeister, H., Battersby, E. J., and Morgan, H. E. 1967. Effects of pressure development on oxygen consumption by isolated rat heart. *Am. J. Physiol.* 212:804–814.

13. Hughes, B. P. 1962. A method for the estimation of serum creatine kinase and its use in comparing creatine kinase and aldolase activity in normal and pathological sera. *Clin. Chim. Acta* 7:597.

14. Crowell, J. W., Jones, C. E., and Smith, E. E. 1969. Effect of allopurinol on hemorrhagic shock. *Am. J. Physiol.* 216:744–748.

15. DeWall, R. A., Vasko, K. A., Stanley, E. L., and Kezdi, P. 1971. Responses of the ischemic myocardium to allopurinol. *Am. Heart J.* 82:362–370.

16. Grøgaard, B., Parks, D. A., Granger, D. N., McCord, J. M., and Forsberg, J. 1982. Effects of ischemia and superoxide radicals on mucosal albumin clearance in the dog intestine. *Am. J. Physiol.* 5:448–454.

Oxygen Radicals and Tissue Damage in Heart Hypertrophy

Carlo Guarnieri, Claudio Muscari, and Claudio M. Caldarera

Istituto di Chimica Biologica
Centro Studi e Ricerche del Metabolismo del Miocardio
Università di Bologna
40216 Bologna, Italy

Abstract. Cyanide-resistant respiration in heart homogenates supplemented with 1 mM NADH was greater in hypertrophied homogenates (60 days banding) with respect to control homogenates, particularly when the homogenates were incubated in 100% oxygen. The intermyofibrillar mitochondria from hypertrophied hearts produced more superoxide radicals than subsarcolemmal mitochondria, and both values were greater than in the unbanded group. H_2O_2 formation was more evident in the intact mitochondria prepared from hypertrophied hearts than in those of the control hearts. Moreover, the perfusion of isolated hearts in anoxic and reoxygenated conditions caused a greater lipoperoxidative and functional damage at the mitochondrial level in hypertrophied hearts than in the control hearts. These results, correlated with the reduction in mitochondrial function found in the overloaded hearts, suggest an involvement of the reactive species of oxygen in the formation of cardiac damage induced by prolonged aortic banding.

INTRODUCTION

Much experimental evidence suggests that "in vivo" processes can produce superoxide ions ($\cdot O_2^-$) and H_2O_2 as intermediates during the progressive univalent reduction of oxygen [1,2]. These intermediates are reactive, and living cells have evolved different defense mechanisms to protect their integrity [3,4]. The heart muscle, which is an organ very rich in mitochondria because of its intense aerobic metabolism, can be the center of the cellular lesions induced by these reactive species. Thus, the structural and functional alterations measured in rat heart muscle after exposure to hyperoxic conditions [5,6] or to a diet deficient in α-tocopherol [7], or following injection of an inhibitor of the enzyme superoxide dismutase (SOD) which scavenges the $\cdot O_2^-$ radicals [8], or consequent to the administration of anthracyclines [9], can be ascribed to an augmented production of oxygen-mediated cellular reactions. Furthermore, perfusion experiments revealed that during reoxygenation of anoxic isolated hearts [10] or during peroxide infusion [11], the cardiac muscle could be impaired by peroxidative reactions. In this chapter, we have investigated the possibility that rabbit hearts subject to acute pressure overload by aortic banding can become more sensitive to oxidative injury, particularly at the mitochondrial level.

METHODS

Surgical Procedure

Supravalvular aortic stenosis was produced in male New Zealand rabbits weighing 2100–2200 g by constricting the aorta with a silk ligature. This operation was accomplished by placing a silk suture around both the aorta and a Teflon calibrated stick, with subsequent removal of the stick. The reduction of the aortic circumference was 60%. This procedure produced after 30 days a left ventricular hypertrophy with a left ventricular/body weight ratio of 2.74 vs. 1.39 in the control. After 60 days of banding, the ratio was 3.27, and occasionally a congestive syndrome characterized by ascites and pleural effusion was also observed.

Tissue Preparation

Heart homogenates were prepared in ice-cold 50 mM KH_2PO_4, pH 7.4. Connective-tissue debris was removed by centrifugation at 3000g for 10 min, and the supernatants were diluted with phosphate buffer. Oxygen consumption was measured polarographically at 25°C using a 1.5-ml water-jacketed cell (Gilson, France) fitted with a Clark oxygen probe.

Mitochondrial Isolation

The mitochondria were prepared from heart muscle according to the method of Williams and Barrie [12]. In some experiments, two populations of heart mitochondria were used. They were isolated using Polytron homogenization (subsarcolemmal mitochondria) and limited Nagarse exposure (intermyofibrillar mitochondria) as described by McMillin-Wood et al. [13]. Electron-microscopic morphology revealed a comparable picture in both rabbit mitochondria populations (results not shown).

Preparation of Submitochondrial Particles

The final mitochondrial pellets were suspended in 2 mM EDTA, pH 8.5 (10 mg protein/ml), and then sonicated at 40 W using a Labsonic Sonifier. The suspensions were centrifuged at 6000g for 10 min, and the sediments were discarded. The particles were separated from the supernatants by spinning at 105,000g for 30 min. The submitochondrial particle pellets were suspended in 250 mM sucrose–10 mM Tris buffer, pH 7.4, centrifuged at 105,000g for 30 min, and resuspended in the same buffer.

Table 1.   Oxygen Consumption of Heart Homogenates Saturated with 21% O_2 (Air) or with 100% O_2 following NADH and KCN Addition[a]

Group	Addition	21% O_2	100% O_2
Control	NADH	26.4 ± 4.6	62.5 ± 6.8
	KCN	0.27 ± 0.06	2.9 ± 1.2
Hypertrophied	NADH	30.8 ± 5.8[b]	76.5 ± 8.4[b]
	KCN	0.34 ± 0.09	9.2 ± 1.9[c]

[a] The heart homogenates were equilibrated with 21% O_2 (air) or with 100% O_2. Oxygen consumption was measured following addition of 1 mM NADH. This measure was repeated after addition of 1 mM KCN. Oxygen consumption represents natoms·min^{-1}·mg $protein^{-1}$. Results are given as means ± S.D. of four experiments.
[b] $p < 0.05$, significantly different from control.   [c] $p < 0.01$.

Biochemical Measurements

Superoxide production by submitochondrial particles was measured by the SOD-inhibitable reduction of succinoyl-cytochrome c according to Kuthan et al. [14]. Cytochrome c reduction was monitored in a double-beam Perkin Elmer (Model 559) spectrophotometer at 550 nm ($E = 20.1$ mM^{-1}·cm^{-1}). Mitochondrial generation of H_2O_2 was quantitated according to Loschen et al. [15] by determining the changes in the fluorescence of reduced scopoletin induced by H_2O_2 in the presence of horseradish peroxidase. Lipid peroxidation was measured by the formation of thiobarbituric-acid-positive material [16]. Protein was estimated by the method of Bradford [17] using bovine serum albumin as standard.

RESULTS

Total and Cyanide-Resistant Respiration of Heart Homogenates

Table 1 shows that the oxygen consumption of control and hypertrophied rabbit heart homogenates supplemented with 1 mM NADH was 26.4 and 35.8 natoms 0/min per mg protein, respectively. These values increased in both control and hypertrophied homogenates when assayed at 100% O_2 saturation. In addition, in response to hyperoxic conditions, the cyanide-resistant respiration of the homogenates particularly increased in the homogenates of the hypertrophied heart.

Superoxide Production by Submitochondrial Particles

The addition of succinate to submitochondrial particles supplemented with succinoylated cytochrome c and antimycin brought about $\cdot O_2^-$ radical formation at rates of 1.98 and 2.60 nmoles/min per mg protein in the subsarcolemmal and intermyofibrillar mitochondria, respectively (Table 2). SOD was able to inhibit cytochrome c reduction, indicating $\cdot O_2^-$ involve-

194   Carlo Guarnieri et al.

Table 2. Production of $\cdot O_2^-$ Radicals in Succinate-Supplemented Rabbit Heart Submitochondrial Particles[a]

Group	Subsarcolemmal		Intermyofibrillar	
	$\cdot O_2^-$ (nmoles/ min·mg prot.)	RCI	$\cdot O_2^-$ (nmoles/ min·mg prot.)	RCI
Control	1.98 ± 0.06	14.0 ± 1.4	2.60 ± 0.05	14.2 ± 1.9
Hypertrophied				
30 Days	2.01 ± 0.4	12.4 ± 2.8	3.01 ± 0.08[b,d]	11.8 ± 2.2[b]
60 Days	2.60 ± 0.04[c]	10.8 ± 1.2[c]	4.28 ± 0.11[c,e]	9.7 ± 1.4[c,d]

[a] The reaction mixture contained 0.2 mg of submitochondrial particles suspended in a 70 mM sucrose buffer containing 50 mM HEPES, pH 7.8, 6 mM succinate, 1 μM antimycin. The reaction was started by the addition of 10 μM succinoylated cytochrome c, which was prepared according to Kuthan et al. [14]. The respiratory control index (RCI) was determined in the intact mitochondria suspended in 250 mM sucrose, pH 7.4, 3 mM KH_2PO_4, 0.5 mM EDTA, 5 mM glutamate. ADP (500 nmoles) was added to obtain State 3 respiration. Results are given as means ± S.D. of six experiments.
[b] $p < 0.05$. [c] $p < 0.01$, significantly different from control.
[d] $p < 0.05$. [e] $p < 0.01$, significantly different from subsarcolemmal mitochondria.

ment. In the subsarcolemmal mitochondria prepared from the banded hearts, there was an increase in the rate of $\cdot O_2^-$ production only after 60 days following the surgical constriction. At 30 days after aortic stenosis, the $\cdot O_2^-$ generation by submitochondrial particles of the intermyofibrillar mitochondria had already augmented. During the following 30 days, the rate of cytochrome c reduction further increased 64% above the corresponding control value. Moreover, the intermyofibrillar mitochondria showed a mitochondrial activity judged by the respiratory control index that decreased inversely with the rate of $\cdot O_2^-$ production; this behavior was less evident in the subsarcolemmal mitochondria (Table 2).

H_2O_2 Production by Mitochondria

Table 3 shows that with the increase in the aortic stenosis period, the H_2O_2 generation from isolated mitochondria increased from an initial rate of 1.85 nmoles/min per mg protein in control hearts to a rate of 2.2 in the hearts banded for 30 days. In the following 30 days, the succinate-induced H_2O_2 production further increased, reaching a rate of 3.4 nmoles/min per mg protein. In the presence of ADP (State 3 respiration), the mitochondria prepared after 60 days of aortic stenosis were able to generate H_2O_2 (0.4 nmole/min per mg protein), and this was contrary to the mitochondria from hearts banded for 30 days and from controls (Table 3).

Experiments with Perfused Hearts

Table 4 shows the mitochondrial function evaluated in mitochondria prepared from control and hypertrophied rabbit hearts after perfusion in anoxia

Table 3.   Formation of H_2O_2 in Rabbit Cardiac Mitochondria in Control and Hypertrophied Hearts

Group	Addition	H_2O_2 (nmoles/min·mg protein)
Control	Succinate	1.85 ± 0.34
	Succinate + ADP	N.D.
Hypertrophied	Succinate	2.20 ± 0.48
30 Days	Succinate + ADP	N.D.
60 Days	Succinate	3.4 ± 0.89^b
	Succinate + ADP	0.4 ± 0.1

[a] Results are given as means $\pm$ S.D. of six experiments. (N.D.) Not detectable.
[b] $p < 0.01$, significantly different from control.

and reoxygenation. The anoxic perfusion caused a reduction of the respiratory control index, and this was more evident in the hypertrophied mitochondria. The reoxygenation further lowered mitochondrial activity, particularly in the hypertrophied perfused hearts. Table 4 also shows that the formation of lipid peroxidation was greater in the mitochondria extracted from hypertrophied–reoxygenated hearts than in those from corresponding control hearts.

DISCUSSION

In this chapter, we provide evidence that hypertrophied rabbit heart muscle shows an augmented ability to produce $\cdot O_2^-$ radicals and H_2O_2 in comparison to control heart muscle. This result was revealed from the

Table 4.   Effects of Hypoxia and Reoxygenation on Succinate-Induced Mitochondrial Respiratory Control Index (RCI) and on Mitochondrial Lipid Peroxidation[a]

Group	Perfusion condition	RCI	TBA-positive material (nmoles/mg protein)
Control	50 min O_2	3.6 ± 0.1	1.18 ± 0.08
Hypertrophied	50 min O_2	3.3 ± 0.2	1.61 ± 0.10
Control	50 min N_2	2.8 ± 0.2^b	1.42 ± 0.07
Hypertrophied	50 min N_2	$2.5 \pm 0.2^{b,c}$	1.38 ± 0.10
Control	30 min N_2 + 20 min O_2	2.4 ± 0.4^b	$2.08 \pm 0.06^{c,d}$
Hypertrophied	30 min N_2 + 20 min O_2	$2.0 \pm 0.6^{c,d}$	$3.98 \pm 0.08^{c,e}$

[a] Hypertrophy was induced by constricting the aorta for 60 days as described in "Methods." The mitochondrial function was measured by using 5 mM succinate as substrate (see Table 2). The hearts were perfused in anoxia and reoxygenated as described elsewhere [10]. Results are given $\pm$ S.D. of four experiments. (TBA) thiobarbituric acid.
[b] $p < 0.05$.   [c] $p < 0.01$, significantly different from 50-min aerobic control.
[d] $p < 0.05$.   [e] $p < 0.01$, significantly different from 50-min aerobic hypertrophied.

greater value of the cyanide-resistant rate of oxygen consumption, an indirect measure of cellular $\cdot O_2^-$ and H_2O_2 production [18], determined in the homogenates of hypertrophied hearts with respect to control heart homogenates. This event was evident, however, only when the homogenates were equilibrated with 100% O_2 in a condition of high oxygen utilization.

From the data reported, it appears that the mitochondria may essentially contribute to $\cdot O_2^-$ and H_2O_2 production. The rate of $\cdot O_2^-$ generation was detected using submitochondrial particles washed free of contaminating SOD.

In this experimental condition, it appears that submitochondrial particles from hypertrophied hearts produced $\cdot O_2^-$ radicals at higher rates, particularly after the more prolonged period of aortic stenosis. Moreover, this elevated production was more evident in the population of intermyofibrillar mitochondria in comparison to the subsarcolemmal mitochondria population. In this respect, it is interesting to note that concomitant with the augmented value of $\cdot O_2^-$ production, a most severe impairment in mitochondrial function was measured in the intermyofibrillar mitochondria after prolonged hypertrophy. In the rat, the two populations of cardiac muscle mitochondria differ not only in cell location, but also in certain biochemical properties [19,20]. The intermyofibrillar mitochondria oxidize substrates 1.5 times faster than the subsarcolemmal mitochondria. This study shows that in control rabbit hearts, the respiratory control index was similar in the Polytron- and Nagarse-prepared mitochondria when glutamate was used as substrate. In contrast long-term hypertrophy seems able to induce a significant difference in mitochondrial function between the two populations of heart mitochondria by reducing particularly the intermyofibrillar respiratory capacity. This result coincides with the observation of Hoppel et al. [21] that State 3 ADP-stimulated respiration was significantly decreased in the intermyofibrillar mitochondria from cardiomyopathic hearts compared to the subsarcolemmal mitochondria. It has been well documented that heart mitochondria can produce $\cdot O_2^-$ radicals accounting for about 1–2% of the mitochondrial oxygen uptake under physiological conditions. Generation of $\cdot O_2^-$ radicals by mitochondria is greatest when the respiratory-chain carriers located on the inner mitochondrial membrane are highly reduced [22]. Endogenous factors that influence mitochondrial radical formation can be the availability of NAD-linked substrates, succinate, ADP, and oxygen [23,24]. Also, heart mitochondria from old rats [25] or from rats exposed to hyperoxia [6] are able to generate greater amounts of $\cdot O_2^-$ radicals. The mechanism or mechanisms reponsible for the augmented production of $\cdot O_2^-$ by mitochondria of hypertrophied hearts are not known. Since in the last phase of developing hypertrophy a severe alteration of the mitochondrial size and morphology has been described [26,27], it is possible that such a modification associated with some metabolic alteration may stimulate the formation of $\cdot O_2^-$ by mitochondrial membranes. In particular, the data of Moravec et al. [28] describing a reduced ability to oxidize NADH, which was not related to oxygen availability, by mitochondria prepared from hearts of rats exposed to severe aortic constriction indicate a metabolic condition that may strongly accentuate mitochondrial $\cdot O_2^-$ radical formation. Accumulation of mitochondrial $\cdot O_2^-$ radicals can be responsible for an augmented production H_2O_2 resulting from the activities of mitochondrial SOD. Our experiments show that in the extramitochondrial space of hypertrophied muscle, there is an increased flux of H_2O_2 from the mitochondria, and this event can be considered dangerous because H_2O_2 can participate with $\cdot O_2^-$ in the formation of the most toxic radical, $\cdot OH$ [29]. Moreover, H_2O_2 inactivation causes a consumption of intracellular GSH by glutathione peroxidase activity [30], and this process, by producing a modification of the GSH/GSSG ratio, can modify the redox state of the cells. For all these reasons, it is expected that hypertrophied hearts should be more sensitive to the damage induced by oxidative stress. The experiments carried out by exposing anoxic perfused hearts to reoxygenation seem to confirm this hypothesis. The hypertrophied hearts are more damaged by the oxidative stress, as shown by a remarkable increase in the mitochondrial lipid peroxidation breakdown. Furthermore, the mitochondrial function of the hypertrophied heart muscle is more injured by the oxidative stress. In conclusion, our results suggest that in the hypertrophied heart muscle, particularly in the late stage of its development, there is an accentuated production of $\cdot O_2^-$ radicals, especially at the mitochondrial level. This event could be linked to the mitochondrial damage produced in heart muscle by prolonged pressure overload or in isolated hypertrophied hearts by reoxygenated perfusions.

ACKNOWLEDGMENTS

The authors thank Dr. C. Cecconi, S. Curello, and C. Ventura for their excellent technical assistance and Miss A. Zarri for her careful secretarial support. Special thanks are due Dr. C. Schallop for his competent assistance. This work was supported by Grant 82.00894.04 from the CNR and by the Ministero Pubblica Istruzione, Rome (Italy).

REFERENCES

1. Halliwell, B. 1978. Biochemical mechanism accounting for the toxic action of oxygen on living organisms: The key role of superoxide dismutase. *Cell Biol. Int. Rep.* 2:113–128.
2. Freeman, B. A., and Crapo, J. D. 1982. Biology of disease-free radicals and tissue injury. *Lab. Invest.* 47:412–426.
3. Fridovich, I. 1975. Superoxide dismutase. *Annu. Rev. Biochem.* 44:147–159.
4. Forman, H. J., and Fisher, A. B. 1982. Antioxidant defenses. In: D. L. Gilbert (ed.), *Oxygen and Living Processes: An Interdisciplinary Approach.* pp. 235–248. Springer-Verlag, New York.
5. Hughson, M., Balentine, J. D., and Daniell, H. B. 1977. The ultrastructural pathology of hyperbaric oxygen exposure: Observations on the heart. *Lab. Invest.* 37:516–525.

6. Nohl, H., Hegner, D., and Summer, K. H. 1981. The mechanism of toxic action of hyperbaric oxygenation on the mitochondria of rat heart cells. *Biochem. Pharmacol.* 30:1753–1757.

7. Guarnieri, C., Ferrari, R., Visioli, O., Caldarera, C. M., and Nayler, W. G. 1978. Effect of α-tocopherol on hypoxic perfused and reoxygenated rabbit heart muscle. *J. Mol. Cell. Cardiol.* 10:893–906.

8. Guarnieri, C., Flamigni, F., Ventura C., and Rossoni Caldarera, C. 1981. Inhibition of rat heart superoxide dismutase activity by diethyldithiocarbamate and its effect on mitochondrial function. *Biochem. Pharmacol.* 30:2174–2176.

9. Doroshow, J. H. 1983. Effect of anthracycline antibiotics on oxygen radical formation in rat heart. *Canc. Res.* 43:460–472.

10. Guarnieri, C., Flamigni, F., and Caldarera, C. M. 1980. Role of oxygen in the cellular damage induced by re-oxygenation of hypoxic heart. *J. Mol. Cell. Cardiol.* 12:797–808.

11. Shattock, M. J., Manning, A. S., and Hearse, D. J. 1982. Effects of hydrogen peroxide on cardiac function and post-ischaemic functional recovery in the isolated working rat heart. *Pharmacology* 24:118–122.

12. Williams, A. J., and Barrie, S. E. 1978. Temperature effects on the kinetics of calcium transport by cardiac mitochondria. *Biochem. Biophys. Res. Commun.* 84:89–93.

13. McMillin-Wood, J., Wolkowiez, P. E., Chu, A., Tate, C. A., Goldstein, M. A., and Entman, M. L. 1980. Calcium uptake by two preparations of mitochondria from heart. *Biochim. Biophys. Acta* 591:251–265.

14. Kuthan, H., Ullrich, V., and Estabrook, R. W. 1982. A quantitative test for superoxide radicals produced in biological systems. *Biochem. J.* 203:551–558.

15. Loschen, G., Flohé, L., and Chance, B. 1971. Respiratory chain linked H_2O_2 production in pigeon heart mitochondrial. *FEBS Lett.* 18:261–264.

16. Ohkawa, H., Ohishi, N., and Yagi, K. 1979. Assay for lipid peroxides in animal tissues by the thiobarbituric acid reaction. *Anal. Biochem.* 95:351–358.

17. Bradford, M. M. 1976. A rapid and sensitive method for the quantitation of microgram quantities of protein utilizing the principle of protein-dye binding. *Anal. Biochem.* 72:246–254.

18. Hassan, H. M., and Fridovich, I. 1979. Regulation of the synthesis of superoxide dismutase in *Escherichia coli. J. Biol. Chem.* 252:7667–7672.

19. Palmer, J. W., Tandler, B., and Hoppel, C. L. 1977. Biochemical properties of subsarcolemmal and interfibrillar mitochondria isolated from rat cardiac muscle. *J. Biol. Chem.* 252:8731–8739.

20. Wolkowiez, P. E., and McMillin-Wood, I. 1980. Respiration dependent calcium ion uptake by two preparations of cardiac mitochondria. *Biochem. J.* 186:257–266.

21. Hoppel, C. L., Tandler, B., Parland, W., Turkaly, J. S., and Albers, L. D. 1982. Hamster cardiomyopathy: A defect in oxidative phosphorylation in the cardiac interfibrillar mitochondria. *J. Biol. Chem.* 257:1540–1548.

22. Turrens, J. F., Freeman, B. A., Levitt, J. C., and Crapo, J. D. 1982. The effect of hyperoxia on superoxide production by lung submitochondrial particles. *Arch. Biochem. Biophys.* 217:401–410.

23. Loschen, G., Azzi, A., and Flohé, L. 1973. Mitochondrial H_2O_2 formation: Relationship with energy conservation. *FEBS Lett.* 33:84–88.

24. Freeman, B. A., and Crapo, J. D. 1981. Hyperoxia increases oxygen radical production in rat lungs and lung mitochondria. *J. Biol. Chem.* 256:10,986–10,992.

25. Nohl, H., and Hegner, D. 1978. Do mitochondria produce oxygen radicals *in vivo*? *Eur. J. Biochem.* 82:563–567.

26. Rabinowitz, M., and Zack, R. 1975. Mitochondria and cardiac hypertrophy. *Circ. Res.* 36:367–376.

27. Wikman-Coffelt, J., Parmley, W. W., and Mason, D. T. 1979. The cardiac hypertrophy process. *Circ. Res.* 45:697–707.

28. Moravec, J., Renault, G., and Hatt, P. Y. 1978. Alterations of mitochondrial function as detected in left ventricular myocardium of rats with acute aortic constriction. *Basic Res. Cardiol.* 73:535–550.
29. Nohl, H., Jordan, W., and Hegner, D. 1982. Mitochondrial formation of OH· radicals by an ubisemiquinone-dependent reaction: An alternative pathway to the iron-catalysed Haber–Weiss cycle. *Hoppe-Seyler's Z. Physiol. Chem.* 363:599–607.
30. Paglia, D. E., and Valentine, W. N. 1967. Studies on the quantitative and qualitative characterization of erythrocyte glutathione peroxidase. *J. Lab. Clin. Med.* 70:158–169.

Disturbances of the Heart Structure and Function in Chronic Hemolytic Anemia, Their Compensation with Increased Coronary Flow, and Their Prevention with Ionol, an Inhibitor of Lipid Peroxidation

F. Z. Meerson and M. E. Evsevieva

Institute of General Pathology and Pathological Physiology of the USSR AMS
Laboratory of Heart Pathophysiology
Moscow 121552, USSR

Abstract. The structure and function of heart muscle were studied in rats with chronic hemolytic anemia induced by phenylhydrazine. Contractural lesions, myocytolysis, fatty dystrophy, and small-focal necrosis were found in the myocardium along with hypertrophy. The disturbances were accompanied by a compensatory increase in the coronary flow by 2.5-fold during myocardial contractions. When the coronary flow of isolated hearts was experimentally decreased to the control level, a great depression of the contractile function developed. Administration of the antioxidant ionol, an inhibitor of lipid peroxidation, simultaneously with phenylhydrazine did not prevent the development of the hemolytic anemia, but decreased by 2 times the degree of hypertrophy and the amount of the lesion foci in the heart muscle. It also significantly inhibited the compensatory increase of coronary flow and completely eliminated depression of the heart contractile function during the normalization of coronary flow. The data allow a suggestion that hemolytic anemia is accompanied by activated lipid peroxidation, this process playing a role in the myocardial damage of anemia. Antioxidants can prevent such damage.

INTRODUCTION

Patients with different hemolytic anemias may have damage of the heart muscle structures [4,10,17] and may develop cardiac insufficiency [13,18]. The mechanism by which myocardial damage remains compensated, the pathogenesis of the damage, and, finally, possible ways of its prevention have been unclear up to now. It has been established that chronic anemia regularly resulted in accumulation of lipofuscin, a final product of lipid peroxidation (LP) in animal myocardium [14] and different human organs [6]; simultaneously, there was a significant increase of coronary flow [2,11]. It is also known that iron-containing products of erythrocyte degradation excessively formed in hemolytic anemia are powerful LP inductors [3]. On this basis, three postulates may be made: First, LP activation may play a role in the structural damage and functional disturbance in the heart muscle dur-

201

ing hemolytic anemia. Second, the increased coronary flow may be an important factor in the compensation of this damage. Third, administration of antioxidants is a possible measure that can prevent anemic damage of the myocardium. The discussed work herein is aimed at verifying these suggestions by a detailed study of disturbances of heart structure, function, and coronary flow in animals with hemolytic anemia and at investigating the therapeutic possibilities of the synthetic antioxidant ionol (4-methyl-2,6-di-t-butylphenol).

METHODS

All experiments were performed on male Wistar rats weighing 200–300 g. Animals intended for the morphological study (39 rats) were divided into four series: I, control; II, hemolytic anemia; III, ionol; IV, ionol + hemolytic anemia. Anemia was induced by an aqueous solution of phenlyhydrazine hydrochloride injected subcutaneously every second day in a dose of 70 mg/kg [8]. With such a dosage of phenylhydrazine, the blood hemoglobin dropped from 16–17 to 6–7% within 12 hr of the first injection and was kept depressed to this level by repeated injections of the drug. Control animals and animals with hemolytic anemia were injected with ionol in a dose of 20 mg/kg intraperitoneally daily for 5 days before the phenylhydrazine injections and for 28 days during the injections. Animals were decapitated and the hearts were extracted at the 28th day after the appearance of anemia. After fixation in 10% neutral formalin, pieces of the myocardium were embedded in paraffin or cut in a freezing microtome with subsequent staining with Sudan [7]. Paraffin sections were stained with hematoxylin–eosin, picrofuchsin, asocarmin according to Heidengein–Selye–Pearls, and with the periodic acid–Schiff (PAS) reaction. Polarization microscopy was used to study the contractile apparatus of cardiomyocytes [12]. To estimate focal damage of the myocardium quantitatively, a combined ocular network for stereometric studies [1] was used to count the number of fuchsinophilous foci in which contractural changes were found by polarization microscopy. To obtain exact data, we measured some 100 squares of the network (1000 points). The results were expressed as percentages of the total number of network points. In the recent literature, this index is designated as volumetric density of the myocardial focal lesions [7].

Physiological experiments were carried out on 44 rats in five series: I, control; II, ionol; III, hemolytic anemia; IV, hemolytic anemia with subsequent normalization of the coronary flow; V, ionol + hemolytic anemia with subsequent normalization of the coronary flow. Cardiac contractile function was studied according to the method of Fallen et al. [5] in a modification that has previously been described in detail [9].

The right auricle was removed, and a latex bulb with a constant volume was placed into the cavity of the left ventricle. The heart performed isovolumetric contractions, pressing this bulb. Contractions at a given rate were paced by an ESL-1 electrostimulator. The pressure in the latex bulb was measured with a Mingograph-34 "Elema" electromanometer. The developed and diastolic pressures and maximal velocities of the pressure development and fall were estimated. The hearts were perfused with Krebs–Henseleit solution through the aorta at 37°C and at a pressure of 600 mm Hg. The solution was oxygenized with a gas mixture containing 5% CO_2 + 95% O_2. The coronary flow was estimated by collecting and measuring the amount of the perfusing solution passing through the coronary bed per time unit. After 60 min of perfusion under normal oxygenation, the oxygenized and glucose-containing Krebs–Henseleit solution was replaced by a nonoxy-genized, glucose-free one. This hypoxic condition was maintained for 20 min and was followed by reoxygenation. In series IV and V, this experimental scheme was changed to take account of the increased coronary flow that occurred during hemolytic anemia. After estimation of cardiac contractile function under spontaneous coronary flow, the perfusion pressure in the aorta was decreased to a level at which the coronary flow in the hearts of animals with anemia was equal to that in the hearts of control animals. Left ventricular contractile function was then estimated under normalized cor-onary flow, and only then was hypoxia with subsequent reoxygenation car-ried out. At all stages of the experiment, the following indices were calcu-lated: developed pressure in mm Hg, velocities of the pressure development and fall in mm Hg, and the intensity of the structure functioning, an index equal to the product of developed tension and the contraction frequency per mass of the left ventricle in milligrams (mm Hg/mg · min).

RESULTS AND DISCUSSION

Figure 1 shows that ionol resulted in some increase in the growth rate of control rats and significantly prevented loss of body mass in rats with hemolytic anemia. The hatched zone characterizes quantitatively the posi-tive effect of ionol. Simultaneously, the antioxidant almost halved the death rate of animals during the 28 days of phenylhydrazine injections (Figure 1B). The wet weight of the ventricles increased by 27.9% during the anemia. This was due to true myocardial hypertrophy because the dry mass of the heart ventricles was also increased by 27%. Ionol reduced the degree of myocar-dial hypertrophy. The ventricular wet mass was increased by only 14.5% in these rats.

In the microscopic study, the myocardium of animals with hemolytic anemia showed Ist–IIIrd degree cardiomyocyte damage of the contractural type [16] (Figure 2A), myocytolysis, vacuolization, and special lesions des-ignated as "central globular decay." These last lesions were characterized by a dark zone of degenerated myofibrils in the center of the fibre, while normally cross-striated myofibrils were preserved in the periphery of the

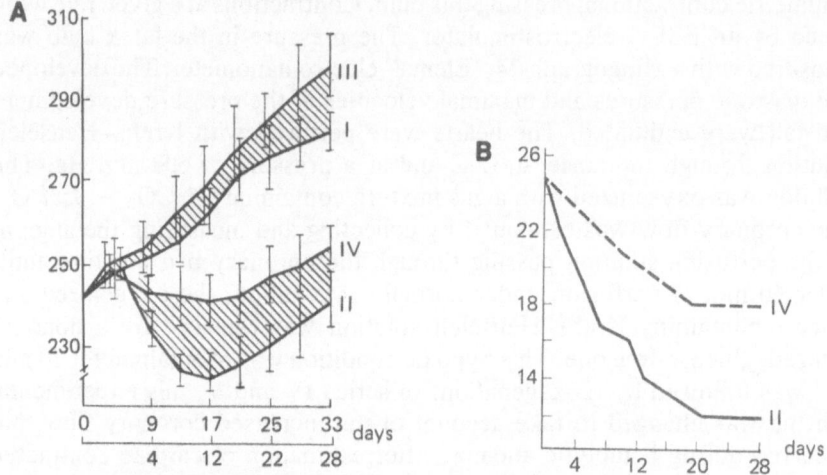

Figure 1.   (A) Effect of ionol on the growth rate of rats with hemolytic anemia. *Upper abscissa:* time from the moment of ionol injection (days); *lower abscissa:* time from the moment of phenylhydrazine injection (days); *ordinate:* body mass (g). (I) Control; (II) anemia; (III) ionol; (IV) ionol + anemia. (B) Effect of ionol on the death rate of rats with hemolytic anemia. *Abscissa:* time from the day of phenylhydrazine injection (days); ordinate: number of animals. Other designations as in (A).

fiber (Figure 2C). The substances of the dark zone lacked anisotropic properties (Figure 2A). In staining after Selye, diffusely distributed foci of fucsinophilous degeneration were seen all through the thickness of the left ventricular myocardium (Figure 2E). Here and there, groups of dead cells were seen.

All these changes were less pronounced or were absent in animals that received antioxidant. The amount of myocardial contractural lesions was significantly less (Figure 2B). Correspondingly, the foci of fucsinophilous degeneration were less widespread (Figure 2F). The phenomena of fatty infiltration and "central globular decay" were absent; many muscle fibers preserved their normal structure (Figure 2D). The data obtained during the counting of focal lesions (Table 1) showed that the volume of myocardium occupied by focal lesions was as little as 2.2 ± 0.10% and 2.1 ± 0.09% in animals injected and not injected with ionol, respectively. In anemia, this value increased 10-fold, reaching 23.2 ± 0.61%. In anemic animals receiving ionol, this value was reduced to 12.6 ± 0.34%. Thus, ionol administration prevented the appearance of half the contractural lesions that usually develop in chronic hemolytic anemia.

The results of physiological studies are presented in Table 2. In hearts of animals with hemolytic anemia, the coronary flow was increased by 2.5 times as compared to the controls at the identical perfusion pressure in the aorta (75 cm H_2O). Under these conditions, the pressure developed by the

Table 1.   Effect of Ionol on the Amount of Myocardial Focal Lesions in Rats with Hemolytic Anemia

Index series	I (control) (N = 10)	II (anemia) (N = 9)	III (ionol) (N = 10)	IV (ionol + anemia) (N = 10)
Amount of myocardial focal lesions [volumetric density of the focal lesions (%)]	2.1 ± 0.09	23.3 ± 0.61	2.2 ± 0.10	12.6 ± 0.34

Significance: $P_{I-II} < 0.001$; $P_{II-IV} < 0.001$.

left ventricle of animals with hemolytic anemia did not differ significantly from that in the controls. The velocities of contraction and relaxation were decreased by one-third and the intensity of the structure functioning (ISF) by 25%. The latter shift was due to left ventricular hypertrophy; the increase in the left ventricular wet weight was approximately the same as the ISF decrease. Myocardial hypertrophy and an increased coronary flow in anemia are well-known events [2,11,15]. Because of the increased coronary flow, disturbances of cardiac contractile function are relatively small in anemic animals, and this explains why a stable compensation without cardiac insufficiency took place in our animals.

The hearts of animals with hemolytic anemia were substantially more resistant to hypoxia then the hearts of control animals. Table 2 shows that at the 20th min of hypoxia, the developed tension and velocities of contraction and relaxation of the anemic animal hearts were approximately 1.5-fold more than those in controls. Thus, under the conditions of spontaneously increased coronary flow, the hearts of animals with hemolytic anemia were characterized by a relatively small depression of the contractile function and an increased resistance to hypoxia.

If the increased coronary flow in hearts of animals with hemolytic anemia was reduced to the level characteristic of that in controls, i.e., from 24.3 to 8.8 ml/min (series IV), a catastrophic depression of the contractile function developed. Developed pressure was reduced by one third; ISF and velocity of contraction, by 40%. The velocity of relaxation was decreased most of all—by approximately 2 times. Moreover, the normalization of the coronary flow in the hearts of anemic rats resulted in the fact that their resistance to hypoxia was not only not increased, but was even reduced as compared to the control level. The values of ISF and velocities of contraction and relaxation under hypoxia were approximately 1.5 times less than in control animals. Thus, increased coronary flow in anemic animals [11], in addition

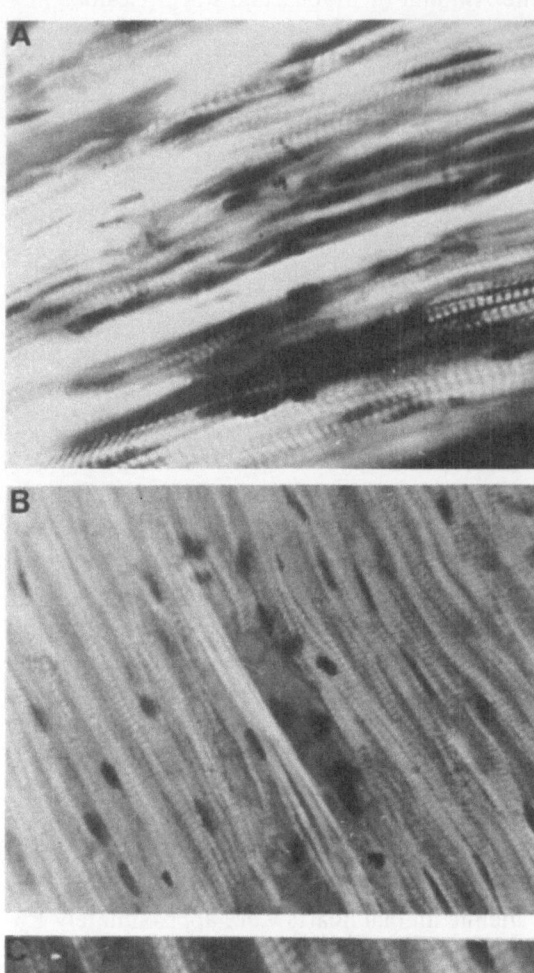

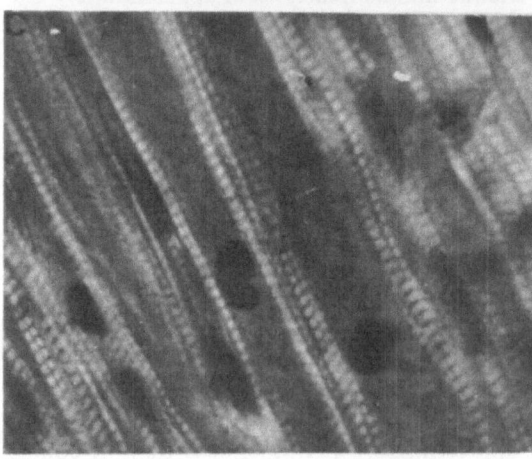

Figure 2.   Effect of ionol on the myocardium of rats with hemolytic anemia. (A, C, E) Anemia; (B, D, F) ionol + anemia. (A) Numerous and (B) single contractures of muscle fibers. PAS reaction, polarized light, ×250. (C) "Central globular decay" and (D) muscle fibers with intact normal structure.   Hematoxylin–eosin, ×600. (E) Numerous and (F) single foci of fucsinophilous degeneration of the myocardium. (Cross section, stained after the Selye method, ×210.

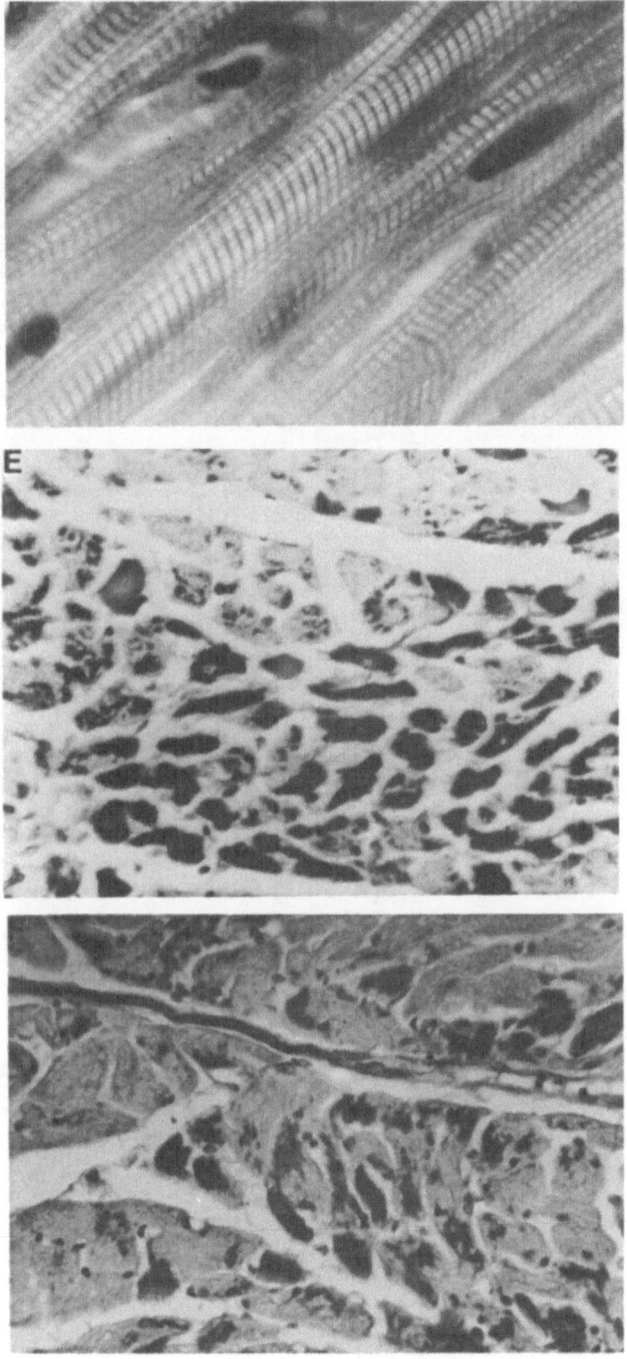

Figure 2.   (*Continued*)

Table 2. Disturbances of the Contractile Function of Isolated Hearts of Rats with Hemolytic Anemia under Spontaneous and Normalized Coronary Flow and Prevention of These Disturbances with the Antioxidant Ionol

Indices	Series (N)	Spontaneous coronary flow	Normalized coronary flow	Hypoxia (20 min)	Reoxygenation (5 min)
Coronary flow (ml/min)	1. Control (14)	9.0–0.4	8.9–0.5	6.4–0.3	8.6–1.2
	2. Ionol–control (7)	10.1–0.5	10.3–0.3	8.8–0.2	9.5–0.7
	3. Anemia (7)	23.1–1.1	23.0–0.8	21.4–2.2	23.3–2.0
	4. Anemia with subsequent normalization of the coronary flow (3)	24.3–1.2	8.8–0.4	6.2–0.2	8.3–1.2
	5. Ionol–anemia with subsequent normalization of the coronary flow (8)	16.2–1.5[b]	8.6–0.3	8.1–0.3	9.2–0.6
Developed tension (mm Hg)	1. Control	104.3–8.7	102.3–8.3	28.4–2.8	81.4–2.6
	2. Ionol–control	105.4–4.2	106.4–0.3	34.8–4.1	87.1–3.3
	3. Anemia	96.8–7.0	95.6–6.0	46.0–4.5	79.0–6.5
	4. Anemia with subsequent normalization of the coronary flow	102.5–5.0	66.4–2.1	23.0–4.1	62.8–3.1
	5. Ionol–anemia with subsequent normalization of the coronary flow	98.5–6.3	93.6–5.3	32.0–3.2	80.1–4.7

Intensity of the structure functioning (mm Hg/mg min)				
1. Control	19.6–1.5	19.5–0.9	5.4–0.8	14.9–1.8
2. Ionol–control	19.2–0.9	19.1–0.7	6.1–0.1	15.4–0.9
3. Anemia	13.5–1.2	13.6–0.9	6.4–1.0	11.8–2.0
4. Anemia with subsequent normalization of the coronary flow	15.2–1.1	9.8–0.8		9.3–0.8
5. Ionol–anemia with subsequent normalization of the coronary flow	15.4–1.6	14.3–0.9^b	4.9–0	12.9–1.2
Velocity of contraction (mm Hg/sec)				
1. Control	2250–147	2245–123	575–47	172
2. Ionol–control	2541–151	2640–140	680–58	1910–181
3. Anemia	1525–100	1574–493	837–81	1775–250
4. Anemia with subsequent normalization of the coronary flow	1640–132	970–86	311–41	920–78
5. Ionol–anemia with subsequent normalization of the coronary flow	1810–151	1776–141^a	553–70	1890–62
Velocity of relaxation (mm Hg/sec)				
1. Control	1557–98	1552–75	311–30	768–80
2. Ionol–control	1748–109	1762–100	390–25	870–74
3. Anemia	1125–50	1136–50	500–62	775–85
4. Anemia with subsequent normalization of the coronary flow	1040–82	540–38	201–24	495–51
5. Ionol–anemia with subsequent normalization of the coronary flow	1240–101	1133–75	303–49	890–68

^{a,b} Significance of differences of data in anemia with subsequent normalization of the coronary flow (series 4). ^{a} $P < 0.05$. ^{b} $P < 0.01$.

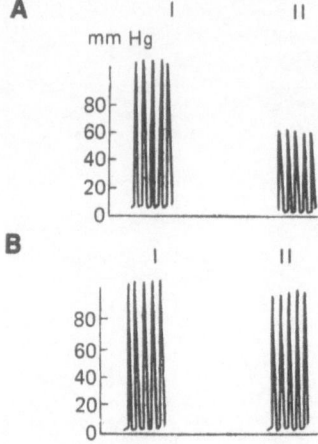

Figure 3.   Effect of normalization of the coronary flow of pressure developed by the heart left ventricle in animals pretreated with ionol. (A) Normalization of the coronary flow in hearts of animals with hemolytic anemia; (B) normalization of the coronary flow in hearts of animals with hemolytic anemia treated with ionol. (I) Spontaneous coronary flow; (II) normalized coronary flow.

to reducing myocardial damage, prevented the depression of the contractile function and increased the resistance of the heart to hypoxia.

The data in Table 2 also show that ionol administration had no effect on cardiac contractile function and coronary flow in control animals and had no significant effect on contractile function in animals with hemolytic anemia under spontaneously increased coronary flow. On the other hand, this LP inhibitor had three important positive effects in the hearts of anemic animals: First, it supported almost normal contractile function of the anemic animal hearts with an increase in spontaneous coronary flow of only 80%, instead of 250%. Second, the hearts of ionol-pretreated anemic animals showed no depression of contractile function when the coronary flow was reduced to the control level. This situation is illustrated by comparison of the curves in Figure 3A and 3B. Third, preliminary administration of ionol eliminated the decrease in resistance to hypoxia observed in the myocardium of animals with hemolytic anemia under normalizing coronary flow.

The physiological effects of ionol may be explained by the morphological data. It would seem that anemia causes myocardial damage, but that this can be compensated for by an increase in coronary blood flow. Ionol prevents the damage and thus reduces the compensatory increase in coronary flow. At the same time, ionol prevents the deleterious effects of hypoxia that are found in the hearts of anemic animals when the coronary flow is reduced to normal.

The results of our experiments indicate that lipid peroxidation plays an important role in the pathogenesis of myocardial damage in anemia and that antioxidants may be valuable in protecting the heart in anemia.

REFERENCES

1. Avtandilov, G. G. 1972. Ocular measuring network for cyto-, histo- and stereometric investigations. *Arkh. Patol.* (6):76–77.

2. Bhatia, M. L., Manchanda, S. C., and Roy, S. B. 1969. Coronary haemodynamic studies in chronic severe anemia. *Br. Heart J.* 31:365–374.
3. Carrel, R. W., Winterbourn, C. C., and Rachmilwitk, J. 1975. Activated oxygen and haemolysis. *Br. J. Haemotol.* 30:259–264.
4. Davydovsky, I. V. 1969. *General Pathology of Human.* Meditzina, Moscow.
5. Fallen, E., Elliot, W., and Yortin, R. 1967. Apparatus for study of ventricular function and metabolism in the isolated perfused rat heart. *J. Appl. Physiol.* 22:836–839.
6. Hyman, C. B., Landing, B., Aefin-Slater, R., Kozak, L., Weitzman, J., Ortega, J. A. 1974. dl-α-Tocopherol, iron and lipofuscin in thalassemia. *Ann. N. Y. Acad. Sci.* 232:211–220.
7. Kaktursky, L. V. 1979. Relation of focal myocardial lesions and coronary atherosclerosis in sudden death. *Arkh. Patol.* 1979(2):10–14.
8. Katekhelidze, M. G. 1979. Experimental anemia. In: B. V. Petrovsky (ed.), *Bolshaya Meditzinskaya Entziklopedia*, 3rd ed. Vol. 1, pp. 523–524, Sovetskaga entziklopedia, Moscow.
9. Meerson, F. Z., and Ustinova, E. E. 1982. Prevention of the heart stress-induced damage and its hypoxic contracture with natural antioxidant α-tocopherol. *Kardiologiya* 1982(7):89–93.
10. Rubber, S., and Fluscher, S. A. 1967. Sickle cell states and cardiomyopathy: Sudden death due to pulmonary thrombosis and infarction. *Am. J. Cardiol.* 19:867–873.
11. Scheel, K. W., Brady, D. A., Ingram, L. A., Keller, F. 1976. Effect of chronic anemia on the coronary and coronary collateral musculature in dogs. *Circ. Res.* 38:553–559.
12. Semenova, L. A., and Tzellarius, Yu. G. 1978. Ultrastructure of the heart muscle cells in focal metabolic damages. Nauka, Novosibirsk.
13. Srivastava, S. C., and Gupta, R. R. 1980. Effect of chronic severe anemia on left ventricular performance. *Jpn. Heart J.* 21:657–663.
14. Sulkin, N. M., and Srivanija, P. 1960. The experimental production of senile pigments on the nerve cell of young rats. *J. Gerontol.* 15:2–7.
15. Swann, J. W., Joseph, F., and Contrera, P. 1976. Depletion of cardiac norepinephrine during two forms of hemolytic anemia in the rat. *Circ. Res.* 38:179–184.
16. Tzellarius, Yu. G., Semenova, L. A., and Nepomnyazhikh, L. M. 1979. Pathologoanatomic diagnosis of pre-necrotic changes and myocardial infarction by polarization microscopy: Methodological recommendations. Sovetskaya Sibir, Moscow.
17. Uszay, N. K. 1964. Cardiovascular findings in patients with sickle cell anemia. *Am. J. Cardiol.* 13:320–329.
18. Zaino, E. C. 1980. Pathophysiology of thalassemia. *Ann. N. Y. Acad. Sci.* 344:284–304.

STRUCTURAL COMPONENTS OF THE
MYOCYTE AND ITS MATRIX

The Role of Actin-Binding Proteins Vinculin, Filamin, and Fibronectin in Intracellular and Intercellular Linkages in Cardiac Muscle

Victor E. Koteliansky, Vladimir P. Shirinsky,
Gennady N. Gneushev, and Michail A. Chernousov

USSR Cardiology Research Center
Academy of Medical Sciences
Moscow 121552, USSR

Abstract. The localization in cardiac muscle and the biochemical properties of fibronectin, filamin, and vinculin were studied. Fibronectin was localized between cardiomyocytes. Filamin was identified in the Z-line region of sarcomeres and in the intercalated disks of heart muscle. Vinculin was found to be present in intercalated disks and near the plasma membrane at the cell periphery between external myofibrils and sarcolemma. It was suggested that fibronectin, filamin, and vinculin play an important role in intercellular and intracellular linkages in cardiac muscle.

An important question in the study of the molecular basis of cardiac muscle functions is how various cellular and subcellular components of the heart are linked. The remarkable constancy of the topography of the various subcellular components suggests the existence of different intracellular and intercellular linkages in the heart muscle (Figure 1).

Cardiac muscle cells contact each other side by side. They also form end-to-end contacts in the regions of intercalated disks that represent complex cell-surface specializations. Within a muscle fiber, actin filaments are anchored to the Z-line and to the plasma membrane. .

Three proteins—fibronectin, filamin, and vinculin—play an important role in the formation and maintenance of these linkages. The properties and localization of these proteins in cardiac muscle will be described below.

Fibronectin is a major extracellular matrix protein [1]. We used monospecific antifibronectin antibodies to localize fibronectin in rat heart sections by indirect immunofluorescence (Figure 2). Cardiac muscle contains fibronectin between the muscle cells. Fibronectin is mainly concentrated around the surfaces of blood vessels and capillaries.

The schematic model for protein interactions in cell–cell contact regions shows how fibronectin could be involved in this process (Figure 3) [1]. According to the model, fibronectin acts as a ligand, connecting the cell to the extracellular matrix. Elongated, multidomain, and dimeric fibronectin

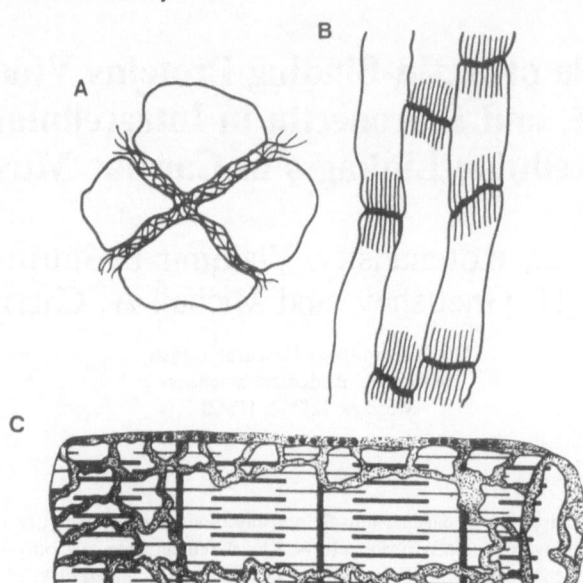

Figure 1. Intracellular and intercellular linkages in the heart muscle. (A) Side-to-side interaction of cardiac-muscle cells; (B) end-to-end contacts of cardiomyocytes in intercalated disk
regions; (C) anchoring of cardiac myofibril actin filaments to Z-lines of sarcomeres.

molecules interact through their N-terminal domains with collagen and
through other binding sites with proteoglycan and with the cells. The
model also shows one possible form of transmembrane interaction between
fibronectin and actin filaments, involving a transmembrane fibronectin
receptor.

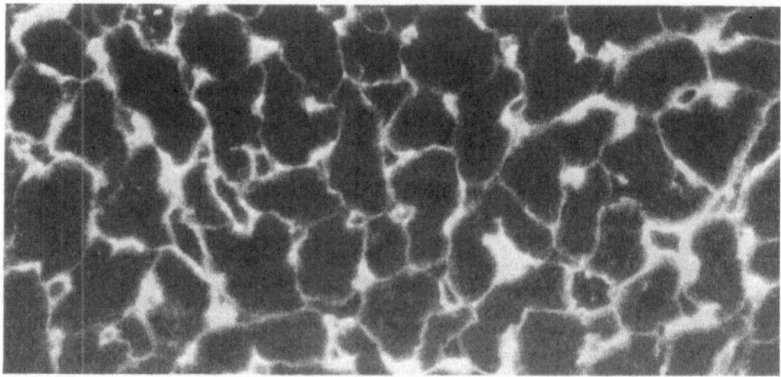

Figure 2.   Localization of fibronectin in cardiac muscle frozen sections by indirect immunofluorescence.

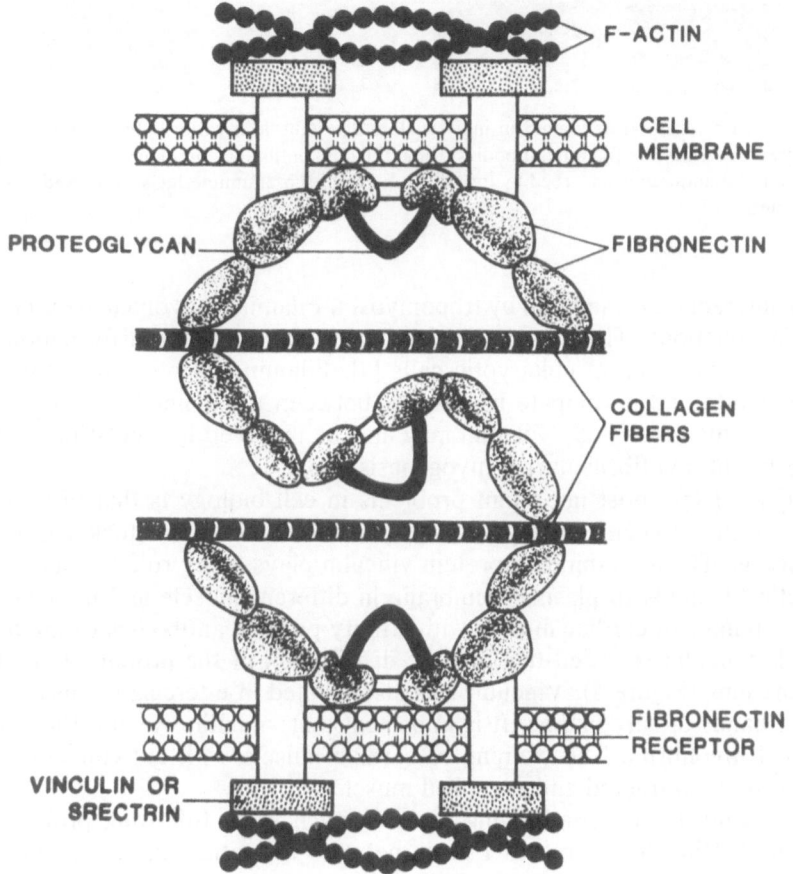

F-ACTIN

CELL
MEMBRANE

PROTEOGLYCAN

FIBRONECTIN

COLLAGEN
FIBERS

FIBRONECTIN
RECEPTOR

VINCULIN OR
SRECTRIN

Figure 3.   Schematic model for protein interactions in cell–cell contact regions.

The myofibrillar Z-line serves as the anchor point for the lattice of actin filaments in a sarcomere. It is responsible for transmitting the forces generated within one sarcomere to other sarcomeres. The Z-line also provides a structural framework on which the actin-filament lattice can be organized. These roles have led to an extensive investigation of the morphology and ultrastructure of the Z-line and its molecular components.

A few proteins have been identified as components of the Z-line: α-actinin, desmin, and actin [2]. Recently, we have identified a new actin-binding protein, filamin, in heart muscle [3]. Immunofluorescence analysis of individual cardiac-muscle myofibrils (Figure 4) shows that filamin is located in one specific region corresponding to the Z-line revealed on phase micrographs (not shown). Filamin was also found to be present in intercalated disk regions between cardiomyocytes.

Filamin has the following properties (Table 1): It induces F-actin gelation and bundling. Filamin accelerates actin polymerization. F-actin–fi-

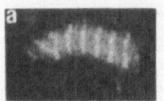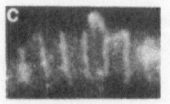

Figure 4. Localization of filamin in individual cardiac-muscle myofibrils by indirect immunofluorescence. (a) Antifilamin antibodies; (b) antifilamin antibodies preincubated with excess of filamin; (c) antibodies adsorbed by myosin and actin; (d) preimmune IgGs were used as first antibodies.

lamin interaction is inhibited by tropomyosin. Filamin is involved in different cellular functions. The most important function is sol–gel transformation of cytoplasm in different eukaryotic cells [4]. Filamin can regulate actin polymerization and participate in linkages between the Z-line of sarcomeres and actin filaments [3,5]. Filamin may also be involved in regulation of the assembly of myofibrils during myogenesis [6].

One of the most important problems in cell biology is that of understanding the molecular mechanism of plasma membrane–cytoskeleton interactions. The actin-binding protein vinculin plays a key role in anchoring of actin filaments to plasma membrane in different muscle and nonmuscle cells. Staining of cardiac muscle with affinity-purified antibodies to smooth-muscle vinculin revealed the periodic distribution of the protein along the cell margins (Figure 5). Vinculin was also located in intercalated disks and near I-bands of sarcomeres. It is important that vinculin was not found on internal myofibrils. The staining of cardiac muscle with antivinculin was identical in contracted and stretched muscles.

Vinculin is an actin-binding protein and has the following properties (Table 2): Vinculin decreases F-actin network formation and the actin polymerization rate [7,8]. It was shown that vinculin stimulates the lateral interactions between F-actin filaments and increases the critical concentration of cross-linking proteins required for F-actin gelation [9]. The most important protein function is anchoring of F-actin at specific membrane sites [10]. Vinculin can regulate the gelation of cytoplasm and participate in linkages between cytoskeleton and extracellular matrix. Phosphorylation of vin-

Table 1.   Properties and Possible Functions of Filamin

Properties	Possible functions
A component of cardiac-muscle myofibrils; located in the Z-line region and intercalated disks.	Plays an important role in sol–gel transformation of cytoplasm. Can regulate actin polymerization.
Induces F-actin gelation and bundling.	
Accelerates actin polymerization.	Participates in linkages between sarcomeres and F-actin filaments.
F-actin–filamin interaction is inhibited by tropomyosin.	May regulate the assembly of the myofibril substructure during myogenesis.

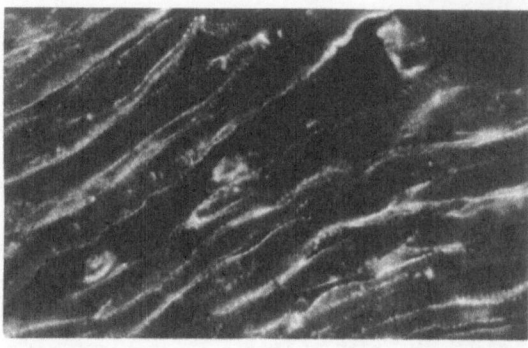

Figure 5. Localization of vinculin in cardiac muscle by indirect immunofluorescence.

culin is under *sarc* gene control and may be important in regulation of cell morphology [11].

Our results and some literature data suggest that in cardiac muscle, vinculin plays an important role in association between contractile apparatus and membranes of sarcolemma [12]. Vinculin is the only nonmembrane component shown to link sarcolemma and myofibrils [12,13]. This means that sarcolemma membranes do not simply cover the myofibrils, but are physically connected with the underlying myofibrils through the periodically distributed structures containing vinculin. These vinculin-containing structures were called "costameres" [13]. The existence of the costameres suggests that sarcolemma being linked with external myofibrils may move during muscle contraction. This movement can be important for regulation of the contraction process.

Figure 6 represents a schematic model for protein interactions in intercalated disk regions of heart muscle cells. At present, six proteins are identified as components of intercalated disks: actin, filamin, α-actinin, vinculin, desmin, and desmoplakin. F-actin cross-linking proteins α-actinin and

Table 2.   Properties and Possible Functions of Vinculin

Properties	Possible functions
In cardiac muscle, present in intercalated disks and between external myofibrils and sarcolemma (periodically over I-bands).	Participates in anchoring of F-actin at specific membrane sites.
Decreases F-actin network formation.	Can regulate the gelation of cytoplasm.
Decreases actin polymerization rate.	May participate in linkages between cytoskeleton and extracellular matrix.
May stimulate the lateral interactions between F-actin filaments.	Phosphorylation of vinculin may be important in control of cell morphology.
Increases the critical concentrations of cross-linking proteins required for F-actin gelation.	

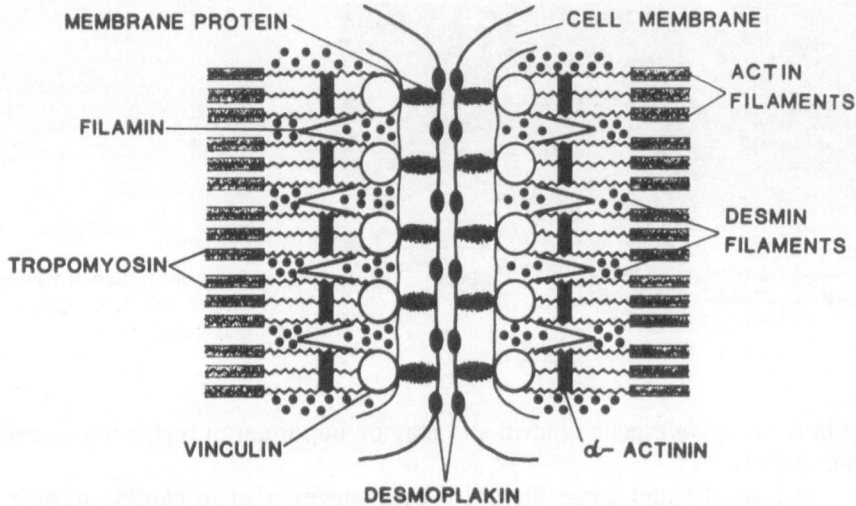

Figure 6.   Schematic model for protein interactions in intercalated disk regions of heart-muscle cells.

filamin induce formation of actin-filament bundles. These bundles are connected to the plasma membrane through vinculin, which is closely associated with the membrane through a hypothetical membrane protein. The ends of actin filaments are free of tropomyosin, probably because of inhibition by filamin and α-actinin of tropomyosin–F-actin interaction [14,15]. A new protein, desmoplakin, is located on membrane external surfaces [16]. It was suggested that desmoplakin is involved in cell–cell contact.

It can be seen that intracellular and intercellular linkages in cardiac muscle are characterized by great complexity. Such complexity raises many questions: How do muscle cells construct their specific cytoarchitecture? Is there a common mechanism of control over spatial order? These questions are likely to provide a fertile field for research in the next few years.

REFERENCES

1. Hynes, R. O., and Yamada, K. M. 1982. Fibronectin multifunctional modular glycoproteins. *J. Cell Biol.* 95:369–377.
2. Granger, B. L., and Lazarides, E. 1979. Desmin and vimentin coexist at the periphery of the myofibril Z-disc. *Cell* 18:1053–1063.
3. Koteliansky, V. E., Glukhova, M. A., Shirinsky, V. P., Babaev, V. R., Kondalenko, V. F., Rucosuev, V. S., and Smirnov, V. N. 1981. Identification of a filamin-like protein in chicken heart muscle. *FEBS Lett.* 125:44–48.
4. Stossel, T. P. 1978. Contractile proteins in cell structure and function. *Annu. Rev. Med.* 29:427–457.

5. Koteliansky, V. E., Shirinsky, V. P., Gneushev, G. N., and Smirnov, V. N. 1982. Filamin, a high relative molecular mass actin-binding protein from smooth muscles, promotes actin polymerization. *FEBS Lett.* 136:98–100.

6. Gomer, R. H., and Lazarides, E. 1981. The synthesis and deployment of filamin in chicken skeletal muscle. *Cell.* 23:524–532.

7. Jokusch, B. M., and Isenberg, G. 1981. Interaction of α-actinin and vinculin with actin: Opposite effects on filament network formation. *Proc. Nat. Acad. Sci. U.S.A.* 78:3005–3009.

8. Wilkins, A., and Lin, S. 1982. High affinity interaction of vinculin with actin filaments in vitro. *Cell* 28:83–90.

9. Koteliansky, V. E., Gneushev, G. N., Shartava, A. S., Shirinsky, V. P., Glukhova, M. A., and Goodman, S. R. 1983. The regulation by vinculin of filamin, α-actinin and spectrin tetramer-induced actin sol–gel transformation. *FEBS Lett.* 151:206–210.

10. Gieger, B. 1982. Involvement of vinculin in contact-induced cytoskeletal interactions. *Cold Spring Harbor Symp. Quant. Biol.* 46:671–682.

11. Sefton, B. M., Hunter, T., Ball, E. H., and Singer, S. J. 1982. Vinculin: A cytoskeletal target of the transformation protein of Rous sarcoma virus. *Cell.* 24:165–174.

12. Koteliansky, V. E., and Gneushev, G. N. 1983. Vinculin localization in cardiac muscle. *FEBS Lett.* 159:158–160.

13. Pardo, J. V., D'Angelo Siliciano, J., and Graig, S. W. 1983. A vinculin-containing cortical lattice in skeletal muscle: Transverse lattice elements ("costamers") mark sites of attachments between myofibrils and sarcolemma. *Proc. Nat. Acad. Sci. U.S.A.* 80:1008–1012.

14. Zeece, M. G., Robson, R. M., and Bechtel, P. J. 1979. Interaction of α-actinin, filamin and tropomyosin with F-actin. *Biochim. Biophys. Acta* 581:365–370.

15. Koteliansky, V. E., Shirinsky, V. P., Glukhova, M. A., Nowak, E., and Dabrowska, R. 1983. The effect of non-muscle tropomyosin on the interaction of filamin with F-actin. *FEBS Lett.* 155:85–87.

16. Franke, W. W., Moll, R., Mueller, H., Schmid, E., Kuhn, C., Krepler, R., Artlieb, U., and Denk, H. 1983. Immunochemical identification of epithelium-derived human tumors with antibodies to desmosomal plaque proteins. *Proc. Nat. Acad. Sci. U.S.A.* 80:543–547.

Intercellular Junctions and the Cardiac Intercalated Disk

N. J. Severs

Department of Cardiac Medicine
Cardiothoracic Institute (University of London)
London W1N 2DX, England

Abstract. Cardiac muscle cells are equipped with three distinct types of intercellular junction—gap junctions, "spot" desmosomes, and "sheet" desmosomes (or fasciae adherentes)—located in a specialized portion of the plasma membrane, the intercalated disk. Gap junctions are responsible for electrical coupling and the transfer of small molecules between cells, whereas the desmosomelike junctions (also known as adherens junctions) provide strong intercellular adhesion. The adhesion sites formed by the "spot" desmosome anchor the intermediate-filament cytoskeleton of the cell; those formed by the fascia adherens anchor the contractile apparatus. An understanding of the ultrastructure of these junctions helps explain how they carry out their functions, and new observations in this field have been made through the application of ultrarapid freezing techniques in conjunction with freeze–fracture electron microscopy. With recent findings from biochemical and immunocytochemical studies, this understanding is now being extended to the molecular level.

INTRODUCTION

Cardiac muscle cells are richly endowed with intercellular junctions. Three distinct types of junction are present—the gap junction (nexus), the "spot" desmosome, and the "sheet" desmosome (fascia adherens). These junctions are not scattered at random over the plasma membrane surface, but are confined to a specialized portion of this surface, the intercalated disk. Within the intercalated disk itself, the pattern of junction distribution is highly specific. To appreciate this pattern, we need to look first at the three-dimensional geometry of the intercalated disk as a whole.

STRUCTURE OF THE INTERCALATED DISK

Intercalated disks are found where the plasma membranes of adjacent cardiac myocytes come into close contact, usually at or near the ends of neighboring cells. Each disk is thus comprised of two apposed plasma membranes and their associated intracellular and extracellular structures. Unlike the smoothly contoured lateral borders of the cells, the membranes at the disk often show highly irregular profiles when viewed in thin-section electron

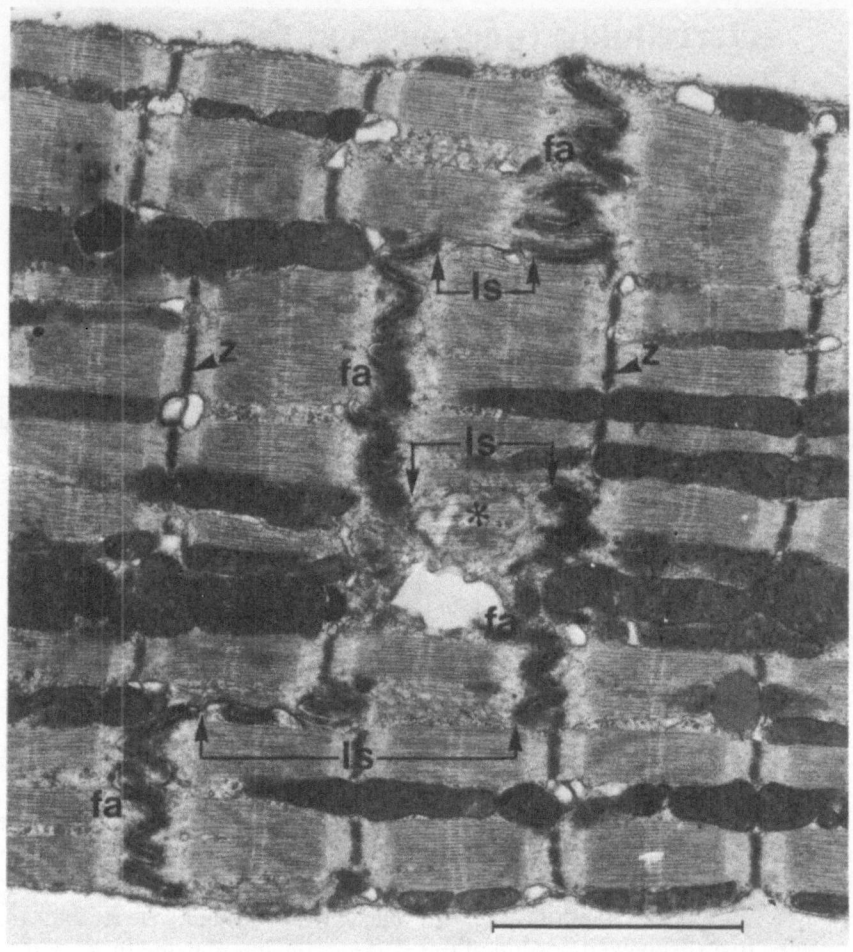

Figure 1.   Thin-section electron micrograph of an intercalated disk between two rabbit cardiac muscle cells. The wavy transverse portions of the disc are rendered especially conspicuous by the electron-dense "filamentous mat" of the fasciae adherentes (fa). The longitudinal segments (ls), by contrast, are more difficult to discern, particularly where the membrane has been sectioned tangentially (*) rather than transversely. (Z) Z-line. Scale bar: 2 μm.

micrographs. This tends to disguise an overall simplicity of design that becomes apparent only when sections are taken in a precise longitudinal plane as in Figure 1. Here it can be seen that individual or grouped bundles of myofilaments terminate at transverse plicate portions of the plasma membrane, always in a position at which their next Z-line would be predicted. However, not all myofilament bundles terminate in register, side by side; instead, they may continue for one, two, or more sarcomeres beyond their neighbors. The transverse portions of membrane are linked to one another by straight longitudinal segments, thus giving the disk as a whole the appearance of a series of irregular steps.

Looking at a survey freeze–fracture micrograph (Figure 2) helps us translate this image into three dimensions. The freeze–fracture technique* splits membranes along their hydrophobic cores, creating extensive en face views which at low magnification reveal with dramatic perspective cellular organization within tissue samples. Exceptionally favorable fractures may travel along both the longitudinal and transverse areas of the same intercalated disk without leaving the membrane. When this happens, it becomes clear that the longitudinal segments seen in thin section represent dorsal, lateral, and ventral surfaces of the myocyte body. In contrast to these smooth surfaces, the transverse membrane bordering the ends of the myofilament bundles appears covered with short, stubby projections. Referring back to the thin-section image in Figure 1, it can be seen that these projections form zones of close interdigitation between adjacent membranes of the disk.

DISTRIBUTION OF INTERCELLULAR JUNCTIONS IN THE INTERCALATED DISK

A schematic view of the pattern of intercellular junction distribution within the intercalated disk is shown in Figure 3. Gap junctions occur predominantly on the smooth longitudinal areas of membrane, where they are often revealed in abundance by freeze–fracture (Figure 4).Fasciae adherentes, by contrast, are found exclusively on the transverse interdigitating portions of the disk (Figure 1). Desmosomes are common over the longitudinal areas, but are also sometimes found associated with fasciae adherentes in the transverse regions.

CLASSIFICATION AND IDENTIFICATION OF INTERCELLULAR JUNCTIONS

The different types of intercellular junction are known by a variety of names, and this can lead to confusion. Cardiac gap junctions, for example, are sometimes erroneously referred to as "tight junctions," and the term "desmosome" may be used both collectively for all adhesive junctions and specifically for the "spot" desmosome. A classification of intercellular junctions is therefore given for reference in Table 1, and their key features of distinction are summarized in Figure 5.

---

* In this technique, specimens are frozen and fractured. A fine platinum–carbon replica is made of the surface exposed by the fracture plane. The specimen is then thawed and digested to release the replica for mounting and examination in the transmission electron microscope.

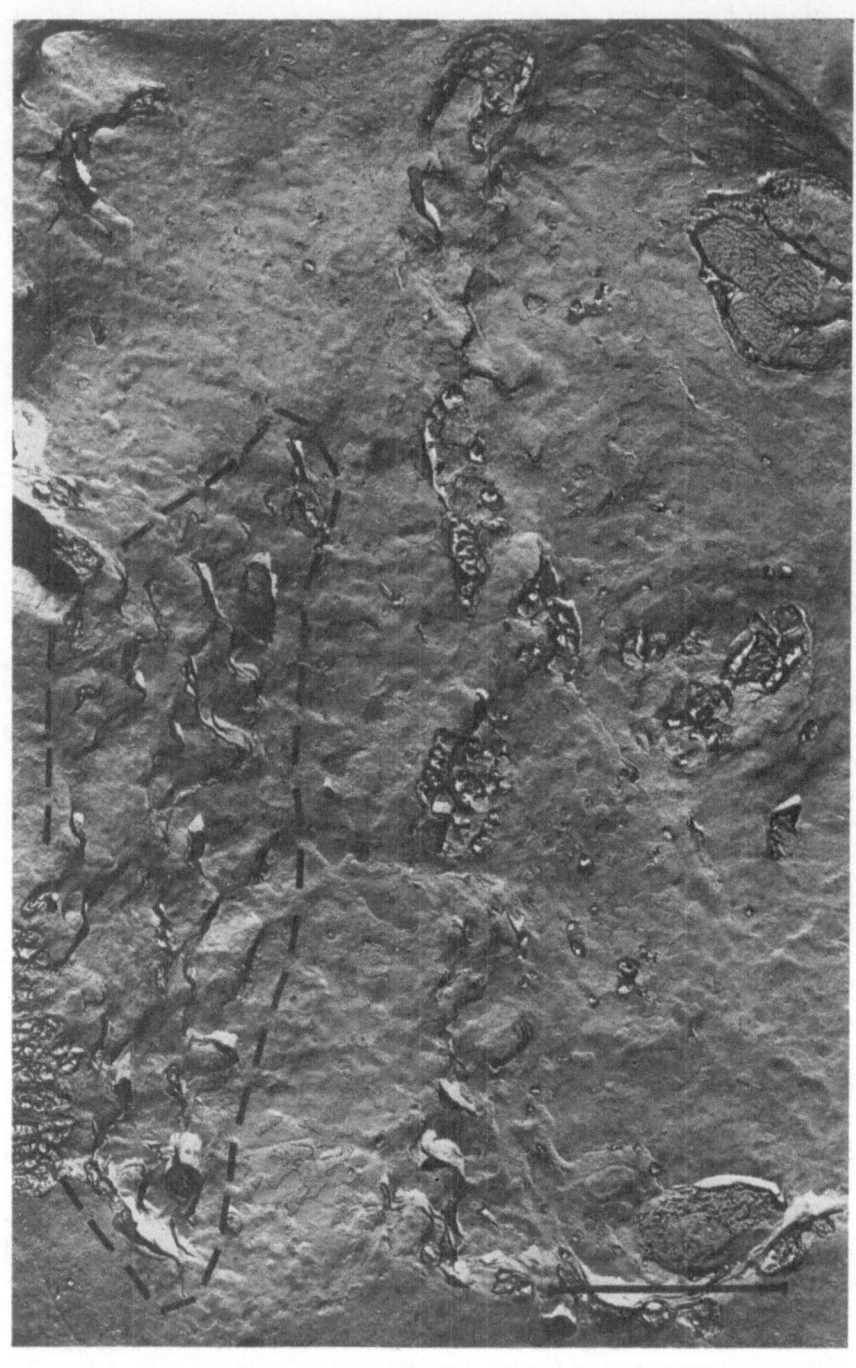

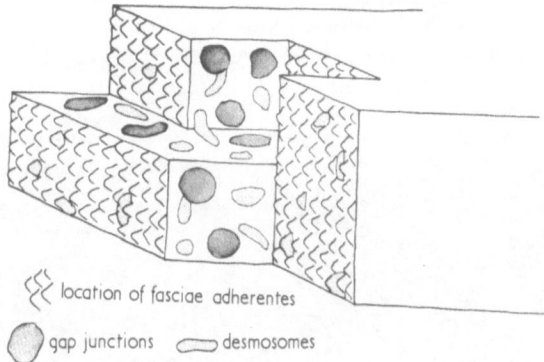

location of fasciae adherentes

gap junctions   desmosomes

Figure 3.   Stylized diagram of the intercalated disk and the characteristic distribution of the different types of intercellular junction within it. Individual fasciae adherentes are not depicted, since information on their size and shape is incomplete.

In this chapter, the intercellular junctions of the heart will be referred to by the terms that are most widely used by cell biologists at present, namely, *gap junction*, *desmosome*, and *fascia adherens*. An illustrated description of the structural components of these junctions will be presented from the functional viewpoint, and particular mention will be made of recent ultrastructural results obtained by myself and my colleagues in this field. Brief reference will also be made to recent biochemical and immunocytochemical findings, especially where these can be correlated with ultrastructurally identifiable components. For further comprehensive information on the structure and function of intercellular junctions in general, the reader is referred to the reviews by McNutt and Weinstein [1] and Staehelin [2].

Gap Junctions

Gap junctions link neighboring cytoplasmic compartments and form low-resistance pathways along which the action potential can spread from one cell to the next [3,4]. To fulfill these functions, the plasma membranes at the gap junction are closely apposed [Figure 6 (inset)], leaving an intercellular gap of only 2 nm. Each junctional membrane contains a collection of integral proteins (connexons) (Figure 6) that project into this gap, meeting halfway across it (Figure 7). When gap junctions are split by freeze–fracture, the connexons remain firmly attached to the protoplasmic membrane-half,

←————————————————————————————————————

Figure 2.   Freeze–fracture electron micrograph illustrating the gross morphology of the intercalated disk. The smooth lateral regions of the disk membrane are seen in face-on view, whereas the transverse regions (example outlined by black dashes) are approximately vertical with respect to the plane of the image. Note the highly irregular surface presented by the latter regions. This example is taken from rat papillary muscle, directly frozen (without pretreatment) by being plunged into propane. Scale bar: 2 µm.

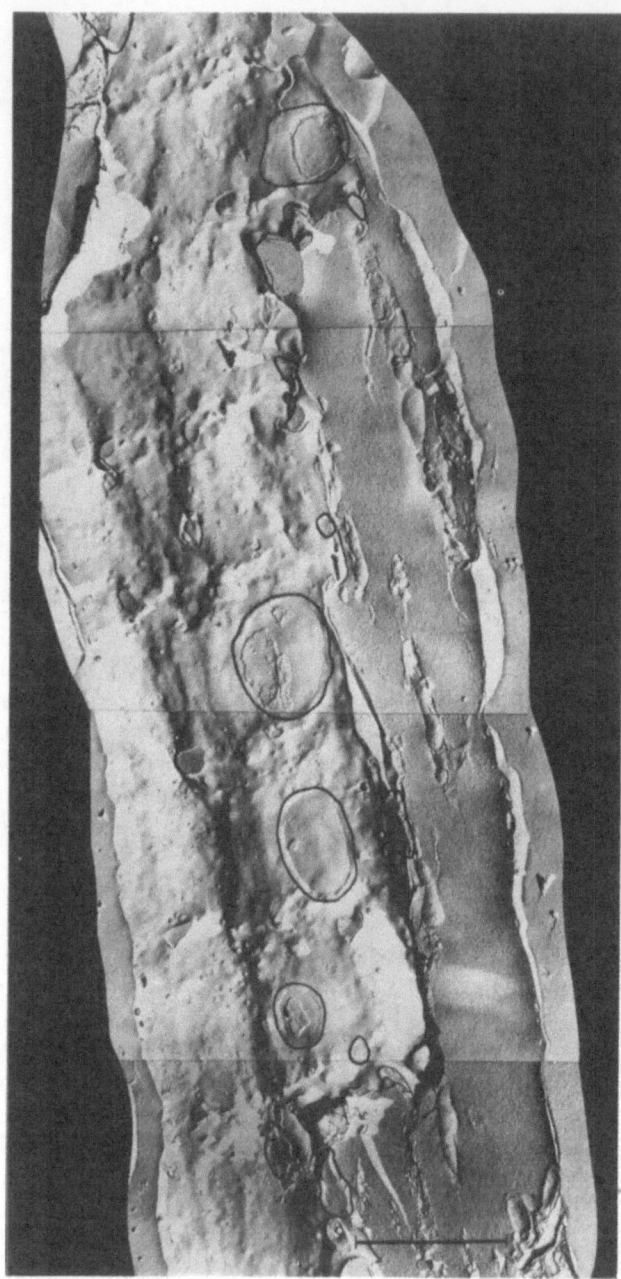

Figure 4.   Survey freeze–fracture view of a lateral portion of the intercalated disk membrane. A large expanse of the lateral membrane has been intercepted by the fracture plane, revealing 12 gap junctions (circled). From fixed and glycerinated rabbit left ventricle. Scale bar: 2 μm.

Table 1.   Classification of Intercellular Junctions, Their Principal Functions, and Their Occurrence in Cardiac Muscle[a]

Type of intercellular junction	Present in cardiac-muscle cells?	Function
1. Adhering junctions		
a. "Spot" desmosome (macula adherens, desmosome)	Yes	
b. "Sheet" desmosome (fascia adherens, intermediate junction)	Yes	Anchorage of cells to one another
c. "Belt" desmosome (zonula adherens)	No	
d. "Half" desmosome (hemidesmosome)	No	Anchorage of cells to basal lamina
2. Communicating junctions		
a. Gap junction (nexus, close junction, macula communicans)	Yes	Electrical and metabolic coupling between cells
3. Occluding junctions		
a. Tight junction—normally found in "belt" form (zonula occludens), but "sheet" (fascia) or "spot" (macula) variants also exist.	No	Vertebrates — Forming permeability barriers across epithelial-cell layers
b. Septate junction	No	Invertebrates —

[a] Note that although tight junctions are not found between cardiac muscle cells, they do occur elsewhere in the myocardium, namely, between endothelial cells in venules and in arterioles and also between endothelial cells and pericytes. Larger blood vessels in the myocardium also contain gap junctions, both in the endothelium and in smooth muscle.

creating pits in the extracellular membrane-half (Figure 8). Often, the fracture plane will jump between the two membranes, thus revealing views both of connexons and of their imprints in the same junction (Figure 6).

As depicted in Figure 7, each connexon is equipped with a narrow channel and is aligned with its partner in the adjacent membrane. This arrangement allows ions and small molecules (molecular weight < 1K) to pass directly between cells without entering the exterior. Gap junction channels do not remain permanently open, however; their opening and closing appear to be under precise cellular control. Calcium and pH have been identified as regulatory factors [5–9], and the possibility that calmodulin mediates the action of calcium has recently been examined [10]. High-resolution electron microscopy and Fourier analysis of hepatocyte gap junctions indicate that each connexon consists of six rod-shaped subunits, and a model by which sliding movements of these subunits could effect opening and closure of the central channel has been proposed [11]. Biochemical analyses of isolated

DESMOSOME
Intermembrane gap — 20 nm

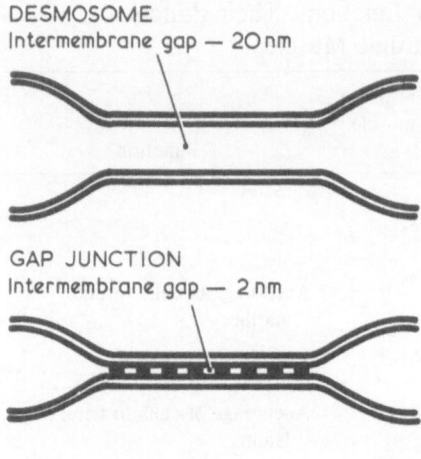

GAP JUNCTION
Intermembrane gap — 2 nm

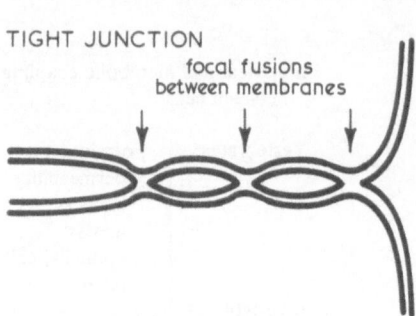

TIGHT JUNCTION
focal fusions
between membranes

Figure 5.   Key to identification of the different types of intercellular junction, based on membrane structure visible by thin sectioning. Each double line represents a single "unit" membrane. The gap between desmosome membranes varies in different tissues; the space of 20 nm given here is applicable to both the cardiac desmosome and the fascia adherens. Electron-dense extracellular tracers are necessary for clear visualization of the 2-nm gap between the gap junction membranes.

gap-junction fractions suggest that in the heart, the junctional subunit is a protein with a molecular weight of 28–29.5K, though a variety of other proteins (possibly contaminants) are present in most preparations [12–15]. Surprisingly perhaps, gap junctions from different tissues seem to differ markedly in protein composition.

Although "open" and "closed" connexons are not readily visualized directly with standard electron-microscopic techniques, it is generally accepted that opening and closing of the junctional channels is accompanied by alterations in connexon size and arrangement that are detectable by freeze–fracture [3,6–8,16,17]. In conventionally fixed and glycerinated cardiac tissue,* gap junctions appear as approximately round or oval-shaped domains with well-circumscribed borders (Figure 6). The connexons are typically arranged in multiple small hexagonal arrays between which lie slightly raised smooth lipid islands. Sometimes, however, a more dispersed

---

* Specimens are routinely treated sequentially in glutaraldehyde fixative and 25% glycerol before being frozen for feeeze–fracture, a procedure referred to as "pretreatment." Glycerol acts as a cryoprotectant to reduce ice-crystal size sufficiently to avoid ultrastructural damage. Glutaraldehyde is used to minimize any alterations in membrane structure that might otherwise arise from the cryoprotectant treatment.

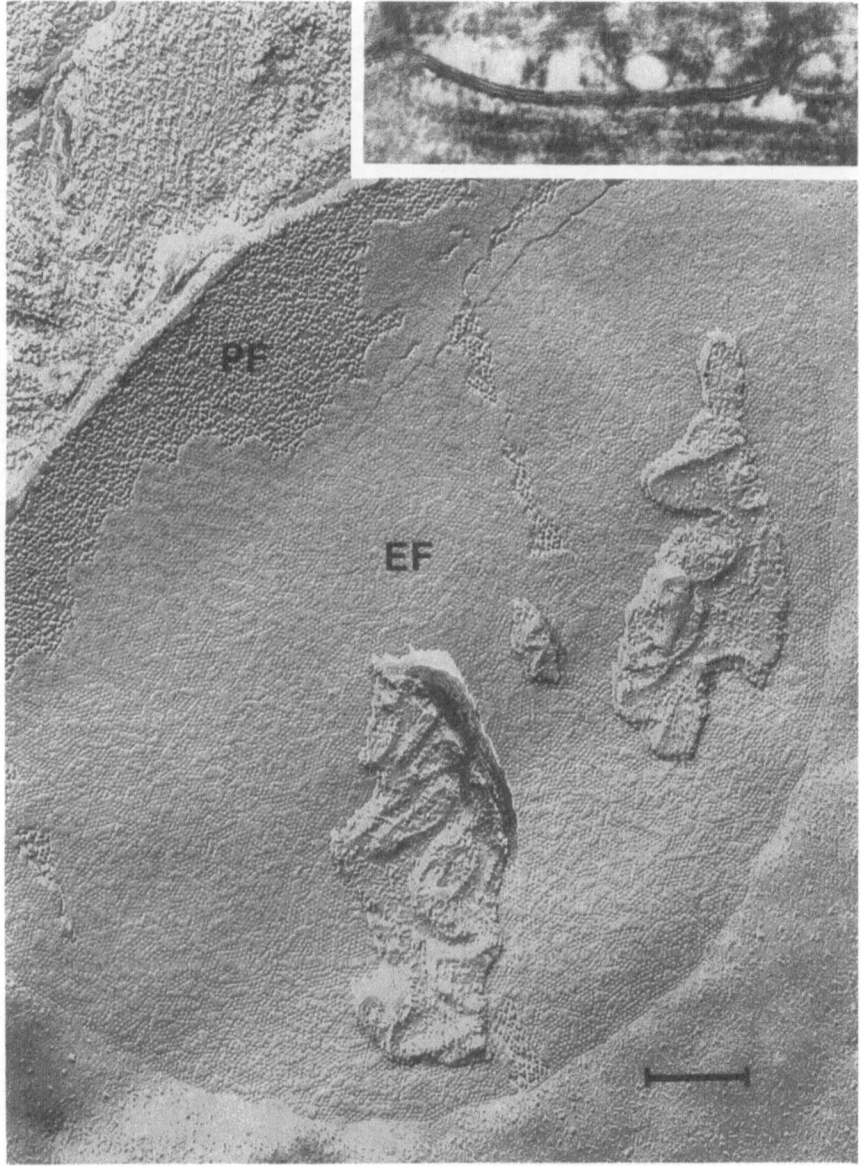

Figure 6.   Ultrastructure of the gap junction in freeze–fracture (main field) and in transverse thin section (inset). (PF) Fracture face of the half-membrane leaflet attached to the protoplasm; (EF) fracture face of the half-membrane leaflet attached to the extracellular space. From rabbit left ventricle, fixed and glycerinated for freeze–fracture, and tannic-acid-treated for thin-sectioning. Scale bar: 200 nm.

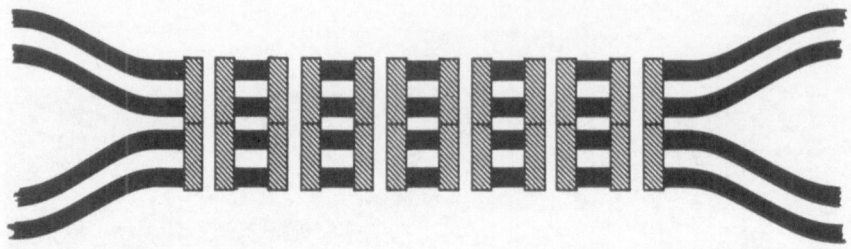

Figure 7.   Diagram of gap-junction structure. Connexons are represented as hatched components in each of the membranes.

connexon configuration is seen (Figure 9). From investigations on a variety of noncardiac cell types, Peracchia [7,8,16,17] advanced the hypothesis that the hexagonal or crystalline connexon arrangement is a characteristic of the uncoupled gap junction, whereas the dispersed or "random" arrangement represents the functionally coupled state. Experimental studies specifically on cardiac muscle have yielded results that apparently accord with this view [18].

By applying new techniques designed to capture cardiac gap junctions in a condition as close as possible to that existing in vivo, however, our own studies raise serious doubts about the universal validity of the Peracchia hypothesis [19]. When rat and rabbit cardiac papillary muscles are directly

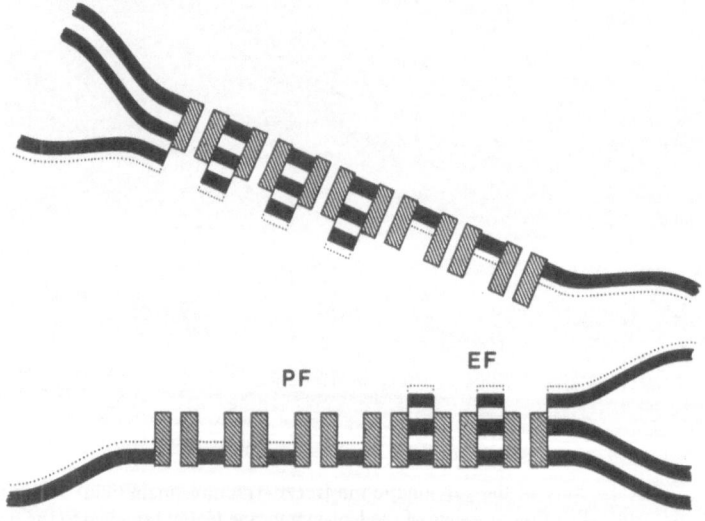

Figure 8.   Diagram showing how gap junctions are split during freeze–fracture (cf. Figure 7). The connexons always remain attached to the protoplasmic half-membrane sheet (PF), leaving pits in the extracellular half-membrane sheet (EF). The PF view in this diagram corresponds to that seen at the top left of Figure 6 and the EF view to that representing the remaining portion of the junction.

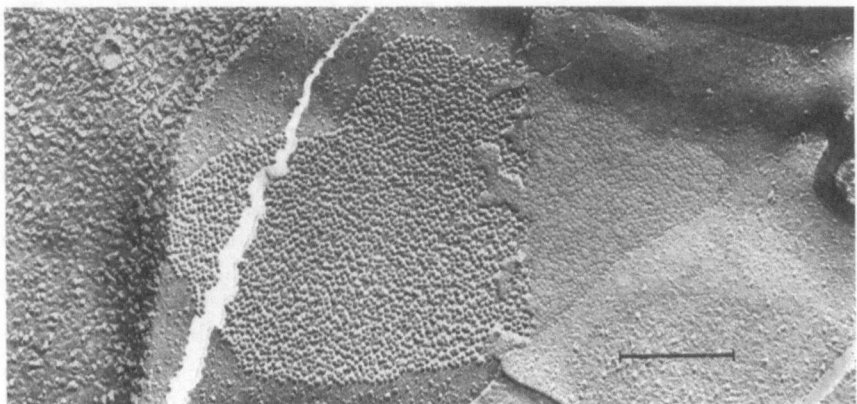

Figure 9.   Freeze–fractured cardiac gap junction with a relatively dispersed arrangement of connexons compared with that seen in Figure 6. The difference in structure between these two junctions is more readily seen by inspecting the EF pits rather than the PF particles. From fixed and glycerinated rabbit septum. Scale bar: 200 nm.

frozen (without the usual chemical pretreatment) by being plunged into propane within 2 sec of excision [20], and when entire hearts are frozen by cold copper block impact in situ in the living animal [21], more than 90% of the gap junctions observed display connexons in a hexagonal arrangement of the type illustrated in Figure 10. Superficially, the structure of these junc-

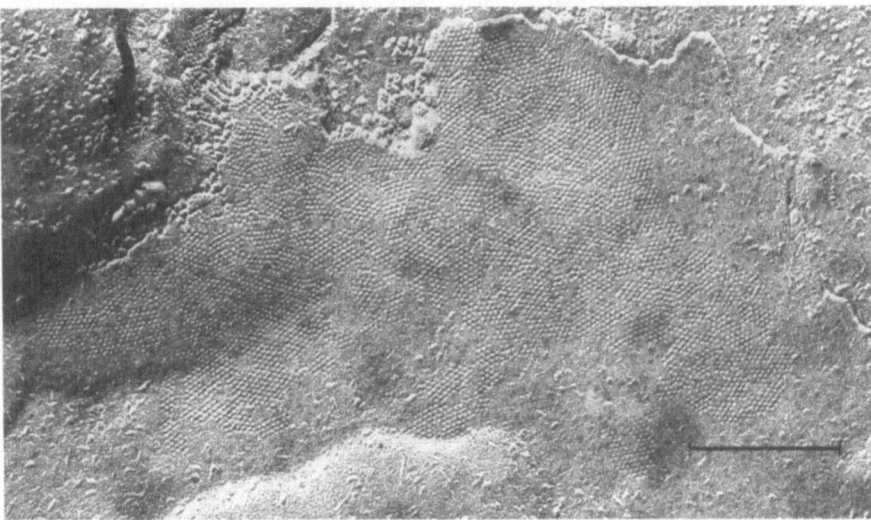

Figure 10.   Gap junction from a freeze–fractured rabbit papillary muscle, frozen directly (without pretreatment) by being plunged into propane [20]. The connexon imprints are seen as multiple small hexagonal arrays. Scale bar: 200 nm.

tions resembles that typically seen in fixed and glycerinated specimens (Figure 6), but it differs in that the junction border is irregular and indistinct, and the lipid regions between the connexon arrays are not raised. This result leads us to conclude that contrary to widespread belief, the functional cardiac gap junction in vivo is comprised of hexagonal arrays of connexons, and that the different connexon arrangements observed may have no bearing on coupling and uncoupling of the junction.

Although interest in gap junctions has quite understandably focused primarily on their role in intercellular communication and electrical coupling, that these junctions also have strong adhesive properties should not be overlooked. Wood and Hageman [22] have argued that since intercellular adhesion must have been a prerequisite for the evolutionary development of communicating junctions, the gap junction is fundamentally multifunctional. In cardiac myocytes, the adhesive property of gap junctions is emphasized by their fate on cell isolation [23]. Using low-calcium solutions containing collagenase [24], the extracellular "cement" material of the desmosomes and fasciae adherentes is removed, separating these junctions in half. Gap junctional membranes tend not to be parted in this manner, however, but are often torn out of the plasma membrane of one cell as it is dissociated from its neighbor. This indicates greater mechanical strength between the adhering connexon pairs across the gap junction than at the boundary between the junction and surrounding membrane.

Desmosomes

Desmosomes are rivetlike structures that fasten adjacent plasma membranes firmly together. They occur widely in multicellular systems, but are most abundant in tissues—like the myocardium—that are subject to severe mechanical stress. The principal components of the desmosome, unlike those of the gap junction, are peripheral membrane proteins, and so thin-sectioning rather than freeze–fracture has supplied the major details of desmosomal architecture. As can be seen in Figures 11–13, the most conspicuous feature of the desmosome is a pair of electron-dense plaques situated close to the cytoplasmic surface of each membrane. The plaques consist predominantly of two large nonglycosylated polypeptides, desmoplakin I and desmoplakin II (molecular weights 250 and 215K, respectively), that occur in equimolar quantities [25]. In contrast to gap junction proteins, these components appear to be identical (or at least very similar) in different tissues and species [26,27]. Intermediate (10-nm-diameter) filaments, which in the cardiac-muscle cell consist of desmin and vimentin [28], are anchored to the desmosomal plaques (Figures 11 and 12). In this way, forces acting on the supportive structural framework provided by the intermediate filament system in the cytoplasm can be distirbuted throughout the tissue as a whole.

The two membranes of the desmosome lie straight and parallel to one another, separated by a uniform space 20 nm in width that is bisected by a

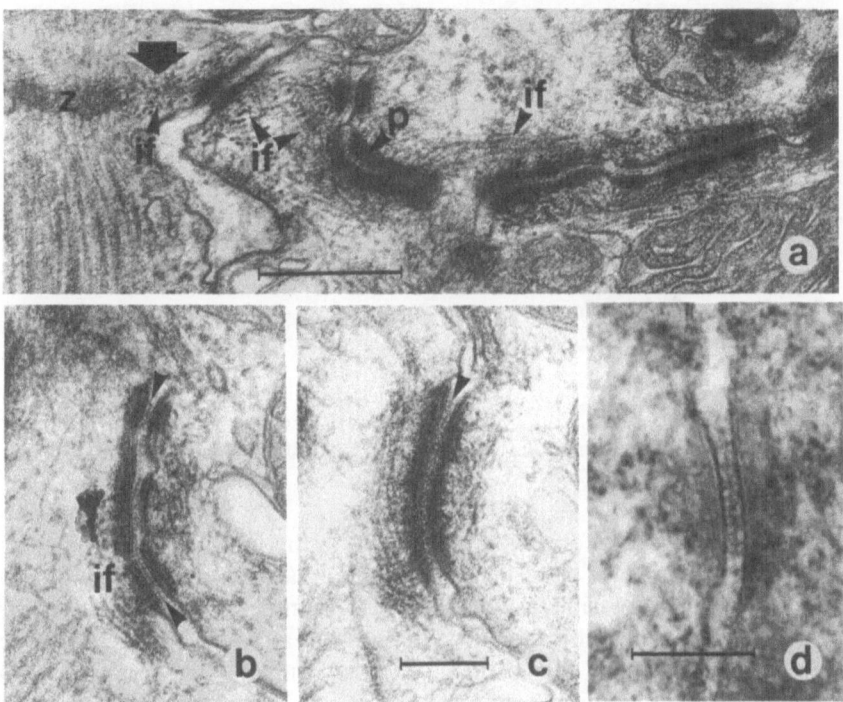

Figure 11.   Ultrastructure of the desmosome as seen in thin sections of rabbit intercalated disk. (a) A series of desmosomes of variable visible diameter. Note the abundance of intermediate filaments (if), which attach to the desmosomal plaques (p) and can also be seen surrounding the Z-line (z) in the area indicated by the large arrow. Scale bar: 400 nm. (b, c) Two sections taken at different levels through the same desmosome. What appears as several desmosomes in (b) is in fact seen to be a single desmosome in (c). A central lamella is visible in the extracellular space (▼). (if) Intermediate filaments. Scale bar: 200 nm. (d) From a tannic-acid-treated specimen. The desmosomal plaques appear less prominent, but the extracellular sides of the desmosomal membranes are densely stained. Details of the central lamella in the extracellular space and of cross-bridges are visible. Scale bar: 100 nm.

central electron-dense lamella. Experiments using extracellular tracers and special staining techniques indicate that the central lamella is linked to the two membranes by a system of staggered cross-bridges [29,30]. Biochemical analysis has shown that these extracellular core components (termed the "desmoglea"), which mediate adhesion between the two membranes, consist of four glycoproteins with molecular weights of 150, 115, 100, and 22K [27,31].

Electron-microscopic evidence suggests that intracellular struts, similar in appearance to the extracellular cross-bridges, may connect the cytoplasmic side of the membrane to the plaques [30]. Freeze–fracture observations are consistent with the idea that the cross-bridges and struts form single continuous units penetrating through the membrane interior. Although

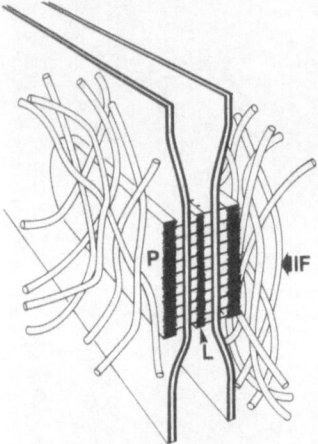

Figure 12. Diagrammatic representation of desmosomal structure. (IF) intermediate filaments; (P) desmosomal plaque; (L) central (extracellular) lamella.

disappointingly little information is gleaned on the intramembranous structure of desmosomes in fixed and glycerinated cardiac tissue, desmosomal domains are readily visible as aggregates of prominent intramembrane particles and fibrils when ultrarapid frozen (unpretreated) tissue is freeze–fractured (Figure 14). The desmosomal particles and fibrils are easily distinguished from gap junction connexons; they are more conspicuous on the extracellular half-membrane leaflet than on the protoplasmic leaflet and are irregular in size, distribution, and shape. Their prominence in the directly frozen specimens is attributed to plastic deformation greater than that normally associated with the fracturing of pretreated specimens.

The improved visibility of desmosomal structure made possible by direct ultrarapid freezing has provided new information on the shape of desmosomes. It is generally assumed, as the names "macula adherens" and "spot desmosome" imply, that the desmosome occupies a disk-shaped domain in the membrane [32,33]. Sommer and Johnson [33], for example, in their comprehensive treatise on cardiac ultrastructure, assert that the desmosome is a "round spot." Our earlier estimates from serial thin section reconstruction had suggested that at least some cardiac desmosomes deviate substantially from this description (Figure 13). Bearing in mind possible errors involved in estimating section thickness, these could nevertheless conform to an oval shape, as recorded in epidermal desmosomes [30,34]. However, our subsequent freeze–fracture studies using ultrarapid freezing disclosed a previously unsuspected and quite remarkable diversity in desmosome shape and size, as illustrated in Figures 14 and 15.

From these observations, the term *macula* (L. "spot") prefixed to adherens is clearly a misnomer so far as cardiac desmosomes are concerned. Strictly speaking, *fascia* (L. "sheet") might be a more accurate description, but a change in the traditional usage of these terms is ill-advised in view of the confusion it would cause.

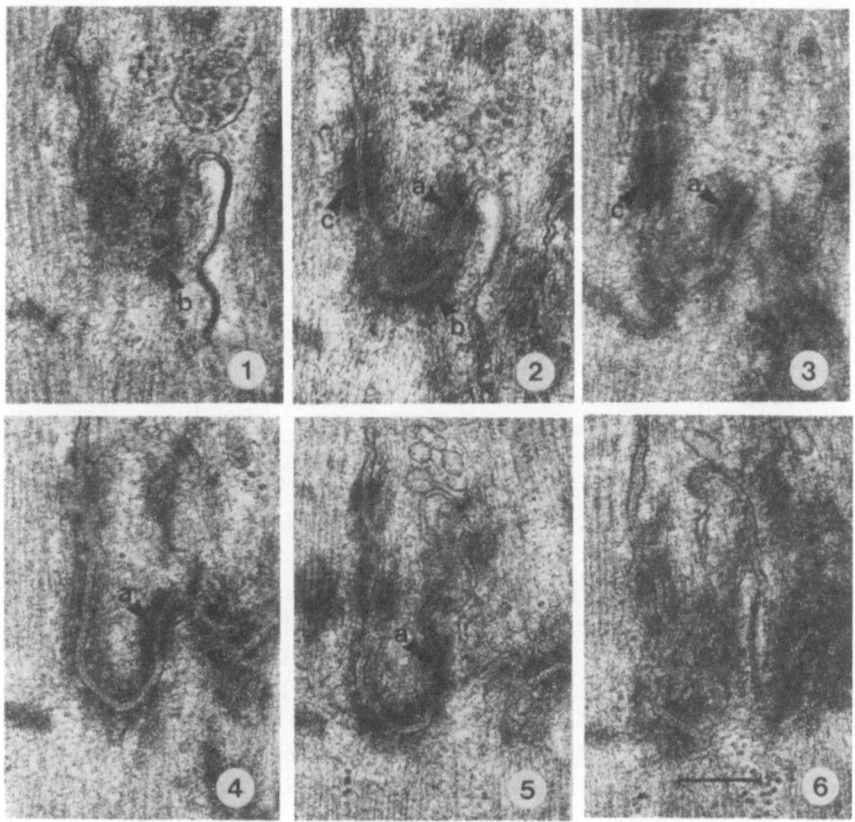

Figure 13. Serial thin sections (1–6) through a desmosome-bearing portion of an intercalated disk from rabbit left ventricle. Three complete desmosomes (a, b, c) can be followed through this sequence. Estimated dimensions of these desmosomes are as follows: (a) 240 × 300 nm; (b) 90 × 150 nm; (c) 205 × 150 nm. Scale bar: 250 nm.

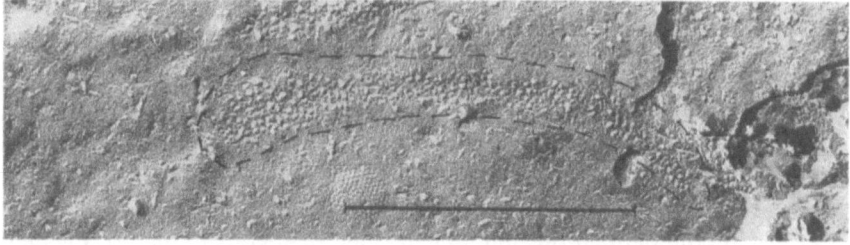

Figure 14. Desmosome (outlined by dashed line) from a directly frozen freeze–fractured rat papillary muscle. This view is of the membrane's E-face (i.e., the fracture face of the half-membrane sheet attached to the extracellular space). Scale bar: 0.5 μm.

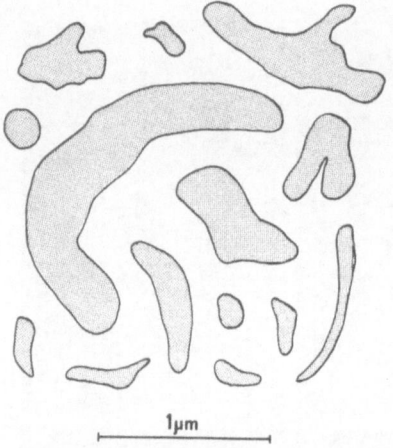

1μm

Figure 15. Representative tracings of desmosomes from directly frozen freeze–fractured rat
papillary muscle. Elongated desmosomes show
no specific orientation in relation to the cell axis.

Fasciae Adherentes

The true fascia adherens resembles the desmosome in ultrastructural appearance and shares with it the function of providing strong intercellular adhesion. However, whereas the desmosome anchors the intermediate-filament cytoskeleton, the fascia adherens performs the equivalent task for the contractile apparatus. Strong attachment of the myofilaments to the plasma membrane and of one plasma membrane to the next is essential for transmission of mechanical tension throughout the tissue.

In place of the electron-dense plaques characteristic of desmosomes, fasciae adherentes are equipped with less compact "filamentous mats" on their cytoplasmic surfaces (Figure 16). This material is ultrastructurally indistinguishable from that of the Z-disk, with which it is sometimes seen in continuity. Z-disks consist of Z-filaments (α-actinin) that link together the actin filaments of adjacent sarcomeres [35], filamin (another actin-binding protein, molecular weight 260K [36]), an amorphous protein, 85K amorphin [37*], and a variety of other protein components [38,*39]. Each Z-disk is surrounded by a network of desmin and vimentin intermediate filaments that tie adjacent sarcomeres together so that they are held firmly in lateral register [40].

The fascia adherens, like the Z-disk, contains actin, α-actinin, filamin, and a range of polypeptides that do not appear to have counterparts in the Z-disk [39,41]. Notable among these is a 130K polypeptide termed vinculin that has been localized using immunochemical labeling in the filamentous mat and is thought to be directly responsible for linking the myofilament bundles to the plasma membrane [41,42]. Intermediate filaments, which occur around the filamentous mat in a manner analogous to the arrangement

* These studies were on *avian skeletal* muscle.

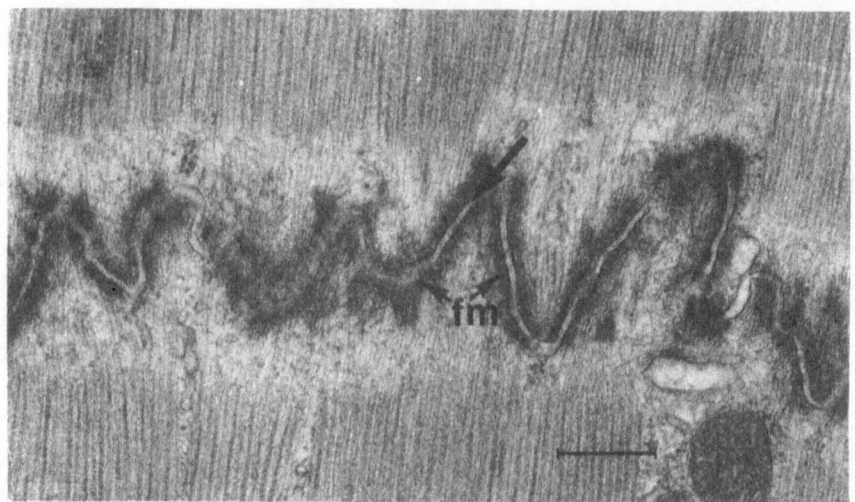

Figure 16.   Ultrastructure of the fascia adherens as viewed in thin section. Actin filaments can be seen approaching and inserting into the dense filamentous mat (fm) of the fascia adherens. An indistinct central lamella is visible at one site (←). Scale bar: 0.5 μm.

found around th Z-disk, attach to desmosomal plaques as described in the preceding section.

The intermembrane gap of the fascia adherens is 20 nm, identical to that of the desmosome. Fasciae adherentes may present curved profiles in thin section, suggesting that their membranes are more flexible than those of desmosomes. The intercellular material of fasciae adherentes usually appears less well organized than does that of desmosomes, and a central electron-dense lamella is sometimes only just discernible (Figure 16). Freeze–fracture demonstrates that in contrast to desmosomes, the fascia adherens membrane contains fewer intramembrane particles than are observed in surrounding regions of membrane. Although it is generally believed that the fascia adherens occupies a larger area in the membrane than does the desmosome, this has so far proved difficult to check. Myofilament bundles appear to divide into subbundles as the membrane is approached; the fascia adherens does not, therefore, correspond in size to an entire Z-disk, but only to a small fraction of one.

Despite some similarity in appearance and chemical composition, recent biochemical studies emphasize that distinct differences exist between desmosomes and fasciae adherentes [26,43]. There now seems to be a good case for dividing adhering junctions (Table 1) into two categories—one to include the desmosome and hemidesmosome, the other to include the fascia adherens and zonula adherens.

CONCLUDING REMARKS

Intercalated disks are highly specialized macrodomains of the plasma membrane the function of which centers on the transmission of both the signal for and the force of contraction from one myocyte to the next. The three distinct types of intercellular junctions that mediate these functions are thus directly responsible for the coordinated contractile response of the myocardium as a whole. Our current knowledge of the structure of these junctions provides a framework for understanding how each is uniquely equipped for performing its function. Biochemical and immunological investigations are now extending this understanding to the molecular level.

ACKNOWLEDGMENTS

Some of the results included herein come from investigations supported by British Heart Foundation grants. I thank Dr. C. R. Green, Mr. A. Slade, Dr. T. Powell, and Mr. V. W. Twist for their collaboration and Mr. G. Storey for help with photography.

REFERENCES

1. McNutt, N. S., and Weinstein, R. S. 1973. Membrane structure at mammalian intercellular junctions. *Prog. Biophys. Mol. Biol.* 26:45–101.
2. Staehelin, L. A. 1974. Structure and function of intercellular junctions. *Int. Rev. Cytol.* 39:191–283.
3. Page, E., and Shibata, Y. 1981. Permeable junctions between cardiac cells. *Annu. Rev. Physiol.* 43:431–441.
4. De Mello, W. C. 1982. Intercellular communication in cardiac muscle. *Circ. Res.* 51:1–9.
5. Turin, L., and Warner, A. 1977. Carbon dioxide reversibly abolishes ionic communication between cells of early amphibian embryo. *Nature (London)* 270:56–57.
6. Dahl, G., and Isenberg, G. 1980. Decoupling of heart muscle cells: Correlation with increased cytoplasmic calcium activity and with changes in nexus ultrastructure. *J. Membr. Biol.* 53:63–75.
7. Peracchia, C., and Peracchia, L. 1980. Gap junction dynamics: Reversible effects of divalent cations. *J. Cell Biol.* 87:708–718.
8. Peracchia, C., and Peracchia, L. 1980. Gap junction dynamics: Reversible effects of hydrogen ions. *J. Cell Biol.* 87:719–727.
9. Burt, J. M., Frank, J. S., and Berns, M. W. 1982. Permeability and structural studies of heart cell gap junctions under normal and altered ionic conditions. *J. Membr. Biol.* 68:227–238.
10. Welsh, M. J., Aster, J. C., Ireland, M., Alcala, J., and Maisel, H. 1982. Calmodulin binds to chick lens gap junction protein in a calcium-independent manner. *Science* 216:642–644.
11. Unwin, P. N. T., and Zampighi, G. 1980. Structure of the junction between communicating cells. *Nature (London)* 283:545–549.
12. Kensler, R. W., and Goodenough, D. A. 1980. Isolation of mouse myocardial gap junctions. *J. Cell Biol.* 86:755–764.
13. Manjunath, C. K., Goings, G. E., and Page, E. 1982. Isolation and protein composition of gap junctions from rabbit hearts. *Biochem. J.* 205:189–194.

14. Manjunath, C. K., Goings, G. E., and Page, E. 1982. Protein composition of cardiac gap junctions: Comparison between mammalian species and between junctions from rat heart and liver. *J. Cell Biol.* 95:88a.
15. Nicholson, B. J., Gros, D., and Revel, J.-P. 1982. Tissue specificity in the gap junctional protein. *J. Cell Biol.* 95:104a.
16. Peracchia, C. 1977. Gap junctions: Structural changes after uncoupling procedures. *J. Cell Biol.* 72:628–641.
17. Peracchia, C. 1980. Structural correlates of gap junction permeation. *Int. Rev. Cytol.* 66:81–146.
18. Baldwin, K. 1979. Cardiac gap junction configuration after an uncoupling treatment as a function of time. *J. Cell Biol.* 82:66–75.
19. Green, C. R., and Severs, N. J. 1983. Structural alterations in cardiac gap junctions captured by ultrarapid freezing. *J. Mol. Cell. Cardiol.* 15(Suppl 3):172.
20. Severs, N. J., and Green, C. R. 1983. Rapid freezing of unpretreated tissues for freeze–fracture electron microscopy. *Biol. Cell* 47:193–204.
21. Severs, N. J., and Green, C. R. 1983. Ultrarapid freezing techniques and connexon arrangement in cardiac gap junctions. *Beitr. Elektronenmikrosc. Directabb. Oberfl.* 16:571–578.
22. Wood, R. L., and Hageman, G. S. 1982. The fine structure of cellular junctions in a marine Bryozoan: Gap junctions. *J. Ultrastruct. Res.* 79:174–188.
23. Severs, N. J., Slade, A. M., Powell, T., Twist, V. W., and Warren, R. L. 1982. Correlation of ultrastructure and function in calcium-tolerant myocytes isolated from the adult rat heart. *J. Ultrastruct. Res.* 81:222–239.
24. Powell, T., Terrar, D. A., and Twist, V. W. 1980. Electrical properties of individual cells isolated from adult rat ventricular myocardium. *J. Physiol.* 302:131–153.
25. Mueller, H., and Franke, W. W. 1983. Biochemical and immunological characterization of desmoplakins I and II, the major polypeptides of the desmosomal plaque. *J. Mol. Biol.* 163:647–671.
26. Franke, W. W., Moll, R. Schiller, D. L., Schmid, E., Kartenbeck, J., and Mueller, H. 1982. Desmoplakins of epithelial and myocardial desmosomes are immunologically and biochemically related. *Differentiation* 23:115–127.
27. Cowin, P., and Garrod, D. R. 1983. Antibodies to epithelial desmosomes show wide tissue and species cross-reactivity. *Nature (London)* 302:148–150.
28. Lazarides, E. 1980. Intermediate filaments as mechanical integrators of cellular space. *Nature (London)* 283:249–256.
29. Rayns, D. G., Simpson, F. O., and Ledingham, J. M. 1969. Ultrastructure of desmosomes in mammalian intercalated disc: Appearances after lanthanum treatment. *J. Cell Biol.* 42:322–326.
30. Kelly, D. E., and Sheinvold, F. L. 1976. The desmosome: Fine structural studies with freeze–fracture replication and tannic acid staining of sectioned epidermis. *Cell Tissue Res.* 172:309–323.
31. Gorbsky, G., and Steinberg, M. S. 1981. Isolation of the intercellular glycoproteins of desmosomes. *J. Cell Biol.* 90:243–248.
32. McNutt, N. S. 1970. Ultrastructure of intercellular junctions in adult and developing cardiac muscle. *Am. J.Cardiol.* 25:169–183.
33. Sommer, J. R., and Johnson, E. A. 1979. Ultrastructure of cardiac muscle. In: R. M. Berne, N. Sperelakis, and S. R. Geiger (eds), *Handbook of Physiology, Section 2: The Cardiovascular System.* Vol. 1, pp. 113–186. American Physiology Society, Bethesda, Maryland.
34. Shimono, M., and Clementi, F. 1976. Intercellular junctions of oral epithelium. I. Studies with freeze–fracture and tracing methods of normal rat keratinized oral epithelium. *J. Ultrastruct. Res.* 56:121–136.
35. Yamaguchi, M., Robson, R. M., and Stromer, M. H. 1983. Evidence for actin involvement in cardiac Z-lines and Z-line analogues. *J. Cell Biol.* 96:435–442.

36. Koteliansky, V. E., Glukhova, M. A., Shirinsky, V. P. Babaev, V. R., Kandalenko, V. F., Rukosuev, V. S., and Smirnov, V. N. 1981. Identification of a filamin-like protein in chicken heart muscle. *FEBS Lett.* 125:44–48.
37. Chowrashi, P. K., and Pepe, F. A. 1982. The Z-band: 85,000-Dalton amorphin and alpha-actinin and their relation to structure. *J. Cell Biol.* 94:565–573.
38. Ohashi, K., and Maruyama, K. 1979. A new structural protein located in the Z-lines of chicken skeletal muscle. *J. Biochem.* 85:1103–1105.
39. Colaco, C. A. L. S., and Evans, W. H. 1981. A biochemical dissection of the cardiac intercalated disk: Isolation of subcellular fractions containing fasciae adherentes and gap junctions. *J. Cell Sci.* 52:313–325.
40. Granger, B. L., and Lazarides, E. 1979. Desmin and vimentin coexist at the periphery of the myofibril Z disc. *Cell* 18:1053–1063.
41. Koteliansky, V. E., Gneushev, G. N., Shartava, A. S., Shirinsky, V. P., Glukhova, M. A., and Goodman, S. R. 1983. The regulation by vinculin of filamin, α-actinin and spectrin tetramer-induced actin sol–gel transformation. *FEBS Lett.* 151:206–210.
42. Geiger, B., Tokuyasu, K. T., Dutton, A. H., and Singer, S. J. 1980. Vinculin, an intracellular protein localized at specialized sites where microfilament bundles terminate at cell membranes. *Proc. Natl. Acad. Sci. U.S.A.* 77:4127–4131.
43. Tokuyasu, K. T. 1983. Present state of immunocryoultramicrotomy. *J. Histochem. Cytochem.* 31:164–167.

Extracellular Structures in Heart Muscle

Thomas F. Robinson

Cardiovascular Center
Department of Medicine
and
Department of Physiology and Biophysics
Albert Einstein College of Medicine
Bronx, New York 10461

Leona Cohen-Gould
Renee M. Remily
and
Joseph M. Capasso

Cardiovascular Center
Department of Medicine
Albert Einstein College of Medicine
Bronx, New York 10461

Stephen M. Factor

Department of Pathology
Albert Einstein College of Medicine
Bronx, New York 10461

Abstract. The extracellular matrix of heart muscle contains a considerable variety of structures. We have systematically studied the morphology of these structures using several methods of fixation and microscopy. Endomysial connections between cells are comprised of struts of collagen [1] as well as combinations of elastin fibers, collagen fibers, and microfibrils. The rest of the extracellular matrix is filled with a polyanionic lattice of unit collagen fibrils, microthreads, and granules. In the course of these investigations, we have observed regions of structural continuity across the sarcolemma, from endomysial collagen struts to Z-bands. We have also correlated the mechanical resistance to stretch with orientation of epimysial collagen fibers and sarcomere lengths in living as well as fixed rat papillary muscles. Our observations suggest that the extracellular skeletal framework plays an important role in normal cardiac function.

INTRODUCTION

The extracellular matrix of myocardium contains a considerable variety of structures. For convenience, the connective tissue is categorized by region within the muscle: epimysium is the sheath of connective tissue that surrounds the entire muscle; endomysium surrounds and interconnects individual myocytes, and perimysium surrounds groups of myocytes and connects epimysium to endomysium.

Classic histological studies of the disposition of collagen fibers have been performed using light microscopy of silver-stained sections [2–4]. More recently, the collagen network of heart muscle has been described with striking images from the scanning electron microscope. Caulfield and Borg used fractured frozen specimens to observe the large perimysial collagen fibers, the weave of collagen that envelops groups of myocytes, and the endomysial struts of collagen, 120–150 nm in diameter, that bridge myocytes to each other or to capillaries [1,5–7]. Several different fibrous substances of the extracellular matrix have also been demonstrated [8–12]. Robinson and coworkers recently described the morphology of elastin, microfibrils, substructure of collagen fibers, and polyanionic lattice and ground substance. They used specialized fixation protocols, light microscopy, conventional and high-voltage transmission electron microscopy, and scanning electron microscopy [13–16].

The purpose of the study presented in this chapter was to structurally characterize the elements of the extracellular matrix of heart muscle in a systematic way and to correlate the dispositions of matrix fibers with mechanical parameters of the muscle. Experiments were carried out primarily on isolated papillary muscles of the rat.

MATERIALS AND METHODS

Muscle Mechanics

The detailed methods for the assessment of mechanical properties of isolated rat papillary muscle and myocardium have been described in a previous publication [17]. The following is a brief description of the methods and materials utilized. Rats were anesthetized with ether. The hearts were rapidly excised and placed in oxygenated Tyrode's solution. Left ventricular papillary muscles were removed and suspended horizontally in a myograph. We used only muscles with relatively cylindrical uniformity and with a cross-sectional area of 1.0 mm^2 or less to ensure adequate oxygenation of central fibers. The muscles were perfused continuously with Tyrode's solution that was maintained at 30°C ($\pm$ 1.0°C) and gassed with 95% O_2–5% CO_2. Stimuli were isolated from ground and delivered to the tissue through bipolar Teflon-coated wires at a frequency of 0.1 Hz.

The nontendinous end of the papillary muscle was inserted into a spring-loaded stainless steel clip mounted at the end of a micrometer assembly that permitted adjustment of external muscle length. The tendinous end was tied to a light steel wire with a short length of wet Ethicon 5-0 braided silk. The wire was attached by a hook to the lever of a servocontrolled galvanometer (Cambridge Technology, Cambridge, Massachusetts), which measured both force and length. Active and passive length–tension curves were obtained after 120 min of equilibration in the tissue bath. During equilibration, the muscle contracted isometrically at a resting tension of 1.0 g/mm². The muscle length associated with maximum peak isometric developed tension (L_{max}) was determined by increasing muscle length in 0.1-mm increments until no further increase in peak isometric tension was detected. The length–tension curve was obtained by reducing muscle length in 0.1-mm decrements from the length associated with maximum developed force (L_{max}) to approximately 80% of L_{max}. Total frictional torque of the servocontrolled lever was calculated at less than 5 mg-cm. Prior to fixation the muscle length was set at a predetermined percentage of L_{max}.

Fixation and Staining

Isolated muscles were dissected and either mounted in the myograph for force and length measurements and subsequent fixation or immediately fixed by immersion. Some papillary muscles were fixed in tetanic contraction induced in a solution containing $BaCl_2$ at a final concentration of 2.4 mM [18] or by rapid stimulation (68 pulses/sec) in the presence of 3 mM caffeine and 5 mM added calcium [19].

Tannic Acid. The use of tannic acid in the fixation protocol improves the preservation of extracellular material and imparts increased electron density both to membranes and to the components of the extracellular matrix [20]. Rat ventricular papillary muscles were fixed for 2 hr at room temperature in a buffer solution that contained 2% glutaraldehyde and 0.5% tannic acid. The samples were then thoroughly rinsed with plain buffer, postfixed with 1% OsO_4, rinsed, dehydrated in graded ethanols, and embedded in epoxy resin.

Cationic Dyes. Several cationic dyes (ruthenium red, alcian blue, and safranin-O) were used. These compounds have been shown to enhance the preservation and contrast of the complex carbohydrates of the extracellular matrix when it is viewed in the electron microscope [21,22]. Rat papillary muscles were fixed in a solution of buffered glutaraldehyde that contained ruthenium red, alcian blue, or safranin-O in a 0.1% concentration. After being rinsed, the samples underwent a secondary fixation with 1% buffered OsO_4 that also contained the appropriate cationic dye, after which all tissues were dehydrated in ethanols and embedded in Spurr's resin. In the case of ruthenium red, some samples were treated with 1% phenylenediamine during dehydration [23]. The phenylenediamine–ruthenium red combination reacts with the same structures as the other cationic dyes. It has the advantage of being visible in both the light and the electron microscope.

Carnoy's Solution. Rat ventricular papillary muscles were isolated and fixed in a modified Carnoy's fixative for rapid fixation of proteins for 3 hr in an ice bath [24]. After fixation, the tissues were rinsed in 0.2% iodine in absolute ethanol for $\frac{1}{2}$ hr (on ice), followed by a brief rinse in plain absolute ethanol. The muscles were then embedded in Spurr's resin and thin-sectioned for electron microscopy.

Silver Reactions. Cryostat sections of formalin-fixed ventricular wall from canine and rat hearts were fixed in a 4% phosphate-buffered formalin solution and were impregnated with silver using a modification of a method developed by Hasegawa and Ravens [25], which is in turn a modified version of a silver carbonate method used by Del Rio Hortega [26]. Most of the tissues impregnated with silver were mounted on glass slides and examined with the light microscope. Some samples of rat ventricular wall were post-fixed with 0.5% OsO_4, dehydrated, and embedded for electron microscopy. Additionally, left and right ventricular papillary muscles from rats were isolated and maintained in oxygenated buffer. Individual specimens of this group were set at slack length, or stretched to a predetermined fraction of L_{max}, and were then fixed with 10% buffered formalin and processed with the modified Del Rio Hortega method.

Light Microscopy

Papillary muscles that were fixed at specific fractions of L_{max} and then impregnated with silver stain were examined by bright-field microscopy on a Zeiss Ultraphot microscope. Photographs were taken on Kodachrome 25 film. Live muscles were studied using differential interference contrast (DIC) microscopy in conjunction with a videocamera connected to a videomonitor and videocassette recorder. The DIC optics permit optical sectioning of the specimen, the thickness of a "section" being equal to the width of one Airy disc [27]. In this way, a thin muscle may be examined in its entirety without physical disruption. The videocamera allows a continuous readout of the position of the connective tissue and cellular structures as the muscle is stimulated to contract, and as it is fixed.

Electron Microscopy

Transmission Electron Microscopy. Muscles embedded in epoxy were sectioned with a diamond knife at a thickness of 0.1 μm. After the compression of the sections was reduced by wafting with xylene vapors, ribbons were mounted on Formvar-coated grids and stained with uranyl acetate and lead citrate. Some sections were cut at $\frac{1}{4}$, $\frac{1}{2}$, 1, and 2 μm for viewing in the high-voltage electron microscope (Department of Molecular, Cellular, and Developmental Biology at the University of Colorado at Boulder).

Scanning Electron Microscopy. Left ventricular papillary muscles were fixed at slack length or at fractions of L_{max} using 6% buffered glutaraldehyde. The tissues were postfixed with 1% buffered OsO_4, dehydrated in graded ethanols, and critical-point-dried using CO_2. The muscles were then immersed in liquid nitrogen and fractured along their lengths using a liquid-nitrogen-cooled razor blade [1]. The resulting pieces were mounted on a

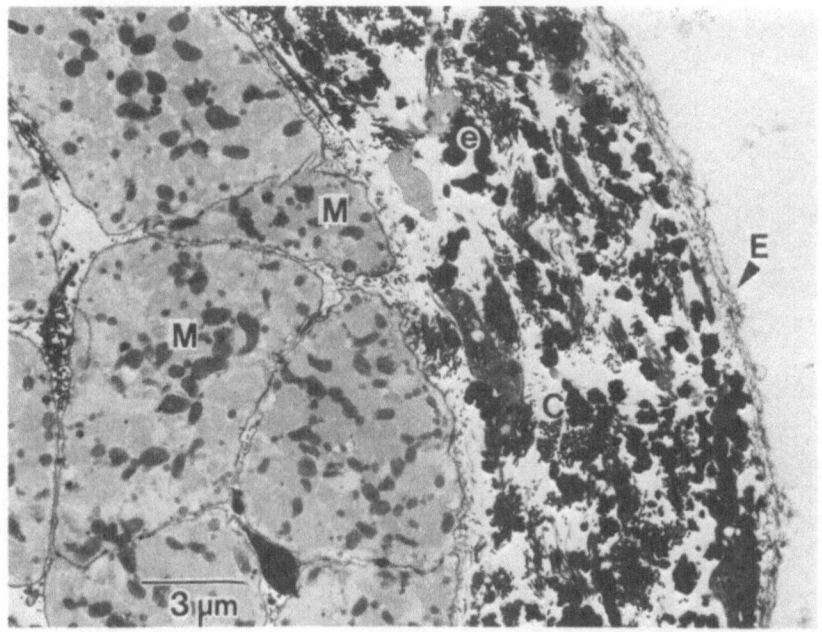

Figure 1. Transmission electron micrograph of a cross section of rat atrial trabecula fixed in a solution containing tannic acid. The collagen fibers (C) and elastic fibers (e) of the epimysium form a sheath around the myocytes (M) and are separated from the heart chamber by the thin layer of squamous endothelium (E).

stub, sputter-coated with a thin layer of gold (about 18 nm), and viewed at 5 or 15 KV.

RESULTS

The epimysium of cardiac muscle is surrounded by a thin layer of squamous endothelial cells and contains relatively large fibers of collagen and elastin that form a sheath around the myocytes (Figure 1). Each collagen fiber is comprised of dozens of striped unit fibrils, 30–70 nm in diameter, and a dense, polyanionic ground substance [28]. Elastic fibers contain the amorphous elastin component and associated microfibrils, 10–17 nm in diameter (Figure 2) [9,29].

The endomysium consists of a weave of collagen fibers around myocytes or groups of myocytes; struts, which are bundles of collagen fibrils connecting the lateral surfaces of myocytes to capillaries and other myocytes (Figure 3A) [1]; and a polyanionic lattice of single collagen fibrils, microthreads, and granules (Figure 3B) [28]. The struts are attached to myocytes tangentially and at various angles relative to the long axes of cells; they

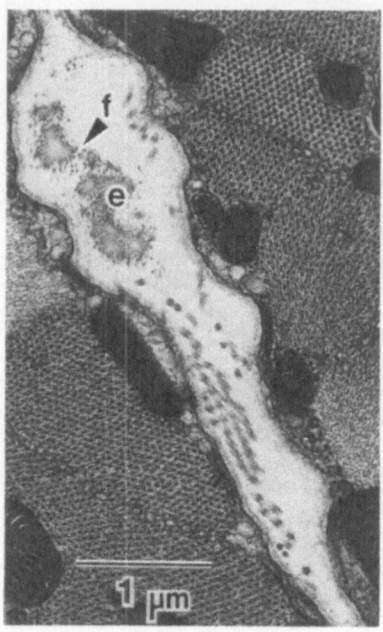

Figure 2.   Transmission electron micrograph of a cross section of rat atrial trabecula. Large elastic fibers with the amorphous elastin component (e) and microfibrillar component (f) are found in the endomysium and often bridge adjacent myocytes.

spread onto the cell surface in a rootlike pattern and are often linked to the membrane slightly lateral to the level of the Z-band [1,5,28]. Many regions of the sarcolemma of the myocyte have a scalloped appearance that is more pronounced if the myocyte has been fixed in a shortened state. The intracellular regions of attachment of the festoons are also slightly lateral to the Z-bands (Figure 4). The possibility of structural continuity between the extracellular struts and intracellular Z-bands was further examined using Carnoy's fixative on contracted papillary muscles. Figure 4B demonstrates the continuity and shows the type of images obtained with this technique.

We have investigated the correlation between the passive mechanical properties, in this case the resistance to stretch of unstimulated muscle, and the orientations of the large collagen fibers of the epimysium. As the papillary muscle is stretched, its resistance to stretch increases gradually from L_{slack} to slightly below L_{max}. Near and above L_{max}, the resistance to further stretch increases sharply (Figure 5). Over this range of lengths, the orientations of the large collagen fibers of the epimysium change dramatically. In silver-stained preparations, the weave pattern of fibers can be seen in muscles that were fixed at slack length (Figure 6A). In muscles fixed near L_{max}, the fibers are essentially coaligned with the long axis of the muscle (Figure 6B). With the light microscope equipped with DIC optics, simultaneous observation of mechanical properties and epimysial fiber alignment of living muscles is now in the early stages of development.

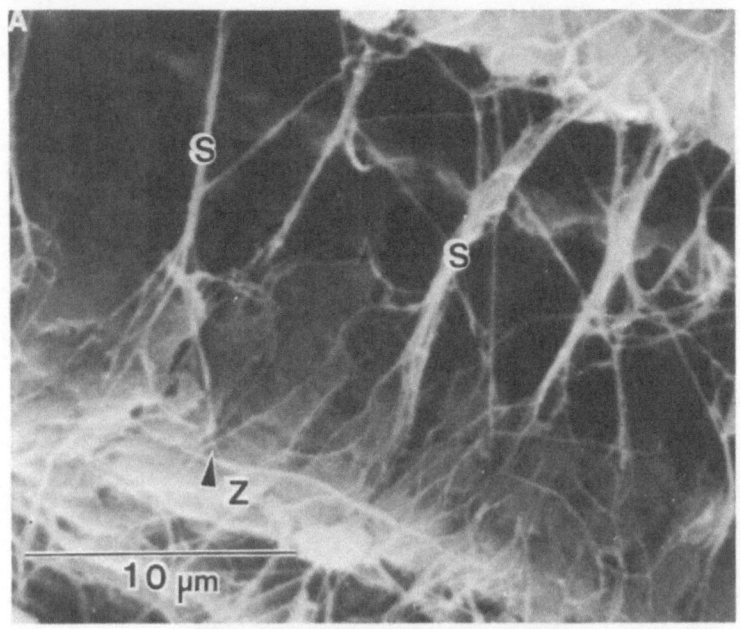

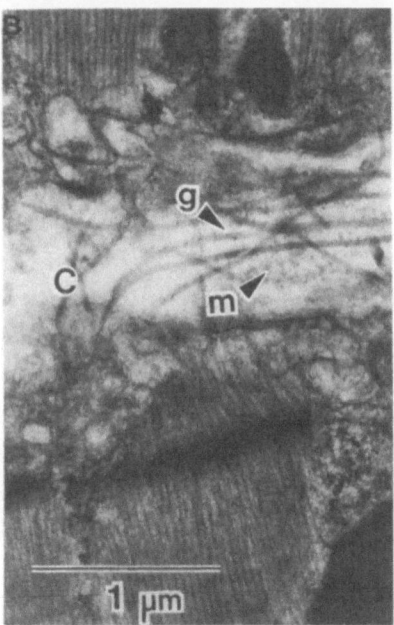

Figure 3. Two prominent structures of the endomysium. (A) Collagen struts (S) that interconnect the lateral surfaces of myocytes, often near Z-band (Z) level. Scanning electron micrograph of rat papillary muscle. (B) Lattice of striated collagen fibrils (C) and polyanionic microthreads (m) and granules (g). Transmission electron micrograph of rat papillary muscle fixed in a solution containing safranin-O.

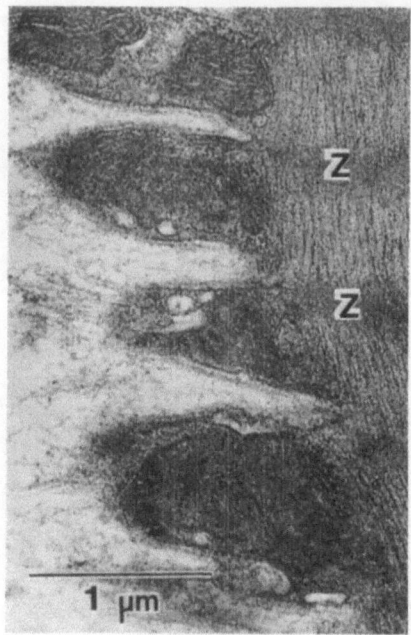

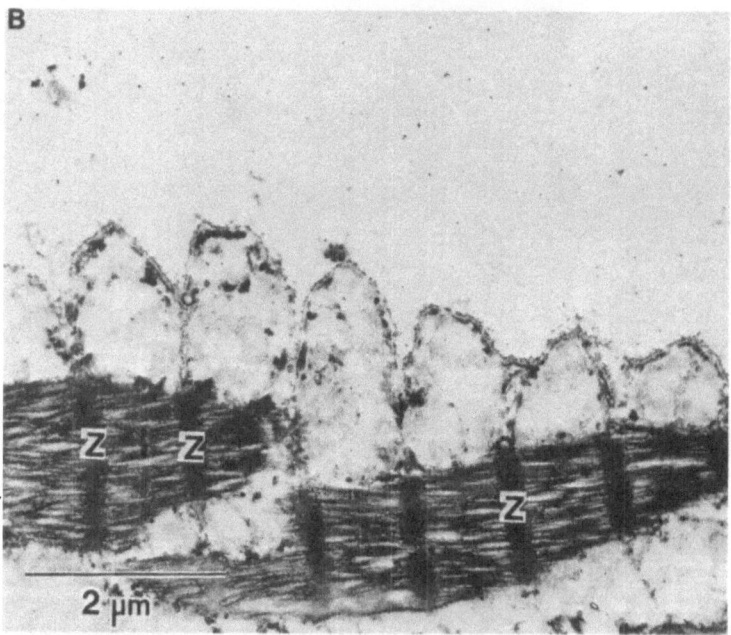

Figure 4. Transmission electron micrograph of a longitudinal section of an actively shortened rat papillary muscle fixed in glutaraldehyde (A) and modified Carnoy's solution (B). The festoons are anchored intracellularly to Z-bands (Z). Continuity of structures can be seen across the sarcolemma. The identification and arrangement of the various structures in the sequence remain to be determined.

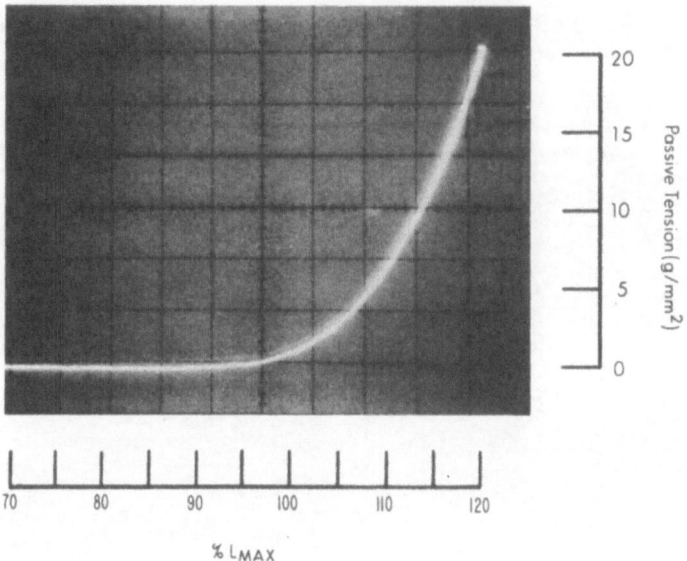

Figure 5. Oscilliscope recording of the passive length–tension curve in rat papillary muscle. Resistance to stretch increases dramatically near L_{max}.

DISCUSSION

The large collagen fibers of the epimysium (Figure 1) of papillary muscle undergo a change in configuration as the muscle is stretched (Figure 6). As the collagen fibers become aligned with the long axis of the muscle near L_{max}, with an average sarcomere length of approximately 2.3 μm, the resistance to stretch increases dramatically (Figure 5). Our working hypothesis is that the essentially inextensible collagen fibers exert little influence on the resistance to stretch of the muscle from 0.8 to 1.0 L_{max} due to their woven disposition. As the muscle is stretched to L_{max} and beyond, the tensile strength of the coaligned collagen fibers produces a sharp increase in resistance to stretch. A convenient analogy is a cargo net. The weave of inextensible ropes can be deformed without much resistance and without damage to the ropes up to the length at which the ropes are coaligned. Beyond this length, resistance to stretch rises sharply. This type of model has been proposed by Bairati [2] for the mechanical properties of the sarcolemmas of frog skeletal myocytes; it is different from the model in which the individual collagen fibers become wavy, as shown in pericardium by Wiegner et al. [30] and in heart valves by Broom [31].

In addition to the correlation of resistance to stretch with epimysial collagen fiber orientations, it is of interest to note their correlation with an

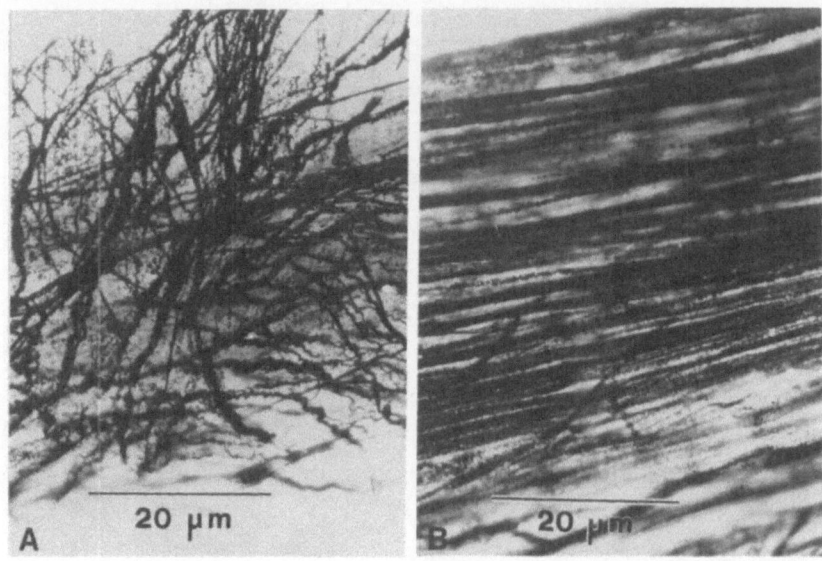

Figure 6.   Light micrographs of silver-stained sections of rat papillary muscles. The epimysial collagen fibers form a criss-cross pattern at slack length (A) and are coaligned beyond L_{max} (B).

important value of sarcomere length. At L_{max}, the average sarcomere length is between 2.2 and 2.3 μm. Robinson and Winegrad [32] have measured the lengths of thin and thick filaments in rat papillary muscle. They have calculated a sarcomere length-developed tension curve with a plateau ending at 2.3 μm. The collagen fibers thus prevent overstretch of the sarcomeres to configurations of thin and thick filament overlap that would be unfavorable to maximal overlap of cross-bridge regions.

The endomysial struts between myocytes appear to tether one cell to another. The suggestion by Caulfield and Borg [1] that struts serve to limit displacement between myocytes is supported by our observations in the light microscope. The struts form a variety of angles with respect to the long axis of the myocyte. Many of these angles are small in highly stretched muscle. The light microscopy and scanning and transmission electron microscopy indicate further that struts not only interconnect endomysial or sarcolemmal collagen but also interconnect intracellular structures near Z-bands of neighboring cells. Such structural continuity is a necessary although not sufficient condition to implicate connective tissue in the transfer of force developed in the sarcomeres to ensuing pressure changes in the ventricular cavity. In skeletal muscle, festoons are anchored at both the Z-bands and M-bands [33]. It is also possible that the struts only limit displacement between cells and play an insignificant role in the transfer of active tension.

The role of the polyanionic collagen fibril–microthread–granule lattice remains speculative. Certainly its ubiquity in the extracellular matrix and the relatively huge water-binding domains commanded by glycosamino-glycans suggests the importance of the lattice in determining viscosity of the extracellular medium [34]. Among continually moving cardiac myocytes, fluid of optimal viscosity would preserve patency of cells as well as influence efficiency of energy use. The abundant negative sites might also play a role in cation binding [35]. The microthread structures studied thus far are similar to those found in other tissues such as cartilage [36], and their substructure and spacing of side chains are consistent with the model used for proteo-glycan monomer [37]. We have also observed the increased branching in preparations fixed with safranin-O or alcian blue relative to those fixed in ruthenium red. Wight and Hascall [38] attribute similar images in cartilage to enhanced fixation by safranin-O. A possible influence on mechanical per-formance of the muscle by the many small links to the cell surface cannot be ruled out [39].

The role of elastin in the recoil of heart-muscle cells during diastole is not yet determined; however, its role must in some ways be complementary to that of the muscle cells themselves. We have found that untethered, en-zymatically isolated myocytes respond to electrical stimulation by contract-ing and then elongating with almost equal speed [40]. This implies that some form of elastic storage of energy resides in the myocyte itself. Whether elastin contributes to elongation of the myocyte after contraction or only has an influence on relative motion between cells and on resistance to stretch is unknown. These latter possibilities are supported by our observation of elastin in the endomysial connections between cells as well as in the epi-mysium. The model of elastin fibers helically wound around myocytes pro-posed by Puff and Langer [11] supports the former possibility in that vectors of stretched elastin could promote return from stretch as well as elongation of a contracted, thickened cell. Their data were generated, however, with a histological stain to elastin that is subject to problems of possible cross-reaction with some types of collagen [41]. The disposition of elasin fibers relative to cardiac myocytes thus merits further investigation.

ACKNOWLEDGMENTS

We thank Dr. E. H. Sonnenblick, Dr. R. Kinne, and Dr. J. B. Caulfield for helpful dis-cussion. For advice and use of facilities, we thank Dr. K. R. Porter, Dr. M. Fotino, Mr. G. Wray, and Mr. G. Charlie of the HVEM Laboratory of the University of Colorado at Boulder; and Dr. R. Terry and Ms. Y. Kress, Ms. J. Fant, and Mr. F. Macaluso of AECOM. We are grateful to Ms. D. Wortsmann Carroll and Ms. R. Dominitz for technical assistance, and to Ms. L. DiDia, Mrs. K. Cohen, and Mrs. M. Abercrombie for translation of articles. This work was supported by NIH Research Grant HL-24336, New York Heart Association Grant-in-Aid, and NIH Research Career Development Award HL-00568 (to T.F.R.); and a Herman Raucher Investigatorship Award of the New York Heart Association (to J.M.C.).

REFERENCES

1. Caulfield, J. B., and Borg, T. K. 1979. The collagen network of the heart. *Lab. Invest.* 40:364–372.
2. Bairati, A. 1937. Struttura e proprietà fisiche del sarcolemma della fibra muscolare striata. *Z. Zellforsch.* 27:100–124.
3. Holmgren, E. 1907. Über die Trophospongien der quergestreiften Muskelfasern, nebst Bemerkungen über den allgemeinen Bau dieser Fasern. *Arch. Mikrosk. Anat.* 71:165–247.
4. Nagel, A. 1935. Die mechanischen Eigenschaften von Perimysium internum und Sarkolemm bei der quergestreiften Muskelfaster. *Z. Zellforsch.* 22:695–706.
5. Borg, T. K., and Caulfield, J. B. 1979. Collagen in the heart. *Texas Rep. Biol. Med.* 39:321–333.
6. Borg, T. K., and Caulfield, J. B. 1981. The collagen matrix of the heart. *Fed. Proc. Fed. Am. Soc. Exp. Biol.* 40:2037–2041.
7. Borg, T. K., Ranson, W. F., Moslehy, F. A., and Caulfield, J. B. 1981. Structural basis of ventricular stiffness. *Lab. Invest.* 44:49–54.
8. Bahr, G. F., and Jennings, R. B. 1961. Ultrastructure of normal and asphyxic myocardium of the dog. *Lab. Invest.* 10:548–571.
9. Battig, C. G., and Low, F. N. 1961. The ultrasturcture of human cardiac muscle and its associated tissue space. *Am. J. Anat.* 108:199–252.
10. Hanak, H., and Böck, P. 1971. Die Feinstruktur der Muskel-Sehnenverbindung von Skelett- und Herzmuskel. *J. Ultrastrct. Res.* 36:68–85.
11. Puff, A., and Langer, H. 1965. Das Problem der diastolischen Entfaltung der herzkammer (Eine Untersuchung über das elastische Gewebe im Myocard). *Gegen. Morphol. Jahrb.* 7:184–212.
12. Renteria, V. G., Ferrans, V. J., and Jones, M. 1976. Striated membranous structures in human hearts. *Am. J. Pathol.* 85(1):85–98.
13. Robinson, T. F. 1980. Lateral connections between heart muscle cells as revealed by conventional and high voltage transmission electron microscopy. *Cell. Tissue Res.* 211:353–359.
14. Robinson, T. F., Factor, S. M., and Sonnenblick, E. H. 1980. The skeletal framework of the heart: The hierarchical arrangement of inter- and pericellular connections. *Circulation* 62:iii–247.
15. Robinson, T. F., and Winegrad, S. 1981. A variety of intercellular connections in heart muscle. *J. Mol. Cell. Cardiol.* 13:185–195.
16. Winegrad, S., and Robinson, T. F. 1978. Force generation among cells in the relaxing heart. *Eur. J. Cardiol.* 7(Suppl.):63–70.
17. Capasso, J. M., Remily, R. M., and Sonnenblick, E. H. 1982. Alterations in mechanical properties of rat papillary muscle during maturation. *Am. J. Physiol. (Heart Circ. Physiol.* 11):242:H359–H364.
18. Saeki, Y., Sagawa, K., and Hiroyuki, S. 1978. Dynamic stiffness of cat heart muscle in Ba^{2+}-induced contracture. *Circ. Res.* 42:324–333.
19. Henderson, A. H., Forman, R., Brutsaert, D. L., and Sonnenblick, E. H. 1971. Tetanic contraction in mammalian cardiac muscle. *Cardiovasc. Res. (Suppl.)* 1:96–100.
20. Simeonescu, N., and Simeonescu, M. 1976. Galloylglucoses of low molecular weight as mordant in electron microscopy. I. Procedure and evidence for mordanting effect. *J. Cell Biol.* 70:608–621.
21. Behnke, O., and Zelander, T. 1970. Preservation of intercellular substances by the cationic dye alcian blue in preparative procedures for electron microscopy. *J. Ultrastruct. Res.* 31:424–438.
22. Luft, J. H. 1971. Ruthenium red and violet. II. Fine structural localization in animal tissues. *Anat. Rec.* 171:369–416.

23. Shepard, N., and Mitchell, N. 1977. The use of ruthenium red and *p*-phenylenediamine to stain cartilage simultaneously for light and electron microscopy. *J. Histochem. Cytochem.* 25:1163–1168.
24. Brown, L. M., and Hill, L. 1982. Mercuric chloride in alcohol and chloroform used as a rapidly acting fixative for contracting muscle fibres. *J. Microsc.* 125(3):319–336.
25. Hasegawa, T., Ravens, J. R. 1968. A metallic impregnation method for the demonstration of cerebral vascular patterns. *Acta Neuropathol.* 10:183–188.
26. Del Rio Hortega, P. 1943. El metodo del carbonato argentico: Revision general de sus tecnicas y aplicaciones en histologia normal y patoligica. *Arch. Histol. Norm. Pathol. (Buenos Aires)* 2:231–243.
27. Allen, R. D., Allen, N. S., and Travis, J. L. 1981. Video-enhanced contrast, differential interference contrast (AVEC-DIC) microscopy. *Cell Motil.* 1:291–302.
28. Robinson, T. F., Cohen-Gould, L., and Factor, S. M. 1983. The skeletal framework of mammalian heart muscle: Arrangement of inter- and pericellular connective tissue structures. *Lab. Invest.* 49:482–498.
29. Ross, R. 1973. The elastic fiber: A review. *J. Histochem. Cytochem.* 21:199–208.
30. Wiegner, A. W., Bing, O. H. L., Borg, R. K., and Caulfield, J. B. 1981. Mechanical and structural correlates of canine pericardium. *Circ. Res.* 49:807–814.
31. Broom, N. D. 1978. Simultaneous morphological and stress–strain studies of the fibrous components in wet heart valve leaflet tissue. *Connect. Tiss. Res.* 6:37–50.
32. Robinson, T. F., and Winegrad, S. 1979. The measurement and dynamic implications of thin filament lengths in heart muscle. *J. Physiol.* 286:607–619.
33. Street, S. F. 1983. Lateral transmission of tension in frog myofibers: A myofibrillar network and transverse cytoskeletal connections are possible transmitters. *J. Cell. Physiol.* 114:346–364.
34. Meyer, F. A., Koblentz, M., and Silberberg, A. 1977. Structural investigation of loose connective tissue by using a series of dextran fractions as non-interacting macro-molecular probes. *Biochem. J.* 161:285–291.
35. Frank, J. S., Langer, G. A., Nudd, L. M., and Saraydarian, C. 1977. The myocardial cell surface, its histochemistry, and the effect of sialic acid and calcium removal on its structure and cellular ionic exchange. *Circ. Res.* 41:702–714.
36. Myers, D. B., Highton, T. C., and Rayns, D. G. 1973. Ruthenium red-positive filaments interconnecting collagen fibrils. *J. Ultrastruct. Res.* 42:87–92.
37. Rosenberg, L., Hellman, W., and Kleinschmidt, A. K. 1970. Macromolecular models of protein polysaccharide from bovine nasal cartilage based on electron microscopic studies. *J. Biol. Chem.* 245:4123–4130.
38. Wight, T. N., and Hascall, V. C. 1983. Proteoglycans in primate arteries. III. Characterization of the proteoglycans synthesized by arterial smooth muscle cells in culture. *J. Cell Biol.* 96:167–176.
39. Jones, R. M. 1975. *Mechanics of Composite Materials.* Scripta, Washington, D.C.
40. Wittenberg, B. A., and Robinson, T. F. 1981. Oxygen requirements, morphology, cell coat and membrane permeability of calcium-tolerant myocytes from hearts of adult rats. *Cell Tissue Res.* 216:231–251.
41. Puchtler, H., and Meloan, S. N. 1979. Orcein, collastin and pseudoelastica: A reinvestigation of Unna's concepts. *Histochemistry* 64:119–130.

Ventricular Collagen Matrix and Alterations

James B. Caulfield, Sun Ben Tao, and Maurice Nachtigal

Department of Pathology
School of Medicine
University of South Carolina
Columbia, South Carolina 29208

Abstract. There is a complex extracellular structural matrix in the heart. This matrix appears to be composed of a variety of fibrils and fibers extending from the cell surface to the basal lamina and from the basal lamina to the matrix. The extensions into the extracellular region interconnect with a system of collagen bundles. The latter are so located that they would tether the myocytes to each other as well as tether the capillaries to the myocytes. There is an extensive weave of collagen analogous to the perimysium of sekletal muscle that separates groups of myocytes. The weave surrounding a group of myocytes is connected to adjacent weave patterns by long, tendonlike structures.

The collagen matrix around cells disappears 2–3 hr after coronary-artery occlusion. In the periinfarct region of viable cells, the matrix is similarly lost and is replaced by scarlike collagen. Encephalomyocarditis virus causes a similar loss of the matrix in necrotic as well as some adjacent nonnecrotic regions. Replacement of the lost matrix is by scar tissue. The long-term appearance of the replacement fibrosis closely resembles the appearance of diffuse fibrosis as seen in a variety of conditions. These observations suggest that diffuse fibrosis can occur secondary to loss of the matrix both with and without myocyte necrosis. This may help explain the diffuse left ventricular fibrosis as seen in a variety of human disease.

CARDIAC EXTRACELLULAR MATRIX

The heart is a displacement-type pump that functions by means of three-dimensional alteration of the ventricular wall. Sarcomeres, the source of motion in the ventricular wall, appear to be in a simple linear array in each cell. For the three-dimensional wall motion to result in displacement, the cells must be arranged in such a way that the simple linear contractile elements result in three-dimensional changes in form. Further, the stress generated by each cell must be delivered to the ventricular cavity. These considerations immediately impose anisotropic nonhomogeneous properties on the ventricle. Anisotrophy has been clearly demonstrated [1,2]. The cellular component of the myocardium has been extensively studied; however, the second component of the nonhomogeneous myocardium, the extracellular matrix, is less well examined or understood.

During isovolumetric contraction, ventricular-wall pressure develops rapidly, and during the ejection portion of systole, pressure to 150 mm Hg

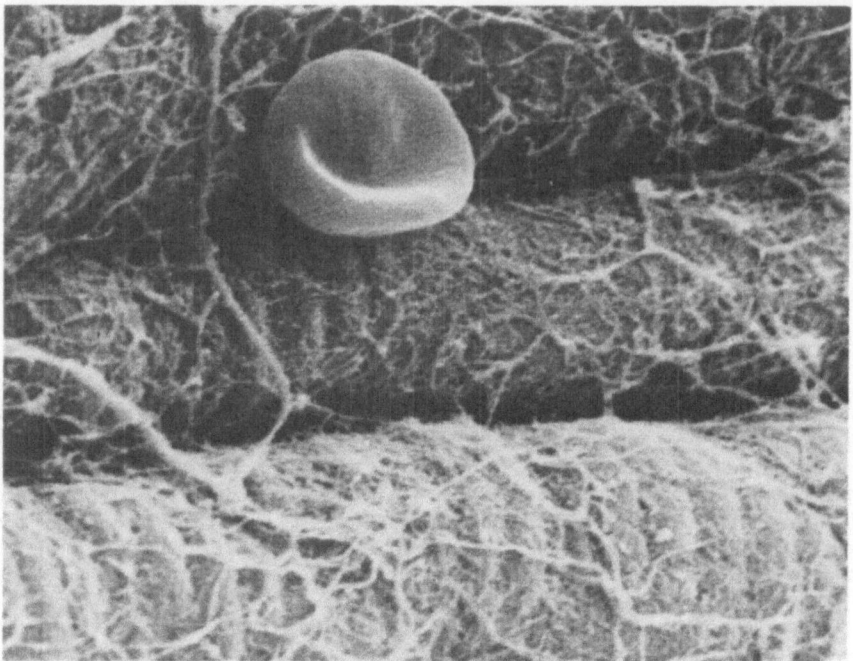

Figure 1.   SEM of dog heart demonstrating the disposition of collagen struts around myocytes. There are numerous interconnections between myocytes as well as bundles of collagen running in the long axes of the myocytes. × 4000.

is transmitted to the ventricular cavity. Associated with ejection, geometric changes occur in the ventricle. Transmission of the force to the ventricle must involve the myocardial matrix. Of the structural proteins in the heart, collagen has the physical properties necessary for force transmission to the ventricle as far as magnitude and rate of development are concerned. One can conclude that a complex system composed primarily of collagen is necessary for at least systolic stress distribution and tethering of myocytes one to another during the spatial translocations that accompny systole. Similarly, one can expect that during systole, some mechanism will maintain the spatial relationships of capillaries to the myocytes. Diastolic pressures of 5–10 mm Hg are sufficient to deform the heart from the end-systolic to the end-diastolic configuration. For proper ventricular function, contiguous myocytes, at least, must be stretched to near the same amount. This again implies a mechanism for distribution of stress throughout the entire ventricular wall as the geometry is markedly changed. The most probable system for such stress distribution involves collagen.

Scanning electron microscopy (SEM) of the ventricles of a variety of species including rats, mice, rabbits, dogs, hamsters, and humans presents a qualitatively similar picture with some quantitative differences [3]. Con-

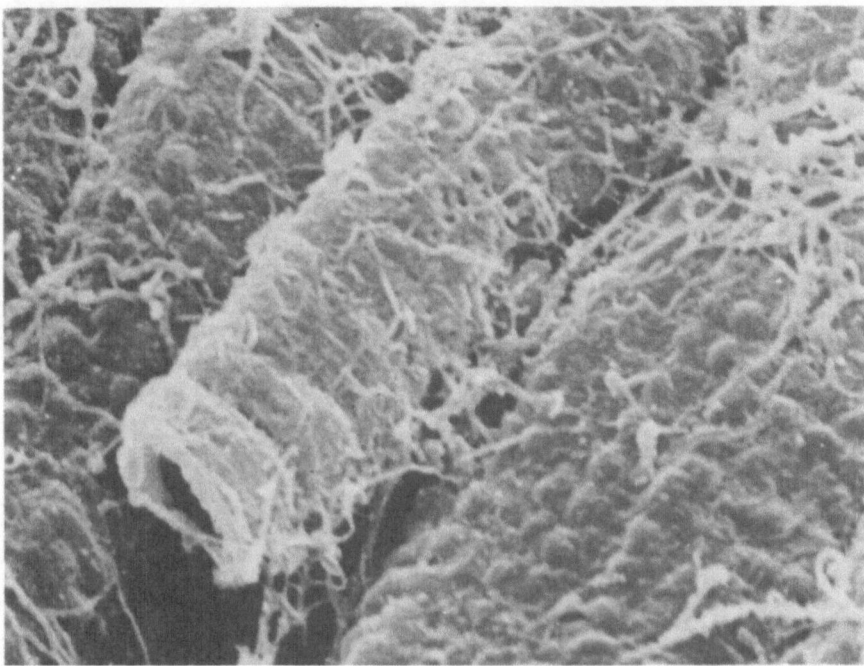

Figure 2.   SEM of rat heart showing the collagen struts that interconnect capillaries with adjacent myocytes. ×4000.

tiguous myocytes are coupled one to another by an extensive array of collagen struts (Figure 1). In small laboratory animals, these struts measure 120–150 nm in diameter and insert near perpendicular into the basal lamina surrounding each myocyte. This system, by the number of struts and their positioning, could assist in maintaining cell-to-cell continuity throughout the cardiac cycle. A second set of struts of similar size extends from the myocytes to all contiguous capillaries (Figure 2). The course followed by these struts is somewhat different from that followed by the struts between myocytes. The collagen struts insert near perpendicular to the basement membrane of the capillary, but course partially around adjacent myocytes and insert tangentially into the basal lamina of the myocyte [4]. The number of struts and their distribution would permit only slight translational movement of the capillary relative to the myocyte throughout the cardiac cycle. The number and course of the struts would assure that capillaries shorten with systole. The observation that blood flow occurs through the myocardium during systole has been made repeatedly [5–8]. This somewhat anomalous situation of flow through vessels subjected to external stresses of 150 mm Hg has provoked numerous investigations, yet a clear understanding of myocardial flow is not at hand. It is possible that the numerous struts that

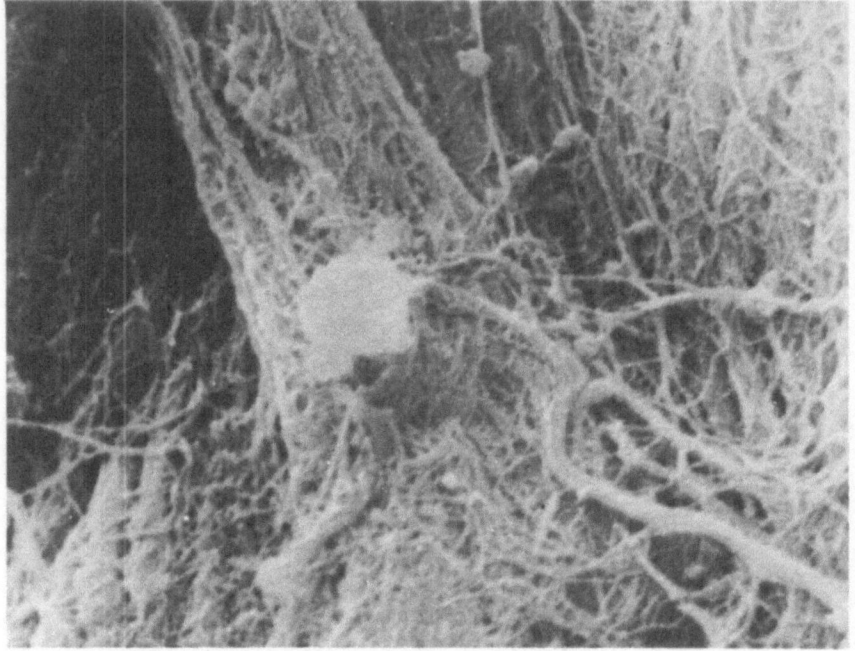

Figure 3.   A small segment of the weave of collagen surrounding groups of myocytes. This area is from the posterior ventricular wall of a dog with an anterior myocardial infarction. × 8000.

connect the myocytes and capillaries result in the coupling of myocardial flow and contraction proposed by Wiggers [9].

   Many of the collagen struts that insert into the basal lamina of the myocyte course parallel to the long axis over two or more sarcomeres to insert into the basal lamina of the same cell. This orientation would assist in preventing overstretch of the cell. The myocytes of the heart occur in groups quite analogous to the fascicles of skeletal muscle [3]. Similarly, the myocyte groups of the heart are encircled by a collagen network that resembles the perimysium and is connected by collagen struts to the enclosed contiguous myocytes (Figure 3). In skeletal muscle, this system has viscoelastic properties and is clearly stress-resistant [10,11]. Comparison of the number of collagen bundles forming the weave of rats and hamsters suggests that this structure can account for the difference in the ventricular elastic modulus between these two animals [12]. Rats from the ages of 1 month to 17 months have an elastic modulus of roughly twice that of hamsters at the same age. SEM of the two species reveals a much more extensive weave of collagen in rats than in hamsters. This difference in weave is the only difference we could demonstrate by light microscopy, SEM, or transmission electron microscopy (TEM) in samples of the left ventricle. Thus, it appears that the weave seen in hearts is similarly located to the perimysium of skeletal muscle and contributes to the elastic modulus of the heart quite analogously to skeletal muscle. If the weave contributes to the diastolic or passive properties of the heart, it is difficult to envision it as the mechanism by which systolic stress is delivered to the ventricle. As yet, no structure in the matrix has been clearly identified as being associated with systolic stress distribution.

Very little collagen is visible by SEM in newborn rats and hamsters [13]. No intermyocyte struts, myocyte-to-capillary struts, or weave are visible at birth. Rats have a mean arterial pressure of 12 mm Hg at birth, but by 20 days of age, it has reached 85 mm Hg [14]. During this period of 20 days, the extensive disposition of collagens has occurred and is indistinguishable from that in the adult. This rapid development occurs as pressure and stroke volume of the heart are increasing, strongly suggesting a relationship. If collagen disposition is blocked during this period, ventricular aneurysms and rupture, among other things, occur [15].

A result of the weave tightly enveloping groups of myocytes would be an extracellular force that could counteract cell swelling. This has been shown in a series of papers by Pine and co-workers [16–19]. Under conditions of isosmotic high potassium or hyposmotic Krebs–Henseleit solutions, the water content of ventricular cells increased 20%, atrial cells 60%, and renal tubular cells more than 100%. The data and discussions in these papers implicate an extracellular hydraulic force that is able to prevent cell swelling. The most likely constituent that varies with the data on cell swelling is the collagen matrix, being most prominent in the ventricle, less so in the atrium, and least in the renal tubular cells. The basement membrane extracellular collagen complex of the renal tubule does inhibit cell swelling to some extent [20].

MATRIX ALTERATIONS

Alterations in the connective tissue of the heart have been implicated in altered compliance in a number of diseases [21]. The precise mechanism by which this comes about is not clear, especially in those conditions with diffuse fibrosis and little actual loss of myocytes. We have been examining two models in which fibrosis is present, both in the form of scars and as a diffuse phenomenon. The first is coronary artery ligation in dogs, the second infection with encephalomyocarditis virus of mice.

The left anterior descending coronary artery was ligated in 12 dogs, and portions of the ventricle with restricted or unrestricted blood supply were examined by light microscopy, SEM, and TEM. Samples were obtained at 2, 3, and 24 hr, 1 week, and 2 weeks after surgery. At 2 hr after coronary-artery ligation, there is extensive loss of the collagen matrix in the ischemic area. Figure 4 is from the posterior wall of the left ventricle of an animal

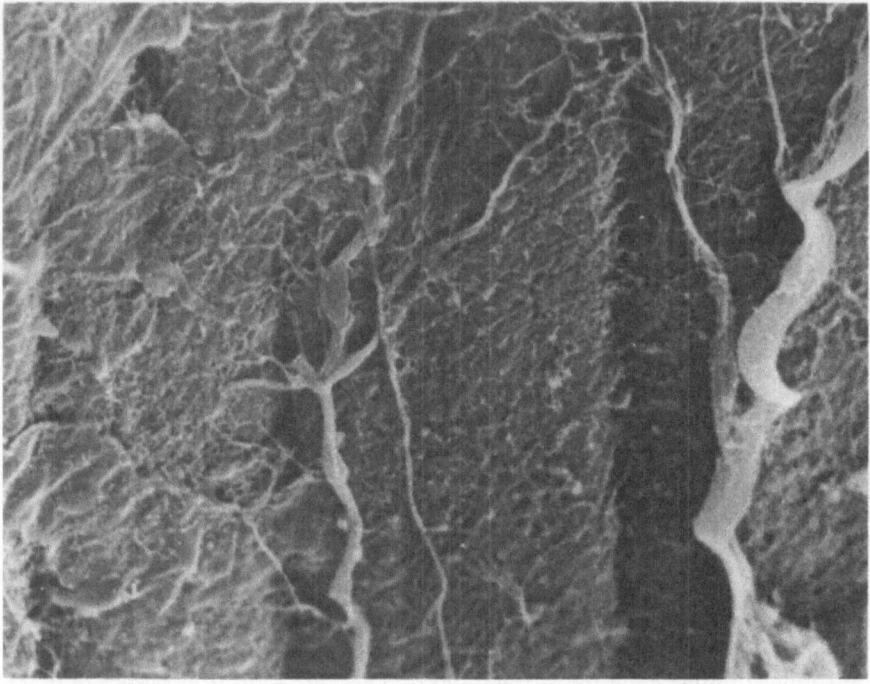

Figure 4.   Normal area of dog left ventricle showing disposition of collagen struts between myocytes. Compare with Figure 5. ×3500.

with coronary artery ligation for 2 hr; Figure 5 is from the anterior ischemic portion of the same animal. At 3 hr, loss is more complete and extends 2–5 mm beyond the bounds of identifiable necrotic cells. Cells with no evidence of rupture of their basal lamina or plasma membrane are free of struts. In these regions of strut loss, both necrotic and viable, the cells are widely separated and have lost lateral connections. The dissolution of the collagen matrix occurring with 2 hr of ischemia precedes invasion of the area by leukocytes. The lack of leukocytes and loss of collagen suggest a collagen-olytic activity actuated by ischemia that is present either in myocytes or in the matrix at the time of vascular occlusion. Alternatively, the ischemic region may permit activation locally of a plasma-derived substance that is delivered to the region, since coronary ligation rarely results in a very extensive area of total loss of blood flow [22].

   At 1 week after the surgery, extensive repair at the margin of the infarct had occurred (Figure 6). The pertinent point is that viable myocytes at the margin that had presumably lost their normal components of struts were now encased in a fine membrane of collagen with no resemblance to the normal collagen distribution expected. By 2 weeks, collagen encircled the

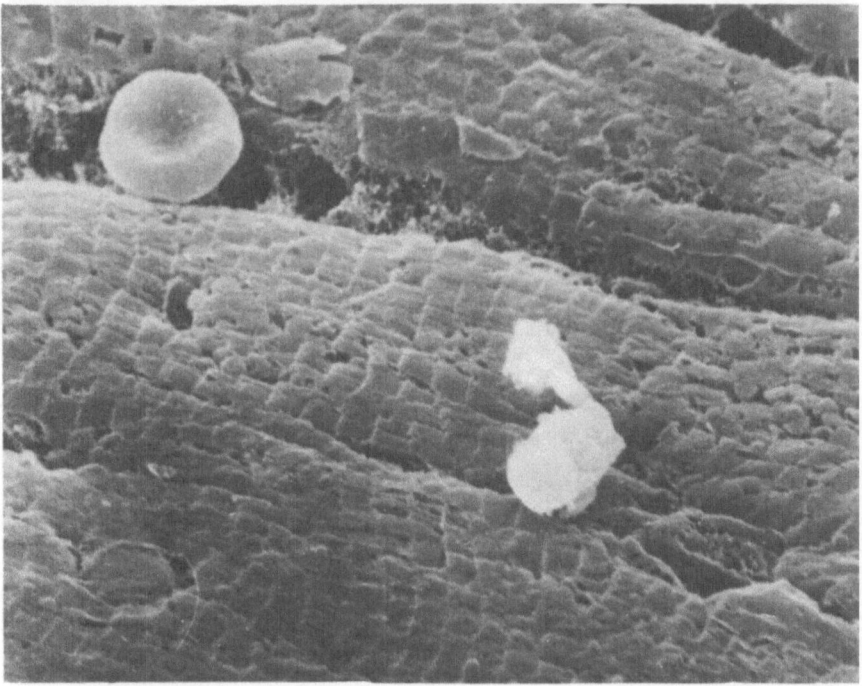

Figure 5.   Area of anterior ventricle of dog with coronary-artery ligation of 2 hr. Marked loss of collagen is evident. × 3500.

cells, especially the Purkinje cells, and clearly isolated them from the contiguous cells (Figure 7). Thus, following loss of the normal collagen matrix, replacement of collagen in a totally abnormal distribution occurs. In the necrotic area, macrophages as well as fibroblasts were evident.

Spontaneous acute infarcts in humans had comparable loss of the collagen matrix at 18 hr after onset of chest pain. This is the earliest time period available to us. It is reasonable to assume a much earlier onset of the collagenolytic activity in humans as is seen in dogs.

If there is a proteolytic activity that can affect the myocardium, it should be demonstrable under other conditions. For this reason, we examined mice following inoculation of encephalomyocarditis virus (EMC), which in the C3H/HeN strain causes an extensive and diffuse reaction. Within 24 hr of the inoculation, evidence of damage to the basal lamina and plasma membrane is evident. These areas are visible by TEM as points of breakdown of the plasma membrane, marked mitochondrial swelling, and partial loss of the basal lamina. The changes become extensive, and at 3 days after infection, large areas of necrotic cells are visible (Figure 8). In these areas, the normal collagen matrix has disappeared. At 1 day after infection, lym-

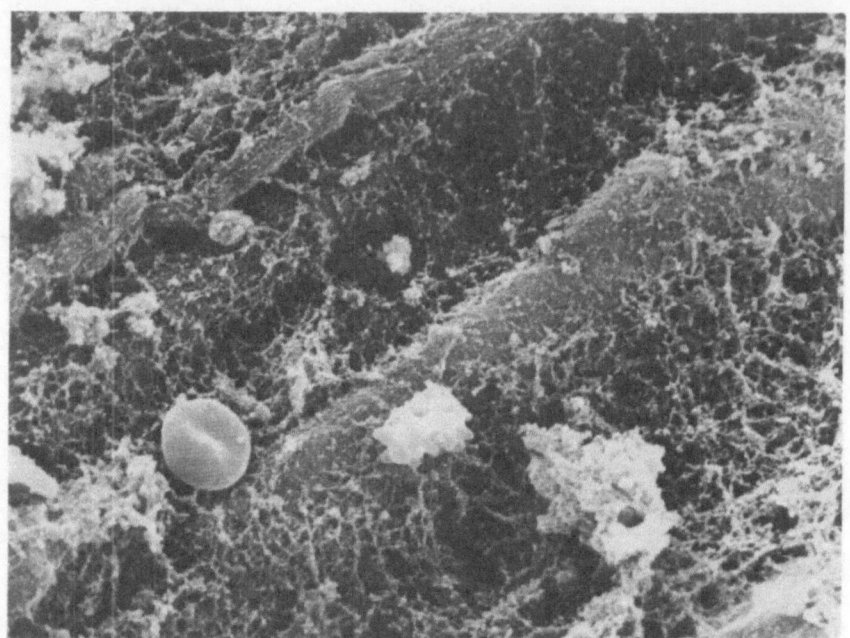

Figure 6. Marginal area of dog ventricle with infarct for 1 week. The normal collagen strut system is gone and is being replaced by a fine filamentous distribution of collagen. ×4000.

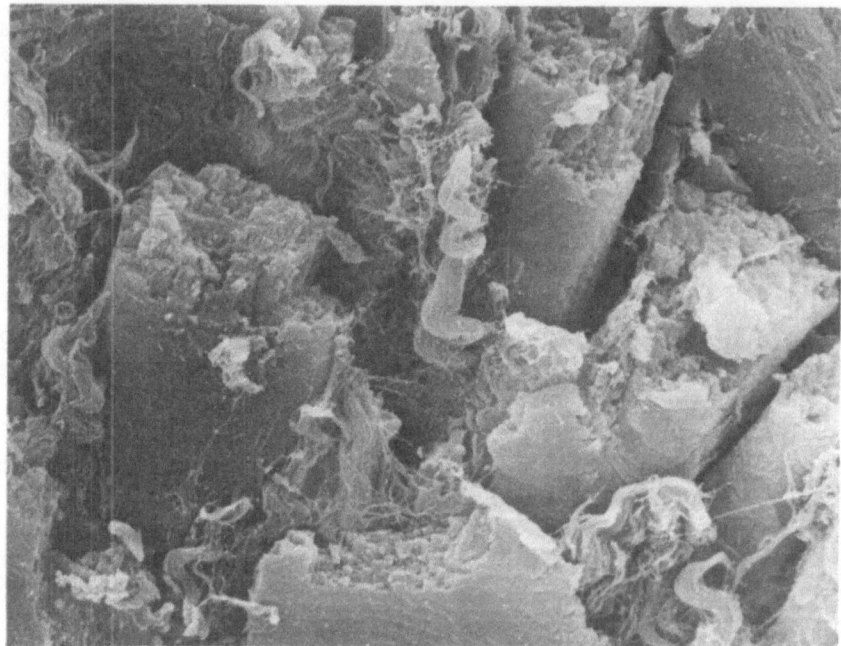

Figure 7. Marginal area of dog ventricle with an infarct of 2 weeks' duration. There is excessive collagen between the myocytes, resulting in separation. ×1000.

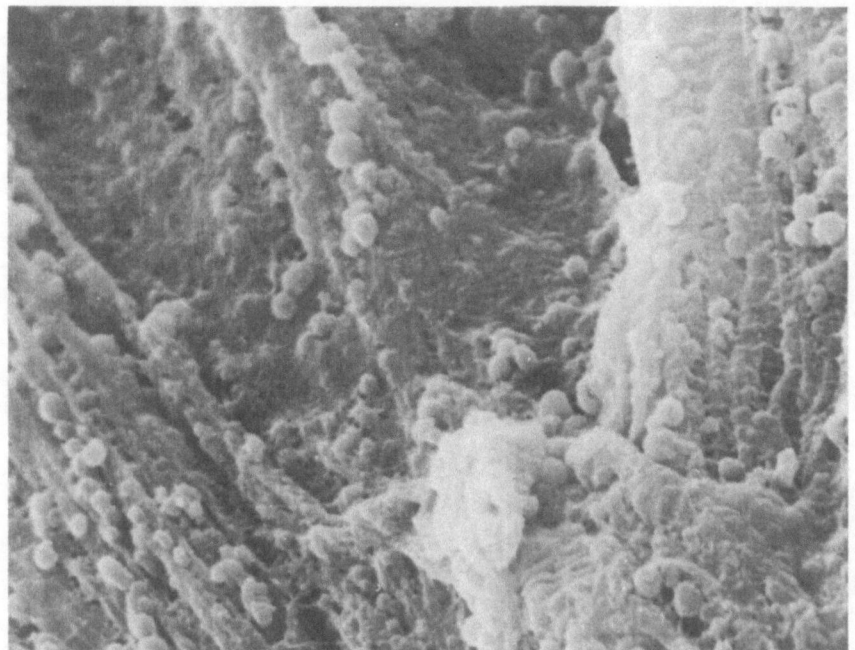

Figure 8.   Mouse heart 3 days after inoculation with EMC virus. The cells are necrotic and the collagen matrix has disappeared. × 3000.

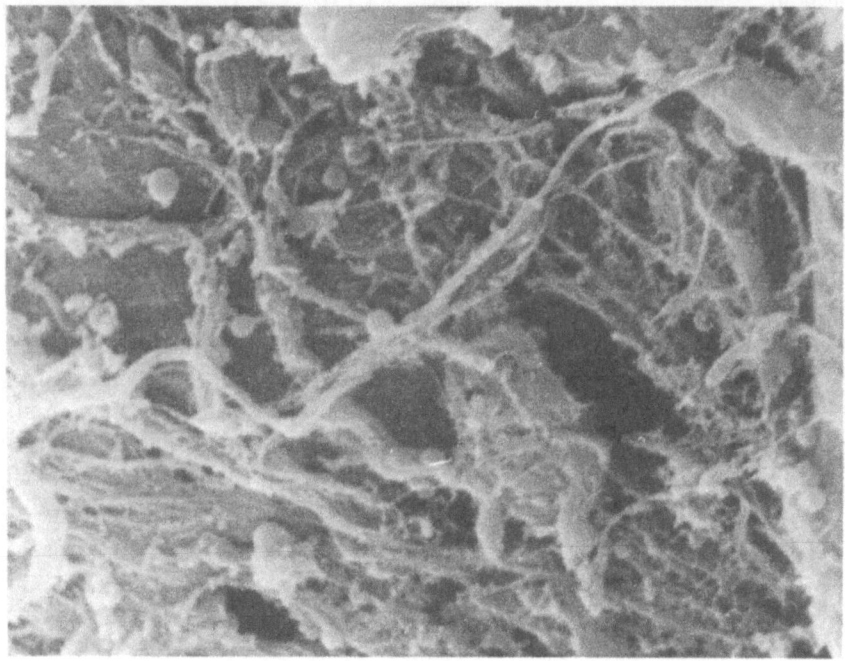

Figure 9.   Mouse heart 5 days after inoculation with EMC virus. The normal matrix is being replaced with thick, dense bands of collagen. × 3000.

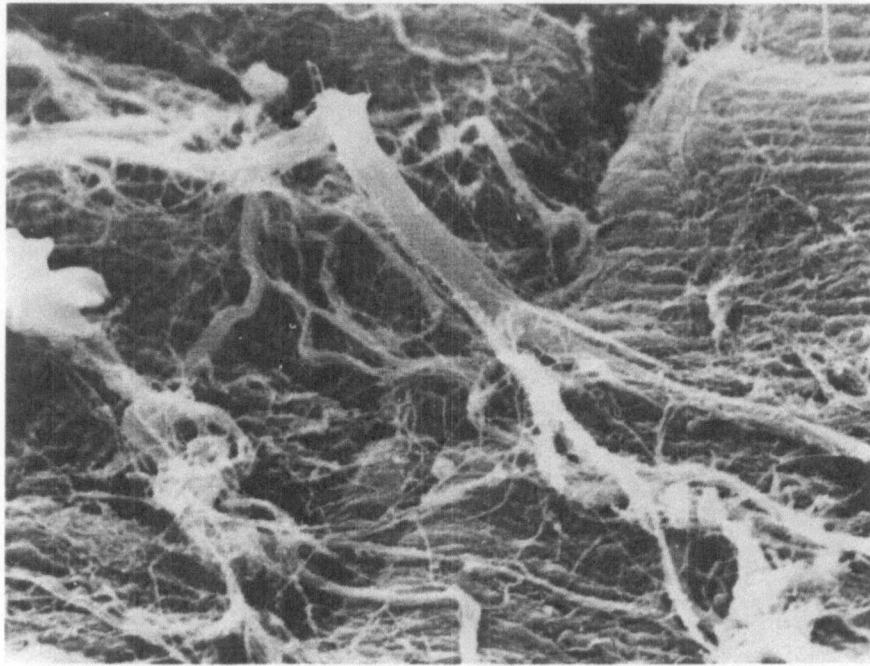

Figure 10.   Mouse heart 1 year after inoculation with EMC virus. Many myocytes are widely separated by thick bundles of collagen that have replaced the normal structures found between cells. ×3000.

phocytes are visible adjacent to damaged areas, and at 3 days, macrophages are present as well. At 4 days, fibroblasts are common in areas of damage and matrix dissolution, and by 5 days, excessive collagen deposition is present (Figure 9).

Animals sacrificed 1 year after EMC inoculation had large areas of scar tissue that replaced the areas of myocyte necrosis. In these animals, there are many areas of excessive collagen deposition in thick bundles that encircle one or more myocytes. The distribution of this collagen is quite abnormal (Figure 10). This process appears to be an extension of the image seen at 5 days, with areas of excessive collagen deposition and abnormal distribution replacing the normal matrix. As with most scars, increase in diameter of the fibril and orientation of the collagen bundles in the lines of stress occur with time.

RELATIONSHIP TO HUMAN DISEASE

The two models of matrix loss and replacement by collagen in the form of scars can be used to interpret some alterations in human disease. Diffuse

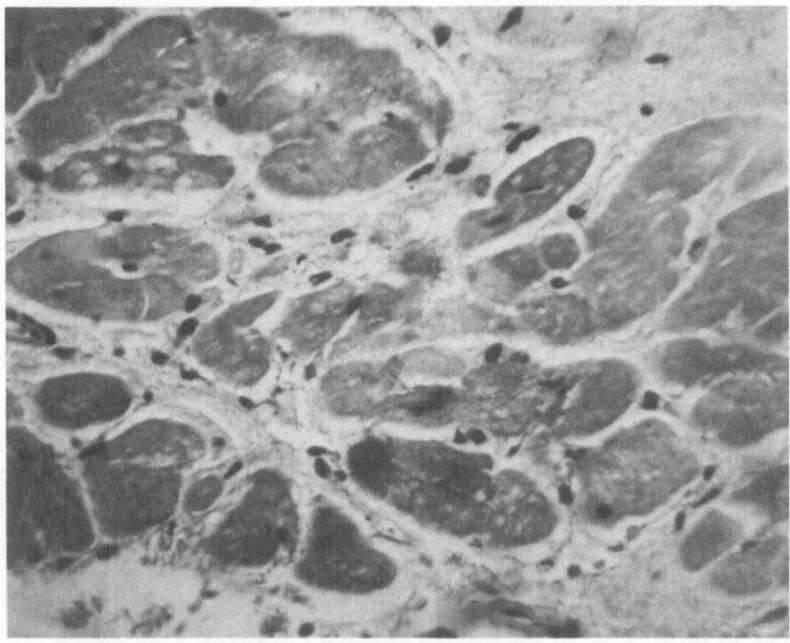

Figure 11.   Light micrograph of subendocardial fibrosis from a human heart. This type of change is commonly seen in various heart conditions. × 400.

fibrosis as seen in atherosclerotic heart disease without infarct, hypertrophic cardiomyopathy, and cardiac hypertrophy secondary to hypertension consist of deposition of collagen around myocytes (Figure 11). By SEM, this change resembles that seen in the periinfarct region of both dogs and humans, i.e., loss of the normal strut complex and replacement by excessive amounts of collagen in an abnormal distribution. In these areas, the myocytes are widely separated and no lateral contacts between cells are visible (Figure 12). The sheath of scar tissue surrounding the myocytes could be the result of reparative processes following matrix damage. In the dog infarct model, the matrix is rapidly lost, apparently secondary to a proteolytic activity. The assumption is that some collagenolytic activity can be exercised in a variety of conditions without necessarily involving myocyte necrosis. The subsequent reparative processes produce diffuse fibrosis.

SUMMARY

There is a complex network of collagen in the heart that is associated with a number of ventricular functions. This system, which is composed of bundles of collagen fibrils that appear to begin and end at the basal lamina,

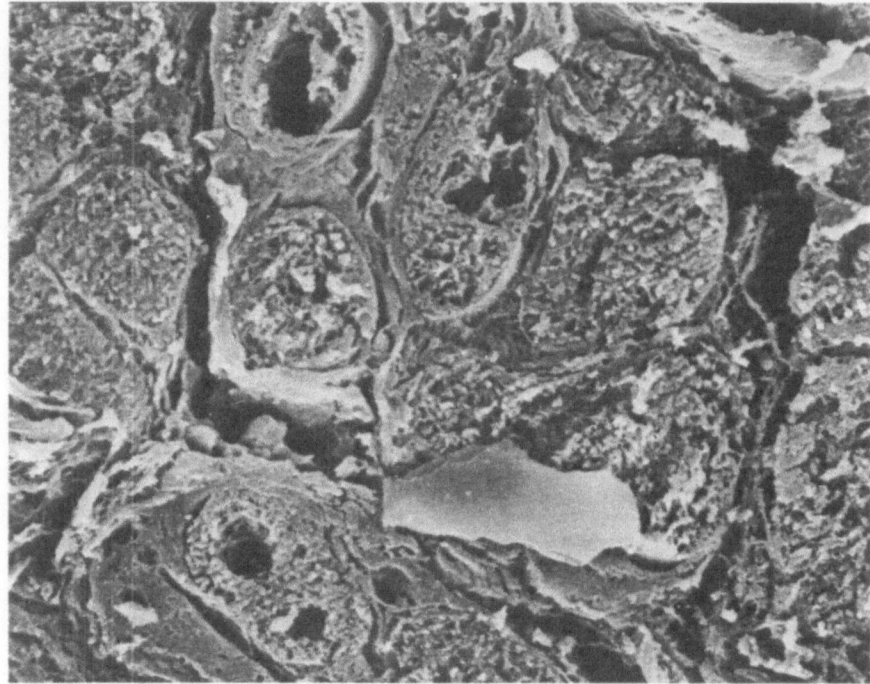

Figure 12.   SEM of subendocardial fibrosis seen near the edge of an old healed infarct. The remaining viable myocytes are encased in fibrous tissue and widely separated. × 1000.

is associated with a series of smaller fibrils extending from the plasma membrane of myocytes to the basement membrane. This network can be damaged or destroyed by ischemic insults and viral myocarditis. In the case of the infarct, loss of matrix occurs before leukocytic infiltration, whereas with the viral myocarditis, areas of damage are associated with the presence of lympyocytes. This loss of collagen does occur in regions of viable myocytes, and subsequent repair in these regions results in excessive and abnormal distribution of collagen, essentially a scar. These areas resemble the diffuse fibrosis seen in a number of disease states, and the mechanism for production of diffuse fibrosis could be similar to that in the two experimental models, i.e., loss of matrix with subsequent deposition of a scar without necessarily involving necrosis of myocytes.

ACKNOWLEDGMENTS

This work was partially supported by NIH grant HL-27533 and by a grant-in-aid from the South Carolina Heart Association.

REFERENCES

1. Lev, M., and Simpkins, C. S. 1956. Architecture of the human ventricular myocardium. *Lab. Invest.* 5:396–407.
2. Mirsky, I. 1970. Effects of anisotropy and nonhomogeneity on left ventricular stresses in the intact heart. *Bull. Math. Biophys.* 32:197–213.
3. Caulfield, J. B., and Borg, T. K. 1979. The collagen network of the heart. *Lab Invest.* 40:364–372.
4. Borg, T. K., and Caulfield, J. B. 1981. The collagen matrix of the heart. *Fed. Proc. Fed. Am. Soc. Exp. Biol.* 40:2037–2041.
5. Caulfield, J. B., Borg, T. K., and Abel, F. L. 1983. The effects of systole on left ventricular blood flow. In: E. Chazov, V. Saks, and G. Rona (eds.), *Advances in Myocardiology.* Vol. 4, pp. 379–393. Plenum Press, New York.
6. Hess, D. S., and Bache, R. J. 1976. Transmural distribution of myocardial blood flow during systole in the awake dog. *Circ. Res.* 38:5–15.
7. Kreuzer, H., and Schoeppe, W. 1963. Das Verhalten des Bruckes in der Herzewand, Pfluegers Arch. 278:181–198.
8. Kreuzer, H., and Schoeppe, W. 1963. Zur Entstehung der Differenz zwischen systolischem Myokard und Ventrikeldruck. *Pfleugers Arch.* 278:199–208.
9. Wiggers, C. J. 1954. The interplay of coronary vascular resistance and myocardial compression in regulating coronary flow. *Circ. Res.* 2:271–279.
10. Nagel, A. 1935. Mechanischen Eigenschaften von Perimysium internum und Sarkolemm bei den quergestreiften Muskelfasern. *Z. Zellforsch. Mikrosk. Anat.* 22:649–704.
11. Banus, M. G., and Zeitlin, A. M. 1938. The relation of isometric tension to length in skeletal muscle. *J. Cell. Comp. Physiol.* 12:403–420.
12. Borg, T. K., Ranson, W. F., Moslehy, F. A., and Caulfied, J. B. 1981. Structural basis of ventricular stiffness. *Lab. Invest.* 44:49–54.
13. Borg, T. K., and Caulfield, J. B. 1979. Collagen in the heart. *Texas Rep. Biol. Med.* 39:321–333.
14. Hopkins, F., McCutcheon, E. P., and Wekstein, P. R. 1973. Post natal changes in rat ventricular function. *Circ. Res.* 32:685–691.
15. Kelly, W. A., Kesterson, J. W., and Carlton, W. W. 1974. Myocardial lesions in the off-spring of female rats fed a copper deficient diet. *Exp. Mol. Pathol.* 20:40–56.
16. Pine, M. B., Caulfield, J. B., and Abelmann, W. H. 1980. Regulation of myocardial cell volume. In G. Bourne (ed.), Hearts and Heart-like Organs. pp. 45–75. Academic Press, New York.
17. Pine, M. B., Brooks, W. W., Nosta, J. J., and Abelmann, W. H. 1981. Hydrostatic forces limit swelling of rat ventricular myocardium. *Am. J. Physiol.* 241:H740–H747.
18. Pine, M. B., Caulfield, J. B., Ring, O. H. L., Brooks, W. W., and Abelmann, W. H. 1979. Resistance of contracting myocardium to swelling with hypoxia and glycolytic blockade. *Cardiovasc. Res.* 12:569–577.
19. Pine, M. B., Borg, T. K., and Caulfield, J. B. 1982. Regulation of atrial myocardial cellular volume during exposure to isosmotic high potassium or hyposmotic media. *J. Mol. Cell Cardiol.* 14:207–221.
20. Linshaw, M. A., and Grantham. J. J. 1980. Effect of collagenase and ouabain on renal cell volume in hypotonic media. *Am. J. Physiol.* 238:F491–F498.
21. Mirsky, I., Cohn, P. F., Leveine, J. A., Gorlin, R., Herman, M. U., Kreulen, T. H., and Sonnenblick, E. H. 1974. Assessment of left ventricular stiffness in primary myocardial disease and coronary artery disease. *Circulation* 50:128–141.
22. Rivas, F., Coble, F. R., Bache, R. J., and Greenfield, J. C. 1976. Relationship between blood flow to ischemic regions and extent of myocardial infarction. *Circ. Res.* 38:439–447.

SARCOLEMMAL SODIUM EXCHANGE

Single Cells and Rapid Inward Sodium Current

Trevor Powell

University Laboratory of Physiology
Oxford OX1 3PT, England

Abstract. This chapter presents a brief review of measurements of rapid inward sodium current in single cardiac cells. It is shown that the simplified morphology of the individual cell, with a lack of restricted extracellular space, has been exploited to provide improved spatial and temporal voltage control, resulting in the first recordings of both the activation and inactivation phases of rapid inward sodium current. It is to be expected that future research will produce much interesting data on this component of membrane current, which will have direct relevance to many processes concerned with cardiac function at the cellular level.

INTRODUCTION

The rapid upstroke of the cardiac action potential is generated by an inflow of sodium (Na) ions[1,2]. Direct measurement of this current is difficult in heart tissue, because the maximum conductance is the largest and the kinetics the most rapid of any cardiac current. Indeed, until recently, it was considered that the complex morphology of cardiac tissue and the inadequacies of voltage-clamp techniques made reliable analysis of rapid inward Na current (I_{Na}) almost impossible [3–6].

Careful use of short rabbit Purkinje fibers and double-microelectrode voltage-clamp has provided the most optimal data from multicellular preparations [7,8], but rapid inward currents were still partially obscured by capacitative transients during the early phases of conductance changes. The two-microelectrode technique has also been applied to spherical clusters of chick embryonic heart cells [9–11], but again, early phases of I_{Na} were obscured by capacitative currents and voltage control was limited by a high external resistance [12]. More marked improvements in the measurement of I_{Na} have been obtained by using single cardiac cells and by applying voltage-clamp with a single suction electrode [13–16] or two suction electrodes [17–19] to isolated rat ventricular myocytes. Recently, single-suction-electrode measurements of I_{Na} have also been made in single bullfrog atrial cells [20] and in segments of cells derived from human atrial tissue [21]. In addition, patch-clamp techniques [22] have been applied to cultured cells from neonatal rat hearts to study both whole-cell recordings of I_{Na} and single-channel Na currents [23].

The purposes of this very brief review are to indicate how the use of single cardiac cells has enhanced our understanding of I_{Na} and to suggest where future research may yield some highly interesting data of immediate relevance to our understanding of heart function.

MAGNITUDE OF I_{Na}

The magnitude of currents recorded under voltage-clamp will be determined by the size of the cell under study and the contribution that I_{Na} makes to the upstroke of the action potential. It is not surprising that the largest I_{Na} is found in isolated ventricular myocytes, measured at 20–22°C [13,17–19]. Brown et al. [17–19] reported that I_{Na} in isolated rat cells was 70–140 nA at a clamp potential of between −30 and −20 mV, with a threshold at −70 to −60 mV. These values are larger than peak inward currents of 50–60 nA in clusters of cardiac cells [9], 10 nA in single rat ventricular cells clamped with a single suction electrode [16], 10–15 nA in segments of human atrial cells [21], and about 5 nA in isolated frog atrial cells [20]. Other than in the cell clusters [9], which were at 37°C, all other measurements were made at ambient temperatures, usually 20–22°C. Hume and Giles [20] noted specifically that unless series resistance compensation was used or the amplitude of I_{Na} was reduced with tetrodotoxin (TTX), I_{Na} was underestimated due to poor voltage control. Similar reasoning had persuaded Lee and co-workers [17–19] to resort to the use of two suction electrodes, even though promising results had been obtained when only one pipette was used [13]. It is still the case that no reliable measurements have been made of I_{Na} in single ventricular cells at 37°C, despite the remarkable advances that have been made in recording techniques.

Translating peak I_{Na} into a peak current density requires a knowledge of the relevant area across which I_{Na} is flowing. This is difficult to determine precisely, since even though cell capacitance might be known, it is not clear what proportion of membrane area contributes to the flow of I_{Na}. Brown et al. [19] assumed an average cell surface area of 8000 μm^2, based on the best morphological evidence then available, to calculate a peak current density of the order 0.9–1.8 mA · cm^{-2}. It is now clear that this was an underestimate of sarcolemmal area and that a value nearer 14,000 μm^2 would have been more appropriate [24], leading to current densities in the range 0.5–1.0 mA · cm^{-2}. It is probably far better to express all currents in terms of preparation capacitance, so that since the cells in this study had capacitances of the order 400 pF [19], peak current density is of the order 175–350 pA · pF^{-1}.

DETERMINATION OF $\bar{g}_{Na}$

Given that due precaution has been taken to ensure that contaminating currents have been eliminated, once the reversal potential for I_{Na} has been determined, then the maximum Na conductance ($\bar{g}_{Na}$) can be calculated from the appropriate current–voltage curves. In isolated rat ventricular cells, $\bar{g}_{Na}$ is of the order of 2 μS/cell [19]. Again, by using an estimated surface area of 8000 μm^2, a maximum conductance of 25 mS · cm^{-2} can be calculated [19]. Direct measurement of single-channel Na conductance in neonatal heart cells [23] gives a value of 15 pS, which when combined with a $\bar{g}_{Na}$ of about 10 nS/cell from whole-cell recordings and a membrane capacity of 5 pF/cell, and assuming a specific membrane capacity of 1 μF · cm^{-2}, gives 670 Na channels/cell or 1–2 channels/μm^{-2}. Cachelin et al. [23] noted that channel densities based on a $\bar{g}_{Na}$ of 25 mS · cm^{-2} were of the order 16 channels/μm^{-2} and suggested that the difference between the values for cultured cells and single myocytes might be due either to cell differentiation during development or to differences in enzyme treatment during the culturing or disaggregation procedures. In fact, the foregoing comparison shows the difficulties encountered when trying to compare conductance estimates based on different assumptions concerning cell surface area. If maximum conductance for ventricular myocytes is expressed in terms of cell capacitance, then $\bar{g}_{Na}$ becomes 5 nS · pF^{-1}, compared to 2 nS · pF^{-1} for cultured cells, so that the difference in magnitude for the two values is not as marked as appears at first sight.

ACTIVATION OF I_{Na}

One great advantage of single cells is that their use has allowed the first estimates to be made of the activation kinetics of I_{Na} over a voltage range of physiological interest. I_{Na} activates, after a delay, with a time constant of about 0.7 msec at −55 mV, decreasing to about 100 μsec on depolarizations positive to +10 mV [19]. These values compare favorably with independent measurements made with a single suction electrode [16], although the voltage dependence of the activation time constant is shifted about 10 mV more positive compared to the data obtained using two suction electrodes [19]. Whole-cell recordings using patch-clamp techniques give activation time constants decreasing from 0.9 to 0.3 msec over the potential range −40 to 0 mV [23].

INACTIVATION OF I_{Na}

The time constant of inactivation of I_{Na} in isolated rat ventricular cells studied with a single suction electrode ranged from 5.2 msec at −58 mV to 0.5 msec at +18 mV and was monoexponential [16]. This contrasts with data from double-suction-electrode clamp, where two time constants were required to describe I_{Na} inactivation during a maintained depolarization, with one time constant 3–4 times as long as the other [19]. The longer time constant was about 2 msec at −50 mV, decreasing to 0.9 msec at −10 mV [19].

The reasons for this discrepancy are not clear, but it has been noted [19] that when only one suction electrode is used to measure I_{Na} and series resistance effects are expected to be substantial [18], I_{Na} relaxes in a mono-exponential fashion.

Steady-state inactivation of I_{Na} is half-maximal at about -75 mV in Purkinje fibers at temperatures of $10-19°C$ and has a reciprocal slope of the order $4-5$ mV [8]. Similar values have been reported for isolated rat cells [16], human atrial cells [21], and cultured rat cells [23], but the steady-state inactivation curve of Brown et al. [19] was shallower. This latter effect was due to the short prepulses used in the experimental protocol, for when longer prepulses are used, steady-state inactivation curves agree with the other studies [25,26]. The overlap between activation and inactivation curves is now small, but still consistent with the hypothesis of a "window current" for I_{Na} [27].

REACTIVATION OF I_{Na}

The time constant for recovery of I_{Na} from inactivation has a value of the order $80-100$ msec in the potential range -60 to -80 mV [19], indicating that reactivation of I_{Na} is a slower process than inactivation. Ebihara et al. [11] have shown that although there are two phases in the reactivation of I_{Na} in embryonic chick heart cells (see also Brown et al. [19]), the observed reactivation time is highly dependent on the pulse protocol used to measure it. When the time course of reactivation is studied by a hyperpolarizing pulse of variable duration from the holding potential, only the fast process is observed. When a depolarizing prepulse is used, two phases of reactivation are seen, depending on the duration of the prepulse. These authors note that further experiments in this area should produce interesting results.

CONCLUSIONS

This very brief survey, which does not do justice to the work already reported in this field and is not intended to be a critical or comprehensive review, does at least indicate that isolated cells are enabling studies to be made in the difficult area of voltage-clamp of I_{Na}. Since marked differences exist between equilibrium binding and binding kinetics of TTX in nerve [28,29] and heart muscle [30,31] (but note similar sensitivity of TTX in frog atrial cells to nerve [20]), and since data are already accumulating on the effects of local anesthetics on I_{Na} [21,25,26], it is confidently predicted that further studies will yield important information on mechanisms involved in membrane Na conductance changes in the myocardium.

REFERENCES

1. Draper, M. H., and Weidmann, S. 1951. Cardiac resting and action potentials recorded with an intracellular electrode. *J. Physiol.* 115:74–94.
2. Noble, D. 1979. *The Initiation of the Heartbeat.* Clarendon Press, Oxford.
3. Johnson, E. A., and Lieberman, M. 1971. Heart: Excitation and contraction. *Annu. Rev. Physiol.* 33:479–532.
4. Beeler, G. W., and McGuigan, J. A. S. 1978. Voltage clamping of multicellular myocardial preparations: Capabilities and limitations of existing methods. *Prog. Biophys. Mol. Biol.* 34:219–254.
5. Attwell, D., Eisner, D., and Cohen, I. 1979. Voltage clamp and tracer flux data: Effects of a restricted extracellular space. *Q. Rev. Biophys.* 12:213–261.
6. Reuter, H. 1979. Properties of two inward membrane currents in the heart. *Annu. Rev. Physiol.* 41:413–424.
7. Colatsky, T. J., and Tsien, R. W. 1979. Sodium channels in rabbit cardiac Purkinje fibres. *Nature (London)* 278:265–268.
8. Colatsky, T. J. 1980. Voltage clamp measurements of sodium channel properties in rabbit cardiac Purkinje fibres. *J. Physiol.* 305:215–234.
9. Ebihara, L., Shigeto, N., Lieberman, M., and Johnson, E. A. 1980. The initial inward current in spherical clusters of chick embryonic heart cells. *J. Gen. Physiol.* 75:437–456.
10. Ebihara, L., and Johnson, E. A. 1980. Fast sodium current in cardiac muscle: A quantitative description. *Biophys. J.* 32:779–790.
11. Ebihara, L., Shigeto, N., Lieberman, M., and Johnson, E. A. 1983. A note on the reactivation of the fast sodium current in spherical clusters of embryonic chick heart cells. *Biophys. J.* 42:191–194.
12. Mathias, R. T., Ebihara, L., Lieberman, M., and Johnson, E. A. 1980. Linear electrical properties of heart cell aggregates. *Fed. Proc. Fed. Am. Soc. Exp. Biol.* 39:2077A.
13. Lee, K. S., Weeks, T. A., Kao, R. L., Akaike, N., and Brown, A. M. 1979. Sodium current in single heart muscle cells. *Nature (London)* 278:269–271.
14. Undrovinas, A. I., Yushmanova, A. V., Hering, S., and Rosenshtraukh, L. V. 1979. Use of the voltage clamp method in single mammalian cardiac cells for ionic current measurement. *Physiol. J. U.S.S.R.* 66:602–606.
15. Undrovinas, A. I., Yushmanova, Q. V., Hering, S., and Rosenshtraukh, L. V. 1980. Voltage clamp method on single cardiac cells from adult rat heart. *Experientia* 36:572–573.
16. Bodewei, R., Hering, S., Lemke, B., Rosenshtraukh, L. V., Undrovinas, A. I., and Wollenberger, A. 1982. Characterization of the fast sodium current in isolated rat myocardial cells: Simulation of the clamped membrane potential. *J. Physiol.* 325:301–315.
17. Brown, A. M., Lee, K. S., and Powell, T. 1980. Reactivation of the sodium conductance in single heart muscle cells. *J. Physiol.* 301:78–79P.
18. Brown, A. M., Lee, K. S., and Powell, T. 1981. Voltage clamp and internal perfusion of single rat heart muscle cells. *J. Physiol.* 318:455–477.
19. Brown, A. M., Lee, K. S., and Powell, T. 1981. Sodium current in single rat heart muscle cells. *J. Physiol.* 318:479–500.
20. Hume, J. R., and Giles, W. 1983. Ionic currents in single isolated bullfrog atrial cells. *J. Gen. Physiol.* 81:153–194.
21. Bustamente, J. O., and McDonald, T. F. 1983. Sodium currents in segments of human heart cells. *Science* 220:320–321.
22. Hamil, O. P., Marty, A., Neher, E., Sakmann, B., and Sigworth, F. J. 1981. Improved patch-clamp techniques for high-resolution recording from cells and cell-free membrane patches. *Pfluegers Arch.* 391:85–100.
23. Cachelin, A. B., De Peyer, J. E., Kokubun, S., and Reuter, H. 1983. Sodium channels in cultured cardiac cells. *J. Physiol.* 340:389–401.

24. Severs, N. J., Slade, A. M., Powell, T., Twist, V. W., and Warren, R. L. 1982. Correlation of ultrastructure and function in calcium-tolerant myocytes isolated from the adult rat heart. *J. Ultrastruct. Res.* 81:222–239.
25. Lee, K. S., Hume, J. R., Giles, W., and Brown, A. M. 1981. Sodium current depression by lidocaine in isolated ventricular cells. *Nature (London)* 291:325–327.
26. Sanchez-Chapula, J., Tsuda, Y., and Josephson, I. R. 1983. Voltage- and use-dependent effects of lidocaine on sodium current in rat single ventricular cells. *Circ. Res.* 52:557–565.
27. Attwell, D., Cohen, I., Eisner, D., Ohba, M., and Ojeda, C. 1979. The steady state TTX-sensitive ("window") sodium current in cardiac Purkinje fibres. *Pflüegers Arch.* 379:137–142.
28. Richie, M. J., and Rogart, R. D. 1977. The binding of saxitonin and tetrodotoxin to excitable tissues. *Rev. Physiol. Biochem. Pharmacol.* 79:1–50.
29. Ulbricht, W. 1981. Kinetics of drug action and equilibrium results at the node of Ranvier. *Physiol. Rev.* 61:785–828.
30. Baer, M., Best, P. M., and Reuter, H. 1976. Voltage-dependent action of tetrodotoxin in mammalian cardiac muscle. *Nature (London)* 263:344–345.
31. Cohen, C. J., Bean, B. P., Colatsky, T. J., and Tsien, R. W. 1981. Tetrodotoxin block of sodium channels in rabbit Purkinje fibers. *J. Gen. Physiol.* 78:383–411.

Influence of Na/K Pump Current on Action Potentials in Purkinje Fibers

David C. Gadsby

Laboratory of Cardiac Physiology
The Rockefeller University
New York, New York 10021

Abstract. Moderate changes in the size of the outward (hyperpolarizing) current that is generated directly by the electrogenic Na/K exchange pump in the surface membrane of cardiac Purkinje fibers can cause substantial alterations in the shape of the action potential, in the level of the diastolic potential, or of the resting potential of quiescent cells, or in the rate of firing of spontaneously active preparations. Transient increments in Na/K pump current, of suitable magnitude, can be elicited experimentally in small canine Purkinje fibers by causing a transient increase in their intracellular Na concentration, $[Na]_i$, and, thereby, a transient increase in the rate of electrogenic Na extrusion. Two techniques were used to increase $[Na]_i$: in the first, the rate of Na extrusion from the cells was temporarily reduced by omitting K ions from the bathing fluid for short periods of time, in the second, the rate of Na entry into the cells was temporarily increased by electrically stimulating the preparations rapidly (e.g., $\geq$ 2 Hz) for brief periods. After the extracellular K concentration was restored, or after electrical stimulation was stopped, respectively, use of a two-microelectrode voltage-clamp technique allowed the resulting increments in pump current to be measured directly, as changes in holding current. Increments in pump current elicited by these two methods in the same preparation decline with the same exponential time–course. In preparations stimulated electrically at a regular, low rate (e.g., $\leq$ 1 Hz) both methods of temporarily stimulating the Na/K pump cause a marked, transient reduction in the duration of the action potential. A closely similar reduction in action-potential duration to that observed during enhanced pump activity can be elicited by injecting, from an external source, a steady hyperpolarizing current of magnitude similar to that of the increment in pump current recorded in the same preparation under voltage clamp.

The preceding chapter deals with the major pathway for Na entry into cardiac cells, namely, the tetrodotoxin-sensitive, voltage-gated Na channels. Na enters through these channels passively (downhill), and the rate of Na entry is governed, in part, by the size of the transmembrane gradient of Na ion concentration. In the face of continuous Na entry, that gradient has to be maintained by active (uphill) extrusion of Na ions, work that is carried out by the Na/K exchange pump. It is well known that the Na/K pump of cardiac cells, as well as of other cells, is electrogenic (for reviews, see Thomas [1], DeWeer [2], Glitsch [3,4] and Gadsby [5]), because it pumps more Na ions out of the cell than it pumps K ions in, and so it directly generates an outward, hyperpolarizing, current across the cell membrane. Present evidence (reviewed in Gadsby [5]) indicates that the coupling ratio of Na/K transport by the pump remains unaltered despite considerable changes in extracellular K concentration ($[K]_o$), intracellular Na concentration ($[Na]_i$), or membrane potential (V_m), and that roughly 3 Na ions are extruded for every 2 K ions taken up [6–8]. This means that the size of the pump current is directly proportional to the pumped rate of Na efflux and, therefore, that changes in pump rate will be mirrored by changes in pump current and, consequently, by changes in resting or diastolic potentials, action potentials, and pacemaker rate [5]. This chapter is concerned with these alterations in the electrical activity of cardiac cells caused by changes in pump rate.

The Na/K pump is well suited to its task of controlling the level of $[Na]_i$ because the pumped rate of Na efflux is itself determined by $[Na]_i$; indeed, over a physiological concentration range, changes in Na efflux are simply proportional to changes in the level of $[Na]_i$ [6,7,9, cf. 10], which may therefore be viewed as exerting a negative feedback influence on itself. This influence can be readily appreciated by considering the relationship in equation (1), describing a simplified system in which the rate of change of $[Na]_i$ is governed by the sum of passive Na influx and active Na efflux terms [cf. 11–13]:

$$d[Na]_i/dt = -s/v \text{ (passive Na influx + pumped Na efflux)} \qquad (1)$$

where s/v is the surface-to-volume ratio of the cells, and the minus sign corrects for the sign convention that defines influx of a cation as negative and efflux as positive. In the steady state, by definition, $d[Na]_i/dt = 0$, so that Na influx must be exactly balanced by Na efflux. If, then, Na influx (negative quantity) were to be suddenly increased to a new level—for example, by raising the frequency of stimulation and so increasing the number of action potentials per unit time—the sum inside the brackets in equation (1) would be negative, $d[Na]_i/dt$ would be positive, and so $[Na]_i$ would rise. That rise in $[Na]_i$, however, would stimulate the Na/K pump to increase Na efflux, so that $[Na]_i$ and Na efflux would both increase, but only until $[Na]_i$ reached the level at which Na efflux could exactly counter the new, elevated Na influx. If Na influx were then suddenly lowered again—by reverting to the original drive rate, for instance—then Na efflux would temporarily exceed influx so that $[Na]_i$ would begin to decline and would continue to fall until it reached the original steady level at which Na influx and efflux were once again in balance. Clearly, the rate of change of $[Na]_i$ is expected to be greatest immediately after making a sudden change in either Na influx or efflux [equation (1)], and to diminish progressively as the resulting change in $[Na]_i$ lessens the difference between influx and efflux. In fact, experiments with Na-sensitive microelectrodes have shown that $[Na]_i$ declines with an exponential time course following either a step increase in Na efflux [6,7,9,14,15] or a step decrease in Na influx [8,16]. Under those conditions, the linear dependence of increments in Na efflux on increments in $[Na]_i$ (mentioned above) requires that Na efflux, and hence pump current, also

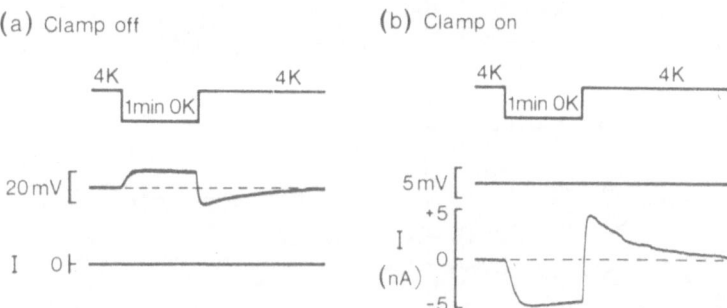

Figure 1. Changes of membrane potential (a) or of net current (I) under voltage clamp (b) recorded consecutively, in the same Purkinje fiber, in response to 1-min exposures to K-free solution, indicated by the upper lines. The dashed line in (a) indicates the steady resting potential in 4 mM K, low-Cl (isethionate) solution, which was at the "lower" level, -33 mV; this was chosen as the holding potential for (b), so that, in the steady state, the holding current was zero ($----$). Note the different voltage calibrations in (a) and (b). Current flowing outward across the cell membrane, i.e., hyperpolarizing current, is defined as positive. From Gadsby and Cranefield [31].

decline exponentially; such parallel, exponential decay of increments in $[Na]_i$ and in pump current has recently been recorded in voltage-clamped Purkinje fibers from sheep hearts [6,7,14]. In the experiments to be reported here, two techniques were used to raise $[Na]_i$ and so cause temporary stimulation of the Na/K pump. In one of these techniques, periods of rapid drive led to a rise in $[Na]_i$, in the manner already described, and in the other, extracellular K was temporarily withdrawn to inhibit the pump, abolishing Na efflux so that continued Na influx would raise $[Na]_i$. On subsequent restoration of $[K]_o$, the pump rate is temporarily enhanced. The effects of this kind of brief exposure to K-free fluid on steady-state membrane current in a voltage-clamped Purkinje fiber are shown in Figure 1. The preparations used in all experiments were small Purkinje fibers, usually less than 2 mm long and less than 200 μm in overall diameter, dissected from the right ventricles of dog hearts, and they were suspended between two fine, stainless steel insect pins in the narrow channel of a modified Hodgkin–Horowicz [17] fast-flow chamber (further details of the rapid superfusion system and its use are given in Gadsby and Cranefield [18]). Each Purkinje fiber was impaled with two microelectrodes filled with 3 M KCl, one at the center of the fiber for injecting current and the other, one third of the distance to the fiber end, for recording membrane potential; the electrodes were connected to a simple voltage-clamp circuit. Figure 1a shows changes in resting membrane potential, with the voltage-clamp amplifier switched off, in response to a 1-min exposure to K-free solution, as indicated by the upper line. Low-Cl solutions, in which the major anion was isethionate, were used in this experiment, and at 4 mM $[K]_o$, the resting potential of this fiber was at the "lower level" (see Gadsby and Cranefield [19]) of -33 mV. Reduction of $[K]_o$ to zero

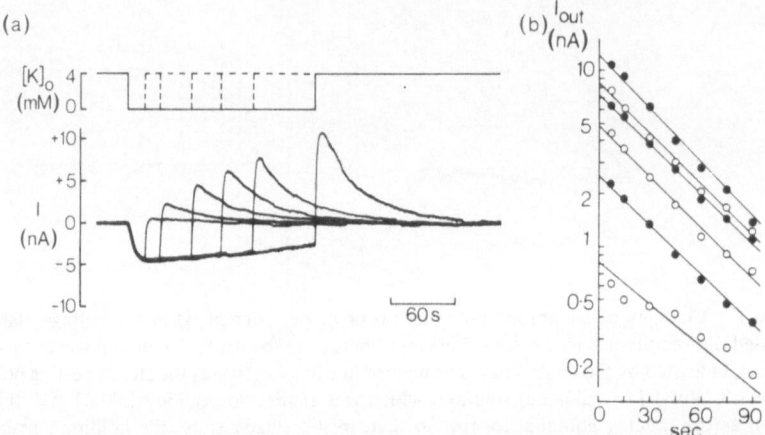

Figure 2.   (a) Superimposed current records showing the approximately linear increase in peak amplitude of increments in pump current with increasing duration of the prior exposure to K-free solution, from 15 to 180 sec, as indicated by the upper lines. Holding and resting potential, −33 mV; low-Cl solutions. (b) Semilogarithmic plots of decaying phases of the pump-current transients shown in (a). Note that despite large changes in the size of the pump-current transients, the rate constant of exponential current decay remains unchanged. From Gadsby and Cranefield [31].

under these conditions caused a depolarization that was complete within a few seconds, presumably the time taken for diffusion equilibration of K ions in the extracellular space, and the subsequent switch back to 4 mM $[K]_o$ caused a hyperpolarization that reached a peak within a few seconds and then slowly decayed over the next minute or two. When the exposure to zero $[K]_o$ was repeated after the voltage clamp was switched on to hold the membrane potential steady as its initial resting, i.e., zero-current, level, as shown in Figure 1b, a net inward current was recorded in the K-free solution, and after $[K]_o$ was returned to 4 mM, a transient outward current was recorded that peaked in a few seconds and then decayed with an exponential time course. Figure 2a shows superimposed records of current changes obtained, in the same experiment as that of Figure 1, in response to six exposures to K-free solution lasting from 15 to 180 sec. The records demonstrate that the inward current caused by K withdrawal was closely similar in all runs and that the transient outward current on restoration of $[K]_o$ was negligibly small following the 15-sec exposure, but following longer exposures, its peak amplitude increased approximately in proportion to the duration of K-free superfusion. These records indicate that the transient outward current is not a direct result of the zero-$[K]_o$ exposure but is, rather, a secondary consequence. Presumably, the inward current on switching to K-free solution (and the depolarization in the absence of voltage clamp) reflects abolition, or diminution, of steady-state outward pump current due to pump inhibition, as well as a possible reduction in outward K current flowing via inwardly rectifying K channels, due to crossing over of K current–voltage relations at different $[K]_o$ levels [e.g. 20]. Restoration of $[K]_o$ after 15 sec, i.e., before $[Na]_i$ could change significantly as a result of pump inhibition, caused a simple reversal of these current changes. At a fixed membrane potential, Na influx is expected to remain approximately constant for the first few minutes of pump inhibition, so that on the basis of equation (1), $[Na]_i$ should begin to rise linearly with time in K-free fluid. The first-order dependence of increments in pumped Na efflux on increments in $[Na]_i$ already mentioned would imply that the increment in Na efflux, and hence the increment in pump current, obtained on reactivating the pump with K should also increase linearly with the duration of the zero-$[K]_o$ exposure. Moreover, this first-order dependence means that as long as Na influx remains unchanged, sudden restoration of $[K]_o$ should cause both Na efflux and pump current to decline with an exponential time–course. The results shown in Figures 1 and 2 are clearly consistent with this interpretation if the transient outward currents illustrated in Figures 1b and 2a are increments in pump current, because these transients increase approximately linearly with time in K-free fluid (Figure 2a) and they all decay with about the same exponential time–course.

Despite this correspondence between expectations and results, however, a number of alternative explanations for the transient outward current should be considered: (1) The increase in $[Na]_i$ during zero-$[K]_o$ exposure might be large enough that the reduced Na gradient causes a reduction in inward Na current, and hence a transient outward shift of net current, until the Na/K pump has restored $[Na]_i$ to its initial steady level. (2) The increment in $[Na]_i$ might enhance Ca uptake via Na/Ca exchange, a process believed to be electrogenic (more than 2 Na ions being extruded per Ca ion taken up [21]), and so generate outward Na–Ca exchange current until the Na/K pump restores $[Na]_i$. (3) A rise in cellular Ca concentration mediated by enhanced Na–Ca exchange might lead to a temporary increase in outward current if any Ca-activated K conductance exists in the surface membrane of cardiac cells [22]. (4) The outward current might be caused *indirectly* by enhanced pump activity as a result of increased outward K current reflecting an increase in the outward driving force on K ions due to temporary, pump-induced, extracellular K depletion. Possibility (4) can be ruled out easily because the records in Figures 1 and 2 show clearly that at such low holding potentials, as $[K]_o$ falls from 4 mM to zero, net membrane current changes monotonically in the *inward*, not the outward, direction. The results shown in Figure 3 allow us to rule out alternative possibilities (1)–(3) by using micromolar concentrations of the cardiotonic steroid acetylstrophanthidin to specifically inhibit the Na/K pump. The time–course of pump block by 5 μM acetylstrophanthidin is illustrated by the rapid inward shift of holding current in the lower trace of Figure 3a, reflecting abolition of the steady-state component of Na/K pump current: pump block appears to be virtually

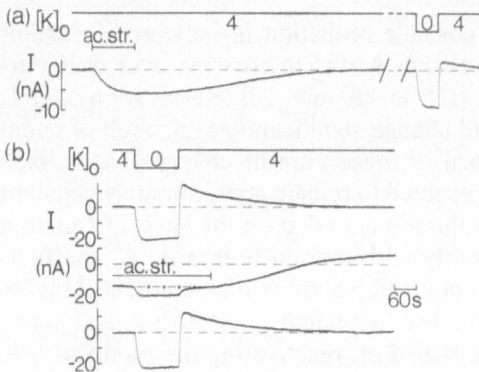

Figure 3. Effects of micromolar concentrations of acetylstrophanthidin [applied during the periods indicated by the bars (ac.str.)] on net membrane current (I) in Purkinje fibers voltage-clamped at the lower resting potential in 4 mM K, low-Cl solution. (a) 2-Minute application of 5 μM acetylstrophanthidin at a holding potential of −32 mV (the subsequent break in the current trace indicates omission of a 5-min section of record), followed by a 1-min exposure to zero [K]$_o$, as indicated by the top line. (b) Net current changes recorded at a holding potential of −40 mV during three consecutive 2-min exposures to K-free fluid as indicated by the upper line. Acetylstrophanthidin, 2 μM, was added 3 min before the start of the second record and was washed out at the end of the bar. The 60-sec time calibration applies to both (a) and (b). (− − −) Zero net current (a, b); (− · −) current level in 4 mM [K]$_o$ in the presence of acetylstrophanthidin (b). From Gradsby and Cranefield [31].

complete by the end of the 2-min exposure to acetylstrophanthidin, and was readily reversible on washing out the drug. Figure 3b shows the effects of 2 μM acetylstrophanthidin on the transient outward current following 2-min exposures to K-free solution (indicated by the top line). The upper current record shows the typical inward shift in holding current on switching into zero [K]$_o$ and the typical transient outward current after returning to 4 mM [K]$_o$. The middle current record starts 3 min after beginning exposure to acetylstrophanthidin, the inward shift of the holding current (with respect to control) presumably reflecting abolition of steady-state pump current. The switch to K-free solution, still in the presence of acetylstrophanthidin, caused a further, smaller inward shift of the holding current, but only to about the same level obtained in the previous and subsequent runs in the absence of acetylstrophanthidin (see below). The important point is that on switching back to 4 mM [K]$_o$ in the presence of acetylstrophanthidin, the holding current returned *monotonically* to the same level that was recorded just before the 2-min exposure to zero [K]$_o$. The acetylstrophanthidin was then washed out and the holding current slowly moved in the outward direction, even becoming net outward for some minutes, presumably reflecting stimulation of unblocked pump sites by the raised [Na]$_i$ resulting from the prolonged pump inhibition in the presence of the drug. Following sudden pump inhibition, [Na]$_i$ is expected to rise at a relatively steady rate for at least several minutes [13] so that the increment in [Na]$_i$ gained during the 2-min exposure to zero [K]$_o$ can be expected to be about the same whether or not acetylstrophanthidin is present. In this case, in the presence of acetylstrophanthidin, any component of net current change due to a change in Na current, or in Na/Ca exchange current, or in any Ca-activated current, should still appear as a difference between the current levels recorded before, and immediately after, exposure to zero $[K]_o$. The fact that these current levels are the same when the Na/K pump is inhibited argues that the outward current shift usually seen on switching back to 4 mM $[K]_o$ from zero $[K]_o$ is generated by enhanced activity of the pump. Since we have ruled out pump-induced K depletion as a mechanism for this outward current shift, the most likely explanation is that it represents an increment in outward current generated directly by electrogenic Na extrusion.

The absence of any outward current shift following exposure to zero $[K]_o$ in the presence of 2 µM acetylstrophanthidin suggests that the Na/K pump was completely inhibited by this concentration of the cardiotonic steroid. Therefore, insofar as indirect effects of pump inhibition can be ignored, the amplitudes of the inward current shifts on applying acetylstrophanthidin in Figures 3a and 3b indicate the sizes of the steady-state pump current in those two preparations. Note that in both cases, a larger inward current shift was recorded on switching to K-free solution than on adding the cardiotonic steroid (Figures 3a,b); the additional inward current presumably reflects reduction of outward K current flowing through inwardly rectifying K channels [e.g., 20]. The records in Figure 3b reveal that the absolute level of the holding current in K-free fluid was similar whether or not acetylstrophanthidin was present, and this suggests that the pump was already completely inhibited by withdrawal of external K.

Temporary stimulation of the electrogenic Na/K pump following a period of rapid drive is indicated by the results illustrated in Figure 4. Action potentials were elicited for 10 min at a rate of 2 Hz in a Purkinje fiber bathed in 6 mM K Tyrode's solution, after which the drive was terminated and the voltage-clamp amplifier was switched on (Figure 4B). A slowly decaying outward current was recorded, which had a single exponential time–course, as shown in the semilogarithmic plot at the right (Figure 4C, lower set of points). When the holding current had become steady, the fiber was exposed to K-free solution for a couple of minutes as shown in Figure 4A. The usual, exponentially decaying increment in pump current was recorded on switching back to 6 mM $[K]_o$, and as the upper points in Figure 4C reveal, its time–course was identical to that of the outward current following rapid drive. This result supports the hypothesis that both decaying outward currents reflect the same underlying process, namely, temporarily enhanced electrogenic Na extrusion during elimination of the increments in $[Na]_i$ induced by the two different experimental techniques.

The effects of such small changes in pump current on the electrical activity of cardiac cells can be quite marked. Vassalle [23] demonstrated that the temporary quiescence and hyperpolarization of spontaneously beating Purkinje fibers that followed brief (e.g., 1-min) periods of "overdrive," i.e., stimulation at rates higher than the intrinsic spontaneous rate, were caused by a transient increase in Na/K pump current. Similarly, it has been shown that brief exposure of Purkinje fibers to K-free fluid is followed, on restoration of $[K]_o$, by temporary abolition of spontaneous action potentials

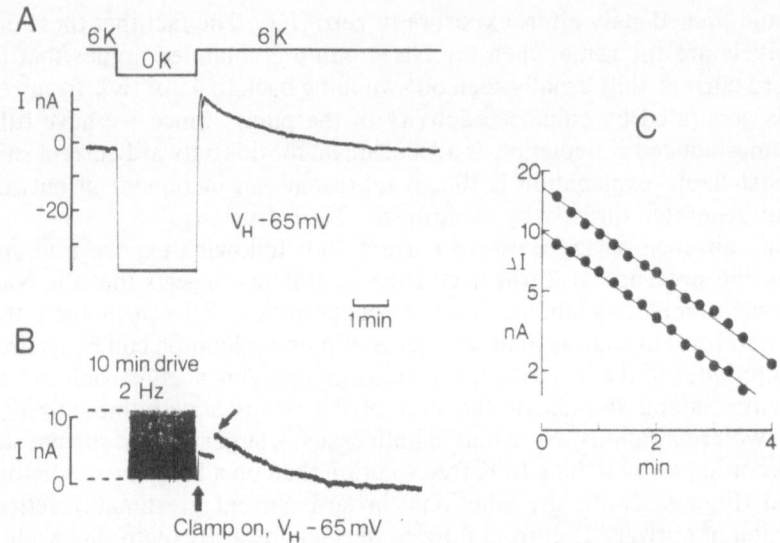

Figure 4. Decline, with the same exponential time–course, of the slowly decaying current transients that follow a period of rapid drive or a brief exposure to K-free fluid. (A) The current record begins 2 min after the end of that in (B) and shows the increment in pump current following a 135-sec exposure to zero $[K]_o$ (the inward current in K-free fluid was off-scale at this holding potential). (B) At the vertical arrow, the voltage clamp amplifier was switched on after a 10-min period of drive at 2 Hz; the diagonal arrow marks a doubling of the sensitivity of the chart recorder to correspond to the current scale at the left. (C) The parallel straight lines were fitted by eye to the semilogarithmic plots of the declining transient currents illustrated in (A) and (B). Cl-containing solutions were used in this experiment; the time calibration is common to (A) and (B). From Gadsby and Cranefield [18].

arising from either the normal, high level of resting potential or the low level of resting potential (slow-response action potentials); in both cases, when spontaneous activity resumes, it does so at a reduced rate and then gradually speeds up to regain the steady control rate [24]. These effects on Purkinje fiber automaticity are readily attributed to increased pump current, rather than pump-induced extracellular K depletion, because experimental reduction of $[K]_o$ is known to enhance, not diminish, spontaneous activity [25].

The question of pump-current influence on the shape of the cardiac action potential was approached by Isenberg and Trautwein [26], who found that sudden inhibition of the Na/K pump in Purkinje fibers with the fast-acting cardiotonic steroid dihydro-ouabain caused marked prolongation of the action potential within 40 sec of its application. This suggests that the pump current plays a significant role in normal repolarization of the Purkinje fiber action potential, a conclusion supported by the shortening of the action potential, illustrated in Figure 5, in response to a temporary increase in pump current induced by a brief period of rapid drive. The chart recording in Figure 5A shows the experimental protocol: Stimulation at the basal rate of 0.67

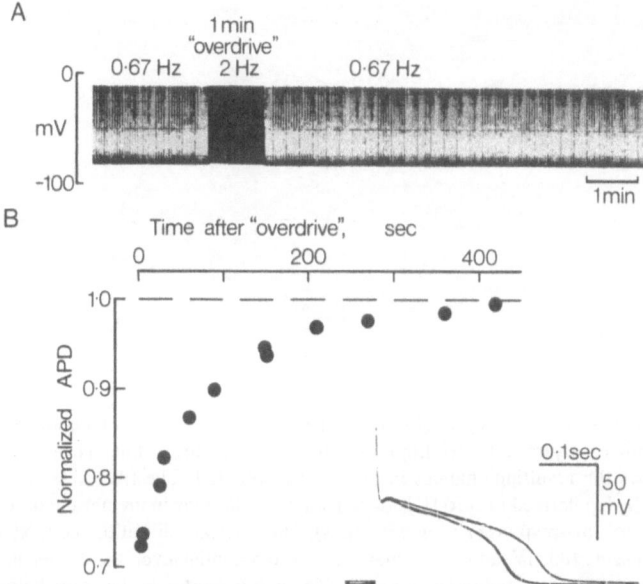

Figure 5. Aftereffects of brief periods of rapid drive ("overdrive") on Purkinje-fiber action potentials elicited at a relatively low rate in 6 mM $[K]_o$, Cl-containing solution. (A) Continuous slow chart recording of action potentials before, during, and after a 1-min period of rapid drive. (B) Time–course recovery of action potential duration (APD), normalized to the steady control duration, in another Purkinje fiber, after 2 min of rapid drive at 2 Hz; the basal drive rate was 0.67 Hz. *Inset:* Superimposed action potentials from this experiment; the longer action potential is a control, photographed 9 min after the rapid drive was stopped, while the shorter action potential, arising from the more negative diastolic potential, was recorded just 25 sec after the drive was stopped. The time calibration for these action potentials marks the zero potential level. From Gadsby and Cranefield [18].

Hz was interrupted by brief periods of drive at 2 Hz, lasting 1 min for the experiment shown in Figure 5A and 2 min for that in Figure 5B, and sample action potentials were photographed from the storage oscilloscope at various times. Following the period of rapid drive, the action potentials at the basal drive rate were temporarily shortened with respect to control, and at the same time the resting potential was slightly increased. These effects are illustrated in Figure 5B, in which action-potential durations, normalized to the control duration before the overdrive, are plotted against time after termination of the 2-min period of rapid drive. Immediately after the overdrive, the action-potential duration was reduced to about 70% of its control value, but it recovered fully along an approximately exponential time–course with a half-time of about 70 sec. The shorter of the superimposed action potentials in the inset was recorded 25 sec after the overdrive, and the longer one, arising from the more positive resting potential, was recorded about 9 min later, after the control duration had been regained. Presumably, both the transient increase in resting potential and the transient abbreviation of the

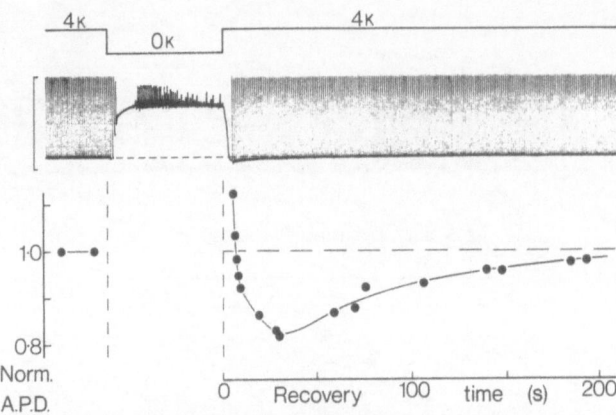

Figure 6.   Changes in action potential duration (A.P.D.) in 4 mM $[K]_o$, Cl-containing solution following a 1-min exposure to K-free fluid, as indicated by the upper line. The continuous chart recording shows the resulting changes in membrane potential. The fiber was stimulated at 1 Hz except while depolarized in zero $[K]_o$ (when small oscillations in membrane potential sometimes gave rise to slow-response action potentials). The vertical calibration bar next to the chart recording represents 100 mV, and its top marks the zero potential level; the dashed line indicates the control level of diastolic potential, -87 mV. The points plotted in the graph below the chart recording, on the same time scale, give the durations of sample action potentials normalized with respect to the control duration (---). From Gadsby and Cranefield [24].

action potential are attributable to a temporary increase in pump current, this increment in pump current decaying as $[Na]_i$ relaxes back to the steady-state level appropriate to the lower rate of drive (cf. Figure 4).

Closely similar effects on the Purkinje-fiber action potential are seen when brief periods of K-free superfusion are used to cause temporary stimulation of the Na/K pump, as illustrated in Figure 6. The chart recording again indicates how the experiments were carried out: action potentials were elicited at 1 Hz except while the fibers were depolarized in K-free solution. In the experiment of Figure 6, the diastolic potential was initially -87 mV, but was -92 mV when stimulation was resumed shortly after the 1-min exposure to zero $[K]_o$, and then slowly returned to -87 mV over the next 2 or 3 min. Normalized action-potential duration is shown plotted against time in the graph below the chart recording. The first two action potentials obtained on resuming stimulation after switching back to 4 mM $[K]_o$ were longer than controls, but subsequent action potentials quickly shortened to about 80% of the control duration within 30 sec and then slowly lengthened back to the control duration over the next 3–4 min. This reduction in action-potential duration was associated with a small increase in diastolic potential, and both effects disappeared along approximately parallel time–courses. Although the increases in diastolic potential in the experiments of Figures 5 and 6 might be attributable to pump-induced extracellular K depletion, this cannot possibly be the explanation for the action-potential shortening observed at the same time, because it is well known that a reduction in $[K]_o$

causes *prolongation* of Purkinje-fiber action potentials [20,25,27]. The reduction in action-potential duration is thus most easily accounted for by an increment in Na/K pump current of the kind illustrated in Figures 1–4, and this also provides a satisfactory explanation for the simultaneous membrane hyperpolarization [24]. However, action-potential prolongation by reduced extracellular K concentration probably does account for the difference between the graphs shown in Figures 5 and 6, because, after sudden switch from zero to 4 mM $[K]_o$ (Figure 6), the K concentration in the innermost extracellular spaces is expected to rise toward 4 mM with a time–course governed by diffusion equilibration, i.e., with a half-time of several seconds (cf. Figures 1–3). In the experiment of Figure 6, therefore, the increment in pump current that shortens the action potential would not be fully activated until diffusion equilibration is complete, and in addition, the passive effects of reduced $[K]_o$ [20,25,27] would tend to increase action-potential duration in the initial seconds, whereas under the conditions of Figure 5, in which no changes in $[K]_o$ were made, the increment in pump current, and hence action-potential shortening, are expected to be maximal immediately on termination of the rapid drive.

The results presented so far suggest that brief periods of K-free superfusion or of rapid drive give rise, subsequently, to transient increments in pump current, lasting for several minutes, which cause a temporary reduction in action-potential duration and a temporary increase in resting, or diastolic, potential. However, to demonstrate that the increment in pump current is of sufficient size to quantitatively account for the observed degree of action-potential shortening requires measurement, in a given fiber, of both the reduction in action-potential duration and the underlying increment in pump current. Figures 7 and 8 illustrate results from this kind of experiment, carried out on a small Purkinje fiber impaled with two microelectrodes and bathed in 6 mM K solution while being regularly stimulated at 1 Hz. In the first part of the experiment, the extent of action-potential shortening was determined following a 2-min exposure to K-free fluid, indicated by the upper line in Figure 7. The chart recording of membrane potential shows that the fiber depolarized and became inexcitable in K-free solution, but rapidly repolarized on restoration of 6 mM $[K]_o$. The two higher-speed chart records (one obtained shortly after switching back to 6 mM $[K]_o$ and the other about 10 min later) verify that as usual, the action potential was transiently shortened after exposure to zero $[K]_o$. The photograph at the lower left, taken from the storage oscilloscope, shows a shortened action potential, arising from the more negative resting potential, recorded about 15 sec after the return to 6 mM $[K]_o$, superimposed on the longer, control action potential recorded much later, after the resting potential had returned to its original, steady-state level. In the second part of the experiment, illustrated by the records at the right-hand side of Figure 7, a hyperpolarizing current was injected to cause hyperpolarization and action-potential shortening similar to that seen during the enhanced pump activity. The photograph at the lower

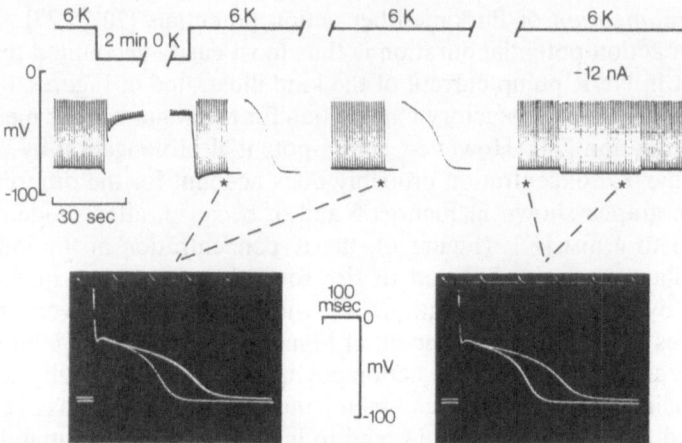

Figure 7. Comparison of action-potential shortening and membrane hyperpolarization caused by enhanced pump activity with that caused by current injection via a second microelectrode in a Purkinje fiber driven at 1 Hz in 6 mM $[K]_o$, Cl-containing solution. The upper line shows the 2-min exposure to K-free fluid and marks the omission of three sections of record of duration 90 sec, 10 min, and 3 min, respectively. Because of the poor frequency response of the pen, action-potential upstrokes are severely attenuated in the chart recording, but the two high-speed chart records (for which the time calibration represents 500 msec) clearly reveal the temporary reduction in action-potential duration following the exposure to zero $[K]_o$. The asterisks indicate when the action potentials, superimposed below, were displayed on the storage oscilloscope. Both the action-potential shortening and the hyperpolarization caused by enhanced pump activity are closely approximated by injection of a steady (i.e., time- and voltage-independent) 12-nA hyperpolarizing current (bar over chart record). From Gadsby and Cranefield [18].

right was obtained a few minutes after that on the left and shows that injection of a steady, i.e., time- and voltage-independent, 12-nA hyperpolarizing current did, indeed, cause effects similar to those seen after the 2-min exposure to K-free fluid. The final part of the experiment, shown in Figure 8, involved measurement, in the same fiber, of the pump-current increment following 2 min of K-free superfusion. The clamp was switched off (first arrow) to allow the fiber to depolarize during the exposure to K-free solution just as it had previously (see Figure 7), but it was switched on again a few seconds after the return to 6 mM $[K]_o$ (second arrow), and a typical, exponentially decaying increment in pump current was recorded with a peak amplitude of roughly 10 nA, i.e., about the right magnitude to account for the action-potential shortening and increase in resting potential illustrated in Figure 7.

SUMMARY AND CONCLUSIONS

The most important conclusion to be drawn from the work discussed in this chapter is that relatively small changes in the size of the Na/K pump current can have pronounced effects on action potentials and on resting, or

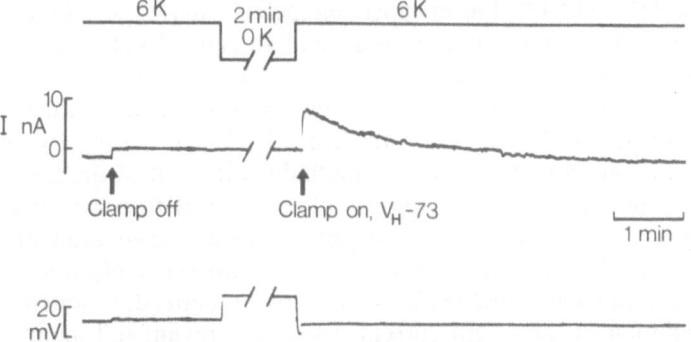

Figure 8.   Direct measurement of pump-current increment in 6 mM K solution following a 2-min exposure to K-free fluid. These records were obtained from the same fiber, but 150 min later than those shown in Figure 7. The upper line indicates the $[K]_o$ changes, the middle trace shows applied current, and the bottom trace shows membrane potential. At the first arrow, the clamp was switched off to allow the fiber to depolarize in K-free fluid as it did previously, in Figure 7 [in this case, the depolarization was off-scale (see bottom trace)]. The voltage clamp was switched on again (second arrow), just after returning to 6 mM $[K]_o$, to record the slowly decaying increment in pump current, which was about 10 nA in total amplitude. From Gadsby and Cranefield [18].

diastolic, potentials of cardiac Purkinje fibers. Pump current seems to vary in proportion to pump rate, which in turn is a sensitive function (approximately linear in the range of interest) of $[Na]_i$ and a saturable function of $[K]_o$ (for a review, see Gadsby [5]). The Na/K pump is half-maximally activated by about 1 mM $[K]_o$ [13] [cf. 12,15], so that at physiological $[K]_o$ levels of 4–5 mM, pump rate is most effectively modulated by changes in $[Na]_i$. The demonstration of a substantial steady component of pump current, even in resting fibers, may have serious implications for interpretation of changes in net membrane current recorded in some voltage-clamp experiments on Purkinje fibers. Since pump-current amplitude is expected to be a virtually instantaneous function of $[K]_o$ and $[Na]_i$, if either concentration changes during voltage-clamp protocols, then allowance must be made for the resulting changes in pump current before any further analysis of the net currents can be made. Because $[Na]_i$ can change only slowly, with a half-time of a minute or so, corresponding changes in pump current will also occur slowly and so would not normally contribute to time-dependent current changes during voltage-clamp pulses, but would appear as slow shifts of holding current whenever Na influx is altered—for example, in response to changes in holding potential [e.g., 14] or in response to pharmacological interventions [e.g., 8,28]. Extracellular K accumulation or depletion, on the other hand, is expected to occur with a much faster time–course and so might modulate pump current even during voltage pulses. In the steady state, however, at a fixed membrane potential, pump current, which is proportional to Na efflux, should be independent of $[K]_o$ and should depend only on the rate of Na influx [12,13]. For instance, an increase in $[K]_o$ would transiently enhance Na efflux, and pump current, and so cause $[Na]_i$ to decline with the usual ($[K]_o$-dependent) exponential time course, until Na efflux had returned to its original magnitude and was once again in balance with Na influx.

A comparison of the size of the current change caused by suddenly inhibiting the pump with acetylstrophanthidin with that of the transient increment in pump current following a brief period of K-free superfusion suggests that the pump current can be roughly doubled in magnitude after about 2 min of Na-loading in K-free solution (e.g., Figure 3) [13,24]. Such changes in pump current have marked effects on action-potential duration in Purkinje fibers: abolition of the pump current can even prevent full membrane repolarization, the membrane potential remaining near the lower resting level [26], whereas after a 2-min exposure to K-free solution, the resulting increase in pump current reduces action-potential duration by about one quarter or one third (e.g., Fig. 7) [24]. Although such large changes might at first sight seem unlikely, it should be borne in mind that as already outlined, steady pump current can be expected to scale with Na influx, which in turn depends on action-potential frequency: if doubling the impulse rate were to roughly double Na influx, then in the steady state (i.e., after about 5 min), the pump current would also be doubled in size. It is well known that an increase in drive rate is associated with a maintained reduction in action-potential duration, at least part of which develops rather slowly, and that a reduction in drive rate causes prolongation of the action potential (for reviews, see Carmeliet [29] and Boyett and Jewell [30]); presumably, changes in the size of the pump current make an important contribution to these alterations in action-potential shape [18,24].

ACKNOWLEDGMENTS

Much of the work discussed here was done in collaboration with Dr. Paul F. Cranefield, to whom I am also indebted for constant advice and encouragement. The preparation of this chapter and the research discussed in it were supported by USPHS Grant No. HL-14899 and by an Established Fellowship of the New York Heart Association.

REFERENCES

1. Thomas, R. C. 1972. Electrogenic sodium pump in nerve and muscle cells. *Physiol. Rev.* 52:563–594.
2. DeWeer, P. 1975. Aspects of the recovery processes in nerve. In: C. C. Hunt (ed.), *Neurophysiology (MTP Int. Rev. Sci., Physiol. Ser. 1)*. Vol. 3, pp. 231–278. Butterworths, London.
3. Glitsch, H. G. 1979. Characteristics of active Na transport in intact cardiac cells. *Am. J. Physiol.* 236:H189–H199.
4. Glitsch, H. G. 1982. Electrogenic Na pumping in the heart. *Annu. Rev. Physiol.* 44:389–400.

5. Gadsby, D. C. 1984. The Na/K pump of cardiac cells. *Annu. Rev. Biophys. Bioeng.* 13:373–398.
6. Eisner, D. A., Lederer, W. J., and Vaughan-Jones, R. D. 1981. The dependence of sodium pumping and tension on intracellular sodium activity in voltage clamped sheep Purkinje fibers. *J. Physiol. (London).* 317:163–187.
7. Glitsch, H. G., Pusch, H., Schumacher, T., and Verdonck, F. 1982. An identification of the K activated Na pump current in sheep Purkinje fibres. *Pflüegers Arch.* 394:256–263.
8. Eisner, D. A., Lederer, W. J., and Sheu, S-S. 1983. The role of intracellular sodium activity in the anti-arrhythmic action of local anaesthetics in sheep Purkinje fibres. *J. Physiol. (London)* 340:239–257.
9. Deitmer, J. W., and Ellis, D. 1978. The intracellular sodium activity of cardiac Purkinje fibres during inhibition and re-activation of the Na–K pump. *J. Physiol. (London).* 284:241–259.
10. Thomas, R. C. 1969. Membrane current and intracellular sodium changes in a snail neurone during extrusion of injected sodium. *J. Physiol. (London).* 201:495–514.
11. Rang, H. P., and Ritchie, J. M. 1968. On the electrogenic sodium pump in mammalian non-myelinated nerve fibers and its activation by various external cations. *J. Physiol.* (London). 196:183–221.
12. Eisner, D. A., and Lederer, W. J. 1980. Characterization of the electrogenic sodium pump in cardiac Purkinje fibres. *J. Physiol.* 303:441–474.
13. Gadsby, D. C. 1980. Activation of electrogenic Na^+/K^+ exchange by extracellular K^+ in canine cardiac Purkinje fibers. *Proc. Natl. Acad. Sci. U.S.A.* 77:4035–4039.
14. Eisner, D. A., Lederer, W. J., and Vaughan-Jones, R. D. 1981. The effects of rubidium ions and membrane potential on the intracellular sodium activity of sheep Purkinje fibres. *J. Physiol. (London).* 317:188–205.
15. Glitsch, H. G., Kampmann, W., and Pusch, H. 1981. Activation of active Na transport in sheep Purkinje fibres by external K or Rb ions. *Pflüegers Arch.* 391:28–34.
16. Cohen, C. J., Fozzard, H. A., and Sheu, S-S. 1982. Increase in intracellular sodium ion activity during stimulation in mammalian cardiac muscle. *Circ. Res.* 50:651–662.
17. Hodgkin, A. L., and Horowicz, P. 1959. The influence of potassium and chloride ions on the membrane potential of single muscle fibres. *J. Physiol. (London).* 148:127–160.
18. Gadsby, D. C., and Cranefield, P. F. 1982. Effects of electrogenic sodium extrusion on the membrane potential of cardiac Purkinje fibers. In: A. Paes de Carvalho, B. F. Hoffman, and M. Lieberman (eds.), *Normal and Abnormal Conduction in the Heart.* pp. 225–247. Futura, Mt. Kisco, New York.
19. Gadsby, D. C., and Cranefield, P. F. 1977. Two levels of resting potential in cardiac Purkinje fibers. *J. Gen. Physiol.* 70:725–746.
20. Noble, D. 1965. Electrical properties of cardiac muscle attributable to inward-going (anomalous) rectification. *J. Cell. Comp. Physiol.* 66:127–135.
21. Mullins, L. J. 1979. The generation of electric currents in cardiac fibers by Na/Ca exchange. *Am. J. Physiol.* 236:C103–C110.
22. Isenberg, G. 1977. Cardiac Purkinje fibres: $[Ca^{2+}]_i$ controls steady state potassium conductance. *Pfluegers Arch.* 371:71–76.
23. Vassalle, M. 1970. Electrogenic suppression of automaticity in sheep and dog Purkinje fibers. *Circ. Res.* 27:361–377.
24. Gadsby, D. C., and Cranefield, P. F. 1979. Electrogenic sodium extrusion in cardiac Purkinje fibers. *J. Gen. Physiol.* 73:819–837.
25. Vassalle, M. 1965. Cardiac pacemaker potentials at different extra- and intracellular K concentrations. *Am. J. Physiol.* 208:770–775.
26. Isenberg, G., and Trautwein, W. 1974. The effect of dihydro-ouabain and lithium ions on the outward current in cardiac Purkinje fibers: Evidence for electrogenicity of active transport. *Pfluegers Arch.* 350:41–54.
27. Weidmann, S. 1956. *Elektrophysiologie der Herzmuskelfaser.* Huber, Bern.

294   David C. Gadsby

28. Colatsky, T. J., and Gadsby, D. C. 1980. Is tetrodotoxin block of background sodium channels in canine cardiac Purkinje fibres voltage-dependent? *J. Physiol.* 306:20P.
29. Carmeliet, E. E. 1977. Repolarization and frequency in cardiac cells. *J. Physiol. (Paris).* 73:903–923.
30. Boyett, M. R., and Jewell, B. R. 1980. Analysis of the effects of changes in rate and rhythm upon electrical activity in the heart. *Prog. Biophys. Mol. Biol.* 36:1–52.
31. Gadsby, D. C., and Cranefield, P. F. 1979. Direct measurement of changes in sodium pump current in canine cardiac Purkinje fibers. *Proc. Natl. Acad. Sci. U.S.A.* 76:1783–1787.

Na–Ca Exchange in Cardiac Tissues

D. Ellis

Department of Physiology
University Medical School
Edinburgh EH8 9AG, Scotland

Abstract.   Our awareness of the importance of Na–Ca exchange in cardiac muscle has progressed from early observations of Na–Ca antagonism in the activation of contractile force. This was followed by demonstrations of actual Na–Ca ion countertransport across cell membranes and later functional studies in which manipulation of intracellular and extracellular Na and Ca concentrations has permitted a better characterization of the exchange process and its contribution to contractile force.

The recent development of vesicle preparations from cardiac sarcolemmal membranes has, despite some drawbacks, produced useful information on the electrogenicity of the exchange mechanism and on the relative affinity of the exchange carrier compared to the ATPase-driven Ca pump. These studies confirmed earlier estimates of the approximate exchange ratio of the Na–Ca countertransport system and have demonstrated its large maximum transport rate capabilities.

The application of ion-sensitive microelectrodes in recent years has enabled measurements of the actual ion-activity gradients across the sarcolemmal membrane. These activity gradients together with the membrane potential control the rate and direction of the Na–Ca exchange. Despite the wide range of techniques employed to tackle the problem, the exchange ratio of Na to Ca movement is still in some doubt, with most estimates ranging between 5:2 and 4:1.

INTRODUCTION

The potentially important role of the Na–Ca exchange system in controlling the Ca supply to the contractile apparatus in cardiac cells has been the subject of considerable experimental work and speculation in the last few years. Due to space limitations, it is not possible to adequately cover all the work that has been produced, but most aspects of the topic have been considered in recent reviews by Chapman [1], Sulakhe and St. Louis [2], Mullins [3], Reuter [4], and Langer [5].

Evidence for the effect of extracellular Na, $[Na]_o$, on cardiac contraction was presented as long ago as 1921 by Daly and Clark [6]. These observations were extended in later functional studies in which antagonism between extracellular Na and Ca on cardiac contractility was demonstrated by Wilbrandt and Koller [7]. This was formalized by Lüttgau and Niedergerke [8] in 1958 into a model wherein Na and Ca ions competed for binding to an anionic receptor at the cell membrane such that the contractile tension produced by the muscle was dependent on the ratio $[Ca]_o/[Na]_o^2$. Once bound to the receptor, Ca could enter the cell and activate contraction. Thus, reduction of the [Na]$_o$ would allow more Ca binding to receptors and result in increased contractile force during the normal contraction (twitch or heartbeat) and result in a contracture (sustained contraction) if [Na]$_o$ was reduced to very low levels.

Langer [9] and Repke [10] introduced in 1964 the concept that intracellular Na, [Na]$_i$, might also be important in affecting Ca influx into cardiac cells, but the mechanism involved could not be specified. The important demonstration of an actual countertransport of Na and Ca across cardiac-cell membranes came in 1968 by Reuter and Seitz [11]. They found that the Ca efflux from guinea pig atrial cells was dependent on external Na. At about the same time, Baker et al. [12] demonstrated, in squid giant axon, a countertransport in the opposite direction, i.e., a Ca influx that was dependent on the [Na]$_i$. This mechanism was also demonstrated in guinea pig atria in 1970 by Glitsch et al. [13].

The Na–Ca countertransport process became readily accepted as a mechanism whereby intracellular Ca could be maintained at a low level by using the energy gradient of Na ions running "downhill" into the cell. This Na would then be extracted from the cell by the action of the Na/K pump. The results obtained from cardiac tissues were consistent with a stoichiometry of 2 Na:1 Ca for this exchange process. At equilibrium, the relationship between the Na and Ca concentrations on either side of the cell membrane would be given by

$$\frac{[Ca]_o}{[Ca]_i} = \frac{[Na]_o^2}{[Na]_i^2} \tag{1}$$

Blaustein and Hodgkin [14] pointed out that such an exchange, if it were electroneutral, would not allow intracellular Ca levels to be reduced to sufficiently low levels, for example, to allow relaxation of muscle cells. In connection with this problem, it has been proposed that the carrier's affinity for Na and Ca is different on either side of the cell membrane and that the carrier may be charged [15]. A simple solution that would result in a lower [Ca]$_i$ was the possibility that more than 2 Na ions move for each Ca ion translocated. This idea has gained increasing popularity (e.g., see Mullins [3] and Blaustein [16]). If this is the case, then the distribution of the two ions is given by the equation

$$\frac{[Ca]_o}{[Ca]_i} = \frac{[Na]_o^n}{[Na]_i^n} \exp \frac{(n-2) FE_m}{RT} \tag{2}$$

and as pointed out by Mullins [17], the electrochemical driving forces for Na and Ca at equilibrium are given by

$$znF (E_{Na} - E_m) = zF (E_{Ca} - E_m) \tag{3}$$

where n is the coupling ratio of Na:Ca ions moved, E_m is the cell membrane potential, E_{Na} and E_{Ca} are the equilibrium potentials of Na and Ca, and z, F, R and T have their usual thermodynamic meanings. This movement of more than 2 Na ions for each Ca ion means that the mechanism is electrogenic and will result in current flow across the cell membrane. It also means that the rate of exchange of the carrier and the direction of movement of the ions will be dependent on the membrane potential of the cells. From equation (3), it can be shown that the direction of net movement of ions will be reversed at a certain membrane potential which is given by

$$E_{rev} = \frac{nE_{Na} - 2E_{Ca}}{n - 2} \tag{4}$$

that is, the direction of net movement of ions is dependent on the Na and Ca electrochemical gradients, and there is no net flux in either direction at the membrane potential, E_{rev}.

Mullins [3,17] has attributed great importance to the Na–Ca exchanger as a controller of contractile force in cardiac muscle (see also Chapman [1]). He suggests that the reversal potential of Na–Ca exchange is about -40 mV. Therefore, during the cardiac action potential, the exchanger reverses direction and carries Ca ions *into* the cell in exchange for intracellular Na, thereby helping to activate contraction. This Ca entry through the exchanger would occur in parallel with the Ca entry through the slow inward current channel. At the end of the action potential, when the cells repolarize past -40 mV, Ca will be transported out of the cell, thereby assisting the relaxation of the muscle in diastole. The Na–Ca exchanger would have to extrude not only the Ca it had carried into the cell during depolarization but also the Ca entering through the slow inward channel. Mullins suggests that the other known mechanism for Ca exit from the cell, the sarcolemmal Ca ATPase pump, plays only a minor role because although it has a higher affinity for Ca binding, its maximum transport rate is much lower than that of the Na–Ca exchanger [18,19].

FUNCTIONAL STUDIES AND ION-FLUX MEASUREMENTS

Perhaps the most dramatic consequences of the presence of an Na–Ca exchange mechanism are found in amphibian heart preparations. This is probably due to the smaller cell size (larger surface area/volume ratio) and the less well developed sarcoplasmic reticulum [20,21]. In a study on the large contracture induced in frog heart by reduction of extracellular Na, Chapman [22] found that the contracture appeared to depend on intracellular Na as well as extracellular Ca. Thus, the Na-free contracture develops rapidly but relaxes spontaneously within a few minutes, probably due to Na efflux from the cells. As the $[Na]_i$ decreases, this reduces the Na_i available

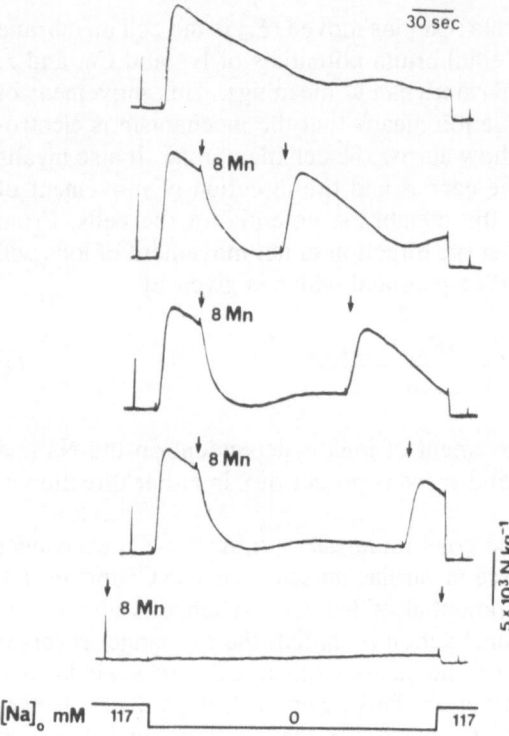

Figure 1. Manganese inhibition of contractures induced in a frog atrial trabecula by removal of extracellular Na (substituted by Tris). *Top trace:* An Na-free contracture in the absence of Mn. The preparations were stimulated at a rate of 4 min^{-1} in the normal Ringer. The last twitch in this sequence is seen prior to the contracture. *Bottom trace:* Mn was applied for 30 sec prior to, and during, the Na-free contracture. *Middle traces:* Mn was added at various times (between the arrows) during the Na-free contracture. From R. A. Chapman and D. Ellis (unpublished).

for exchange with extracellular Ca. As Ca influx is reduced, this allows internal Ca uptake systems to reduce [Ca]$_i$ and permit relaxation. Following the spontaneous relaxation, the muscle needs to be returned to a normal [Na]$_o$ for about 3 min before it can redevelop a similar-sized contracture on exposure to a low-[Na]$_o$ solution for a second time. This recovery process is aided by electrical stimulation or by inhibition of the Na/K pump, i.e., conditions likely to increase [Na]$_i$. Contractures could be produced by relatively small reductions of [Na]$_o$ if the Na/K pump was inhibited by strophanthidin [23], again illustrating a dependence on [Na]$_i$.

Manganese ions inhibit Ca fluxes across a wide variety of cell membranes. Manganese produces a large inhibition of the contractures initiated by reduction of [Na]$_o$ in frog heart [24,25]. Figure 1 illustrates this point. The top trace shows the contracture induced in a frog atrial trabecula by Na-free solutions. When 8 mM Mn was applied for 30 sec prior to, and during, the removal of Na$_o$, the Na-free contracture was almost completely blocked (bottom trace).

Addition of manganese ions after the development of the Na-free contracture caused a rapid relaxation (middle traces) consistent with an inhibition of Ca influx. Figure 2 shows the results of an experiment carried out on a sheep heart Purkinje fiber that had been penetrated with an Na-sensitive

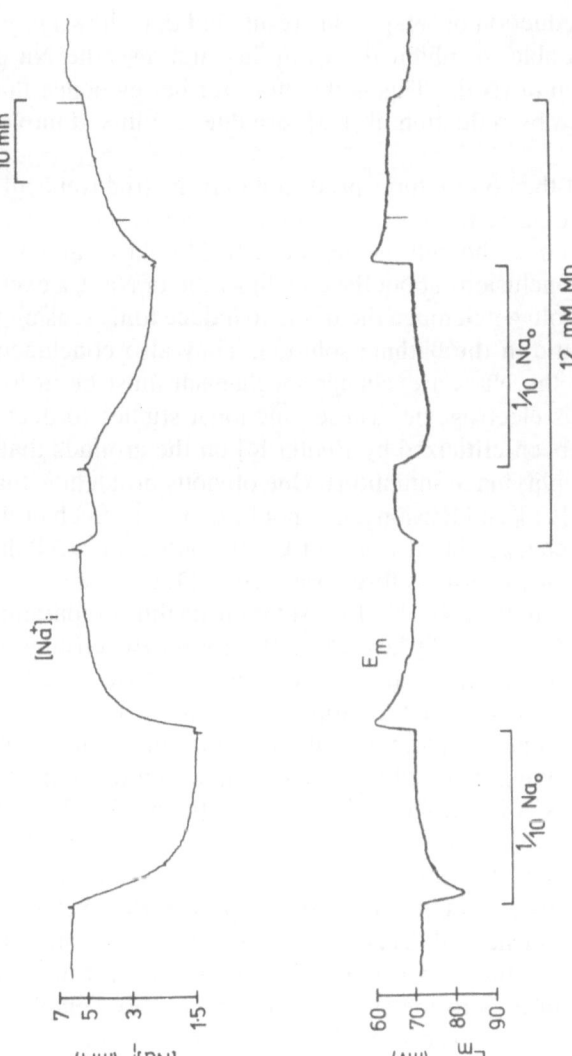

Figure 2.   Inhibition by Mn of the decrease in intracellular Na activity produced by reduction of $[Na]_o$ (substituted by lithium) in a sheep heart Purkinje fiber. All solutions that did not contain 12 mM Mn had an extra 18 mM lithium added to maintain isotonicity. All solutions contained 2 mM Ca. Levels of Na are expressed as Na *ion* concentration, $[Na]_i$. This can be converted to Na activity by multiplying by 0.75. From Ellis [26].

microelectrode to measure changes in the levels of intracellular Na. The first part of the record shows the effect of reduction of $[Na]_o$ to 10% of its normal concentration (substituted by lithium). This induces a large rapid decrease of intracellular Na that is not mediated via the Na/K pump [26,27]. The right-hand part of the record shows that manganese greatly inhibits the decrease of Na_i produced by reduction of $[Na]_o$. This result and that shown in Figure 1 suggest that Mn is able to inhibit the Ca influx and also the Na efflux produced by reduction of $[Na]_o$. This is therefore further evidence that the contractures produced by reduction of $[Na]_o$ are due to a linked movement of Na_i and Ca_o.

The amplitude of the contractures produced in frog atrial trabeculae by low-$[Na]_o$ solutions could be fitted by a model that involved an exchange of 1 Ca for 3 Na ions across the cell membrane [23]. Horakova and Vassort [28] reached similar conclusions about the coupling ratio of Na–Ca exchange in frog atrium. They voltage-clamped the tissue to induce tonic tension while altering the Ca/Na ratio in the bathing solution. They also concluded that the coupling ratio of the Na–Ca exchange mechanism must be at least 3; i.e., the mechanism is electrogenic. These functional studies to determine coupling ratios have been criticized by Reuter [4] on the grounds that they involve too many simplifying assumptions. One obvious problem is that the relationship between $[Ca]_i$ and tension might not be constant. Such problems could occur because changes in intracellular Ca also affect intracellular pH [29,30] and intracellular pH affects force production [31].

The contractures induced by Na-free solution in thin preparations of amphibian heart muscle are usually larger than the normal twitch contraction produced by an action potential [e.g., Figure 1 shows a twitch contraction induced 15 sec prior to the contracture (top trace)]. The reverse is normally true in mammalian cardiac preparations. If, however, intracellular Na activity is raised, e.g., by inhibition of the Na/K pump, then the amplitude of low-$[Na]_o$ contractures is increased and a contracture can develop even at normal levels of $[Na]_o$ [e.g., 29].

Functional studies by Langer and co-workers (e.g., see Langer [5]) on mammalian cardiac muscle emphasize another aspect of the exchange process that needs to be considered. This is the availability of Na and Ca ions at the external surface of the sarcolemma. The authors suggest that there is considerable binding of ions to the sarcolemmal glycocalyx complex. It is suggested that this acts as a reservoir of ions for the transport systems in the cell membrane. Thus, the degree of binding of any particular ion species will affect its availability for transport. When $[Na]_o$ is altered, in experiments designed to investigate Na–Ca exchange, it cannot be assumed that the *effective* $[Ca]_o$ remains constant. There appears to be a good, but perhaps unexpected, linear correlation between the contractility (maximum rate of force developed) of cardiac muscle and the amount of Ca bound to the sarcolemma [32,33]. Na and Ca ions may display part of their long-known antagonistic behavior in this respect and thus the need to investigate the binding properties of the tissue at these extracellular sites.

Tillisch et al. [34] found that in rabbit ventricle, lowering the $[Na]_o$ produced a transient increase in the force of the twitch contraction, while raising $[Na]_o$ produced a transient decrease. These transient changes were followed by a return to control levels. The transient nature of these changes was suggested to be due to an initial change in the amount of Ca bound at the membrane, i.e., increased Ca binding when Na_o is reduced. This would give increased Ca entry on the exchange carrier initially and increased contractile force. The carrier transport would slow as intracellular Na became depleted. This would return force production to control levels. This result would also be predicted if the competition between Na and Ca binding occurred at the actual exchanger site rather than at the sarcolemmal glycocalyx complex. This is unfortunately the case for most of the evidence cited in favor of an important role of the glycocalyx in controlling ion entry into the cells. It is of course conceivable that selectivity and competition for binding are similar at the glycocalyx and at the exchanger site. The problem does not appear to be feasibly amenable to experimental testing.

One interesting aspect of these studies [35,36] was that Ca efflux via the Na–Ca exchange system appeared to be fully saturated as long as the $[Na]_o$ was greater than 30 mM. Thus, Langer [5] is forced to attribute the large changes that do occur in cardiac contraction when $[Na]_o$ is varied between the normal level and 30 mM to effects on Ca binding and thus influx. This would also mean that the *effective* affinity for $[Na]_o$ on the Ca efflux system is high and has a K_m for $[Na]_o$ of about 10 mM or less. The external Na affinity has been suggested from previous results [11,13] to be higher than the internal Na affinity. Values of 40 and 60 mM for the K_m for Na at the external and internal sites, respectively, are indicated from the results of the latter authors.

Cultured chick heart-cell preparations have been demonstrated to produce ion fluxes similar to those occurring in adult hearts and are indicative of an Na–Ca exchange mechanism. Fosset et al. [37] found that veratridine stimulated Na uptake and that this was followed by a Ca uptake. Tetrodotoxin and local anesthetics inhibited both processes. Murphy et al. [38] described large, rapid changes in Na_i $(t_{\frac{1}{2}} = 13$ sec$)$ and Ca_i $(t_{\frac{1}{2}} \leqslant 30$ sec$)$ on reduction of $[Na]_o$. When $[Na]_o$ was reduced to 20 mM, there was an increase of $[Ca_i]$ by 3 to 5 fold. The effect appeared to be saturated at relatively low $[Na]_o$, since only small Ca uptakes were apparent if the $[Na]_o$ was greater than 30 mM. The use of such cultured heart-cell preparations has the advantage that rapid exchange times are possible for extracellular solution changes.

Since 1979, there have been considerable advances in another technique for intestigating Na–Ca countertransport, i.e., the preparation of vesicles prepared from cardiac-cell membranes. Various techniques have been used to produce these vesicles, but they normally involve disruption of cardiac cells via homogenization. This is followed by centrifugation to isolate the sarcolemmal fraction, and some form of salt extraction. The vesicles can be loaded during the preparation procedure with desired amounts of Na and Ca or other ions. A number of problems are likely to arise from the preparation procedure: (1) The purity of the membrane fraction is crucial. If there is substantial contamination of the sarcolemmal fraction by other membrane fractions or microsomes, then interpretation of ion-flux data will be subject to error. (2) In any vesicle preparation, there are likely to be some damaged or leaky vesicles. The effects of ion uptake or loss from these vesicles may alter the normal flux values. (3) When the sarcolemma forms vesicles, some procedures appear to yield predominantly right-side-out vesicles (the extracellular membrane surface of the sarcolemma becomes the outside of the vesicle), while others result in inside-out vesicles or an equal mixture of both (see Sulakhe and St. Louis [2] for a discussion of this and other problems). There appears to have been good progress in devising techniques for separating the two types of vesicles from a mixed population using affinity chromatography for various intracellular and extracellular membrane markers [39,40].

The first demonstrations of Na–Ca exchange in cardiac sarcolemmal vesicles were made by Reeves and Sutko [41], using dog ventricle, and by Pitts [42], also using dog ventricle. These vesicle preparations were shown to be capable of accumulating Ca, if they had been previously Na-loaded. These ion movements could occur in the absence of ATP. From a comparison of the rates of Ca efflux from, and Na influx into, dog ventricle vesicles, it was concluded that more than 2 Na ions moved for each Ca. It was suggested that the coupling ratio was 3 Na to 1 Ca [42]. Additional evidence that the Na–Ca exchange in vesicles was electrogenic was obtained by Reeves and Sutko [41] by addition of tetraphenylphosphonium ions. These are very lipid-soluble and positively charged. Their distribution across cell membranes acts as an indicator of membrane potential. It was found that the tetraphenylphosphonium ions accumulated in the vesicles when there was an Na loss coupled to a Ca uptake, i.e., the Na–Ca exchange must have created an internal negative charge. Similar conclusions were reached by Bers et al. [43] and Philipson and Nishimoto [44]. They found that the Na_i-dependent Ca influx into vesicles was enhanced by an inside positive membrane potential and inhibited by an inside negative potential. These changes in vesicle potential were induced by use of the K ionophore valinomycin and a K gradient. Caroni et al. [45] found a similar relationship between Na–Ca movement and charge generation across cardiac sarcolemmal vesicle membranes.

Caroni and Carafoli [18] and Caroni et al. [19], using dog heart vesicles, have also described the properties of an ATPase-driven Ca pump similar to the better-known Ca pump of dog red blood cells [46,47]. They found [18,19] that the ATP-dependent system had a higher affinity for Ca ($K_m = 0.3$ μm) than the Na–Ca exchanger ($K_m = 1.5$ μm), but that the maximum Ca transport rate of Na–Ca exchange was more than 30 times higher than that of the Ca ATPase system. They suggested that the K_m of the Na–Ca exchanger might be even lower on the sarcoplasmic side of the sarcolemma and that ATP might decrease it even further, as is the case in squid giant axon. The Na–Ca exchange in these vesicles was inhibited by chlorpromazine, an antagonist of calmodulin. The exchange also appears to be inhibited by acidic conditions and stimulated by alkaline conditions [48].

In the few years that sarcolemmal vesicles have been used to investigate membrane-transport processes in cardiac tissues, much useful information has accumulated. No doubt sarcolemmal purification procedures and methods for production of vesicle populations of uniform sidedness will improve. In the same way that studies of ion transport across red blood cells have now reached high levels of exactness, the ability to readily manipulate both the internal and the external media across cardiac-cell membranes should add greatly to our understanding.

ION-SENSITIVE ELECTRODE MEASUREMENTS

Ion-sensitive microelectrodes permit direct measurements of intracellular Na and Ca ion activities (a_{Na}^i and a_{Ca}^i, respectively). They can therefore provide us with our best estimates of the transmembrane Na and Ca electrochemical gradients on which the Na–Ca exchanger operates. Traditional methods of ion analysis (e.g., flame photometry or atomic absorption spectroscopy) can give information only about the total Na or Ca content of cardiac tissues. This will include an unknown amount of intracellular ion buffering and an unknown amount of Na and Ca tightly bound either intracellularly or extracellularly to membranes. Continuous measurements of changes in intracellular ion levels are possible with ion-sensitive microelectrodes, so that the time–course of internal ion changes can be discerned.

The first measurements of a_{Na}^i in cardiac muscle were made by Lee and Fozzard [49] in rabbit papillary muscle. They found that a_{Na}^i was 6.4 mM and much lower than measurements of the total Na content of cardiac tissue. This low value has subsequently been confirmed in a wide variety of cardiac preparations (see Table 1) and indicates a large concentration gradient for Na entry ($E_{Na} \geqslant +70$ mV). Measurements of a_{Ca}^i indicate that the free Ca ion concentration, $[Ca]_i$, is about 2×10^{-7} M (see Table 2).

The effects of altering $[Ca]_o$ on a_{Na}^i have been examined in sheep heart Purkinje fibers by Ellis [26] and Deitmer and Ellis [50]. An 8-fold increase of $[Ca]_o$ was found to decrease a_{Na}^i by 1–3 mM. Coray et al. [51] found that similar increases of $[Ca]_o$ produced an approximate doubling of a_{Ca}^i in sheep heart Purkinje fibers. Similar results have been found in ferret papillary muscle [52] and sheep ventricle [53]. These results can be explained by an Na–Ca exchange mechanism. However, these Na measurements are probably affected by an influence of $[Ca]_o$ on the Na permeability of the cell membrane. Thus, an increase of $[Ca]_o$ will decrease the passive inward leak of Na, allowing the Na/K pump to reduce the level of a_{Na}^i to a lower value at which the new leak rate approximately equals the new pump rate. As a result of this problem, it was necessary to investigate the effect of $[Ca]_o$ on a_{Na}^i when the Na/K pump had been inhibited.

Inhibition of the Na/K pump either by removal of extracellular K or by application of cardioactive steroids produces an increase in a_{Na}^i. Under these conditions, when $[Ca]_o$ is altered, there are larger changes of a_{Na}^i [30,50], presumably due to an increased contribution of Na_i–Ca_o exchange. For a given increase in $[Ca]_o$, the resultant decrease of a_{Na}^i was linearly related to the initial a_{Na}^i [50]. No saturation of the process was apparent at a_{Na}^i values in excess of 20 mM. This confirms the high K_m measurements for Na_i on the Na–Ca exchanger [13]. The reduction of a_{Na}^i on raising $[Ca]_o$ would be an "uphill" movement of Na, against its electrochemical gradient, at a time when the Na/K pump is inhibited. This movement of Na therefore appears to be caused by the increase in the inward transmembrane Ca gradient. Other divalent cations like Mn and Mg appear to act like Ca in reducing the Na permeability of the cell membrane. They are able to slow the rate of increase of a_{Na}^i on inhibition of the Na/K pump. However, high concentrations of Mn or Mg were unable to produce a reduction of a_{Na}^i [50]. It is interesting that Sr and Ba were able to act like Ca and produce decreases of a_{Na}^i, and this suggests that they might be able to be transported on the exchanger. It was also found that with the Na/K pump inhibited, a 10-fold increase in $[Ca]_o$ resulted in a decrease of a_{Na}^i by approximately 50%. This would suggest that the coupling ratio of the Na–Ca exchange is just over 3 [from equation (2)], but again, this does not take into account effects of $[Ca]_o$ on the passive Na permeability.

The results also indicate that when the Na/K pump is inhibited, another mechanism, i.e., the Na–Ca exchanger, is able to keep a_{Na}^i at reasonably low levels. This may be related to the ability of cells to regulate their cell volume in the presence of high concentrations of cardiac glycosides [54].

Attempts to perturb the Na–Ca exchanger by reduction of $[Na]_o$ produce changes of intracellular ion activities consistent with its previously suggested mechanism of action. Thus, a decrease of $[Na]_o$ produces a rapid fall of a_{Na}^i [26,27,29,53,55]. This is associated with a small increase of a_{Ca}^i [29,52,53,56]. The increase of a_{Ca}^i would of course be small due to the large buffering capacity of the cells for intracellular Ca changes. Lee et al. [56] described a 3-fold increase in a_{Ca}^i in rabbit ventricle when $[Na]_o$ was reduced to 20 mM. This rise of a_{Ca}^i was sufficient to induce a contracture. Marban et al. [52] reported that complete removal of $[Na]_o$ could produce a rise of a_{Ca}^i in ferret papillary muscle of just over 40% and that this was just above the threshold for tension production. Bers and Ellis [29] also found only small increases of a_{Ca}^i and tension when $[Na]_o$ was reduced to 14 mM in sheep heart Purkinje fibers. However, when the Na/K pump was inhibited with strophanthidin, there was a slow rise of a_{Ca}^i and a contracture developed. If

[Na]$_o$ was reduced under these conditions, there were extremely large rises of a_{Ca}^i and very large contractures were produced. These large contractures could be attributed to an increased rate of Na$_i$–Ca$_o$ exchange and perhaps also to a reduction in the number of intracellular buffering sites available to prevent further large increases of a_{Ca}^i. It was suggested that under conditions of severe Ca loading of the cells, changes of intracellular pH also become apparent because Ca and H ions show some common intracellular buffering sites [57]. An interaction of Ca and H ions at the mitochondrial membrane is to be expected. This probably contributes to the intracellular acidification observed under conditions of Ca loading. Vaughan-Jones et al. [30] also describe changes of pH$_i$ associated with changes in [Ca]$_i$ that were initially induced by manipulation of the Na–Ca exchange system.

The ability of raised levels of [Na]$_i$ to increase the [Ca]$_i$ was suggested as a mechanism for the therapeutic action of cardiac glycosides [12]. Thus, digitalis-like compounds should inhibit the Na/K pump, causing a rise of [Na]$_i$ and a subsequent increase of [Ca]$_i$ resulting in increased force production. That therapeutic doses of cardiac glycosides have their action by this mechanism is not proven, since there are conditions in which Na/K pump inhibition and positive inotropy appear to be dissociated. There is some evidence for apparent stimulation of the Na/K pump at low glycoside concentrations. Noble [58] has recently reviewed the literature on this topic. Regardless of the mechanism for producing positive inotropy by low doses of cardiac glycosides, there seems to be general agreement that the effects of high doses occur as a result of Na/K pump inhibition and raised levels of [Ca]$_i$ via the Na–Ca exchange mechanism. Thus, the contracture that develops and other toxic signs are probably due to a raised level of [Ca]$_i$. This may well induce other damaging effects by causing intracellular acidification [30,57]. The apparently contradictory evidence on the action of cardiac glycosides may therefore be due to more than one mechanism of action, which will depend on the concentration of the glycoside as well as other factors [58].

The large reduction of a_{Na}^i that occurs on reduction of [Na]$_o$ [26] is difficult to inhibit. Note that in Figure 2, a high concentration of Mn produced only partial inhibition. It has also been found that the a_{Na}^i decrease appears to have a relatively low sensitivity to reduction of [Ca]$_o$ (D. Ellis, unpublished). It may well be that the Na substitute used in these experiments (lithium) was able to exchange for intracellular Na. Thus, some of the Na loss from the cell would not be coupled to a Ca uptake. Some evidence for this idea comes from the observation that the low-[Na]$_o$ contracture is small when Li is used as an Na substitute compared to its amplitude with some other Na replacers, e.g., tetramethylammonium, K, or sugars. Ponce-Hornos and Langer [59] studied the effects of Ca fluxes and tension from rabbit interventricular septum on the reduction of [Na]$_o$ together with inhibition of the Na/K pump. They concluded that Li can inhibit Ca binding at the external surface of the cell, and this prevents the contracture that develops if sucrose is used as an Na substitute.

Recently, Chapman et al. [55] have measured the decrease of a_{Na}^i on reduction of [Na]$_o$ in ferret ventricular muscle preparations. They used very thin preparations and a fast-flow system. They point out that to use larger preparations would result in diffusion-limitation problems. They observed large rapid decreases of a_{Na}^i. The rate of decrease of a_{Na}^i in these experiments was probably up to 10 times faster than that in corresponding experiments in sheep heart Purkinje fibers (rate constant 3.3 min) [26]. This, they calculate, could be adequately accounted for by the larger cell size in Purkinje fibers. Chapman et al. [55] assumed that the Na was leaving the cell on the Na–Ca exchange carrier and plotted the rate of Na efflux against the level of a_{Na}^i. The results were then fitted by the equation

$$J = J_{max} \frac{[Na]_i^n}{(K_m)^n + [Na]_i^n} \tag{5}$$

where J is the Na efflux (pmole/cm^2 sec) and J_{max} is the maximum rate of Na efflux estimated from their data. The curve appeared to be S-shaped and was best fitted by a line with $n = 3$. The K_m for [Na]$_i$ was 9 mM.

One other interesting aspect from this paper was that the normal a_{Na}^i was more than 11 mM, i.e., about 65% higher than the average a_{Na}^i measured from a variety of cardiac preparations (Table 1), even though a higher level of [Ca]$_o$ was used. They attributed this high level of a_{Na}^i to the low temperatures at which these experiments were carried out (22–26°C). Presumably, there would be some inhibition of the Na/K pump at these temperatures. As yet, there has been no ion-sensitive microelectrode study to investigate the relationship between a_{Na}^i and temperature in cardiac muscle.

Na–Ca EXCHANGE AT REST AND DURING ELECTRICAL ACTIVITY

Tables 1 and 2 show that in a wide variety of cardiac preparations, the levels of a_{Na}^i are very similar, as are the values for [Ca]$_i$. Some of the small differences could be accounted for by differences in the [Na]$_o$ and [Ca]$_o$ used in the various studies. Marban et al. [52] pointed out that the rather low value for [Ca]$_i$ obtained by Lee et al. [56] would in fact be identical to their own measurement if the same effective stability constant for Ca–EGTA had been used; i.e., the difference is due to the problem of calibrating Ca electrodes.

Taking values for E_{Ca}, E_{Na}, and E_m from the data given in the papers quoted in Tables 1 and 2 and using equation (3) to calculate the coupling ratio of Na–Ca exchange gives a value for n of 2.6. Similar values were found from simultaneous measurements of a_{Na}^i and a_{Ca}^i in sheep heart Purkinje fibers ($n = 2.4$–2.9) [29] and in sheep ventricle ($n = 2.5$) [53]. These

Table 1.   Intracellular Sodium Activity in Cardiac Tissues

a_{Na}^i (mM)	Preparation	Reference
6.4	Rabbit papillary muscle	Lee and Fozzard [49]
7.2	Sheep Purkinje fiber	Ellis [26]
6.6	Sheep Purkinje fiber	Deitmer and Ellis [50]
7.8	Guinea pig atrium	Glitsch et al. [63]
6.4	Sheep Purkinje fiber	Lee et al. [64]
8.1	Sheep Purkinje fiber	Glitsch and Pusch [65]
6.6	Sheep Purkinje fiber	Sheu et al. [66]
5.8	Guinea pig papillary muscle	Cohen and Fozzard [67]
6.4	Sheep Purkinje fiber	Eisner et al. [68]

values would be correct for a coupling ratio only if the Na gradient and Ca gradient are linked in the way assumed in the derivation of the equations with the system near to equilibrium. This might be the case if other forms of Ca entry, i.e., Ca "leak," are compensated for by the ATPase-driven Ca pump [18,55]. In a recent study, Sheu and Fozzard [53] have shown that when the [Na]$_o$ or the [Ca]$_o$ is varied over a wide range of values (giving rise to large changes in a_{Na}^i and a_{Ca}^i), the value for n remains remarkably constant at about 2.5. Only when the Na/K pump was inhibited did n begin to rise to about 3. It was suggested that as a_{Ca}^i rose to high levels, the mitochondria might take up Ca and thus limit the reduction in the transmembrane Ca gradient.

The attractive model discussed by Mullins [3,17] (see the Introduction) suggests that Na–Ca exchange might help to activate contraction by taking Ca into the cell when the membrane potential depolarizes past -40mV and then assist in relaxation by extruding Ca when the cell is repolarized. For the exchange to reverse direction at this potential requires that values for

Table 2.   Free Intracellular Calcium Ion Concentration in Cardiac Tissues[a]

[Ca^{2+}]$_i$ (M)	Preparation	Reference
2.1×10^{-7}	Sheep Purkinje fiber	Sokol et al. [69]
2.6×10^{-7}	Sheep Purkinje fiber	Dahl and Isenberg [70]
1.7×10^{-7}	Sheep Purkinje fiber	Coray et al. [51]
3.6×10^{-7}	Sheep ventricular muscle	Coray et al. [51]
2.6×10^{-7}	Ferret ventricular muscle	Marban et al. [52]
1.2×10^{-7}	Rabbit ventricular muscle	Lee et al. [56]
2.8×10^{-7}	Sheep Purkinje fiber	Bers and Ellis [29]

[a] Where authors have quoted values of Ca activity, a_{Ca}^i, rather than Ca ion concentration, [Ca^{2+}]$_i$, these have been converted for uniformity. Although Ca electrodes measure activity, they are calibrated in buffered solutions of known ion concentration. The Ca activity coefficient in complicated mixed solutions is not known with accuracy, but is approximately 0.32.

[Na]$_i$ and [Ca]$_i$ be chosen carefully. Values of about 20 mM [Na]$_i$ and 10^{-8} M [Ca]$_i$ were suggested [3]. These figures are not substantiated by actual experimental data, as shown in Tables 1 and 2. If we take mean values from Tables 1 and 2 and apply equation (3) with $n = 3$, there should be a reversal of the Na–Ca exchange at a membrane potential of about -8 mV. If $n = 4$ (as Mullins suggests), then the reversal would be at about $+33$ mV. There would therefore be a very short time of reversal during the Purkinje-fiber action potential because of the relatively low plateau. In ventricular muscle, however, because of its longer sustained plateau, there could be a significant amount of time for Ca entry on the Na–Ca exchange mechanism. However, much less Ca would enter than if the reversal potential was more negative. Similar values for the reversal potential (between -2 and -25 mV, assuming $n = 3$) were obtained from studies in which simultaneous measurements of a_{Ca}^i and a_{Na}^i have been made in a particular tissue [29,53,60]. Clearly, in the absence of further information on the Na–Ca exchanger and on other mechanisms that affect intracellular Ca, such manipulation of figures must be regarded with some caution. The attractive ideas put forward by Mullins [3,17] are obviously rather speculative. Their importance, however, lies in the great deal of interest and experimental work that they have initiated in this field.

   The ion activities discussed so far have been obtained from quiescent preparations. The normal electrical activity of the heart will affect both passive movements of Na and Ca (due to the change in electrical gradient during the action potential) and the flow of these ions through channels that are activated by membrane depolarization. Recently, Cohen et al. [61] and Lado et al. [62] have described changes of a_{Na}^i and a_{Ca}^i, respectively, in cardiac muscle during electrical stimulation at various frequencies. There is a significant rise of a_{Na}^i at a stimulation rate of only 0.2 Hz, and at 3 Hz, a mean increase of a_{Na}^i of about 30% was demonstrated in Purkinje fibers [61]. The size of the a_{Na}^i rise is rather variable. I have confirmed the a_{Na}^i measurements, and find that at 3 Hz, a_{Na}^i rises by more than 40% in sheep heart Purkinje fibers (D. Ellis, unpublished). The probable reason for this higher value is that longer periods of stimulation (15 min) were employed than in the experiments of Cohen et al. [61] (3 min) in order to measure the new steady-state level of a_{Na}^i. Lado et al. [62] found that at 3 Hz stimulation (for 3 min), the a_{Na}^i increased from 93 to 162 nM in sheep Purkinje fibers.

   The recovery of a_{Ca}^i after cessation of stimulation was exponential with a time constant (80–120 sec) similar to that for a_{Na}^i recovery [61]. Thus, the Ca gradient appears to be controlled by the Na gradient, which in turn is controlled by the activity of the Na/K pump. The increase of a_{Na}^i during electrical stimulation would lead to a rise of a_{Ca}^i. The measured rise of a_{Na}^i would be expected to give the measured rise of a_{Ca}^i if the coupling ratio [n in equations (2) and (3)] was 2.5. This is in excellent agreement with previous results described above, but may be fortuitous. As Lado et al. [62] point out, a rise of a_{Ca}^i would be expected due to the Ca entry of the slow inward current. The fact that the coupling ratio appears to be constant in quiescent and in stimulated preparations means that the reversal potential of the Na–Ca exchange [E_{rev} in equation (4)] is not altered in beating cardiac muscle.

Lee and Dagostino [60] have measured the changes in a_{Na}^i and a_{Ca}^i that occur when the stimulation of dog-heart Purkinje fibers is temporarily interrupted. Their results indicate that stimulation at a frequency of 1 Hz causes a rise of a_{Na}^i of about 20% and a rise of a_{Ca}^i of approximately 11–43%. These results are consistent with those of Cohen et al. [61] and Lado et al. [62].

CONCLUSIONS

Information obtained using a wide variety of experimental techniques, i.e., functional studies of contractile force, flux experiments, sarcolemmal vesicles, and ion-sensitive microelectrodes, indicates the presence of an Na–Ca exchange mechanism in cardiac-cell membranes. This process appears to be electrogenic; i.e., more than 2 Na ions are translocated for each Ca ion in the exchange. The exact coupling ratio is still in some doubt, since the experimental data suggest values between 2.5 and 4. The system might be near to equilibrium in resting muscle, with the level of Ca_i controlled by the transmembrane Na gradient. This might not be the case if the membrane Ca ATPase pump makes a larger contribution to the control of intracellular Ca than is currently thought. Reversal of the Na–Ca exchange mechanism during the cardiac action potential could play an important role in assisting the activation of contraction, but the case is not yet proved.

ACKNOWLEDGMENTS

I am very grateful to Dr. K. T. MacLeod for valuable comments on this manuscript. The experiments described herein that were carried out by the author were funded by grants from the Medical Research Council and the British Heart Foundation.

REFERENCES

1. Chapman, R. A. 1979. Excitation–contraction coupling in cardiac muscle. *Prog. Biophys. Mol. Biol.* 35:1–52.
2. Sulakhe, P. V., and St. Louis, P. J. 1980. Passive and active calcium fluxes across plasma membranes. *Prog. Biophys. Mol. Biol.* 35:135–195.
3. Mullins, L. J. 1981. *Ion Transport in Heart.* Raven Press, New York.
4. Reuter, H. 1982. Na–Ca countertransport in cardiac muscle. In: A Martonosi (ed.), *Membranes and Transport 1980.* Vol. 1, pp. 623–631. Plenum Press, New York.
5. Langer, G. A. 1982. Sodium–calcium exchange in the heart. *Annu. Rev. Physiol.* 44:435–449.

6. Daly, I. de Burgh, and Clark, A. J. 1921. The action of ions upon the frog's heart. *J. Physiol.* 54:367–383.

7. Wilbrandt, W., and Koller, H. 1948. Die Calciumwirkung an Froschherzen als Funktion des Ionengleichgewichts zwischen Zellmembran und Umgebung. *Helv. Physiol. Pharmacol. Acta* 6:208–221.

8. Lüttgau, H. C., and Niedergerke, R. 1958. The antagonism between Ca and Na ions on the frog's heart. *J. Physiol.* 143:486–505.

9. Langer, G. A. 1964. Kinetic studies of calcium distribution in ventricular muscle of the dog. *Circ. Res.* 15:393–405.

10. Repke, K. 1964. Über den biochemischen Wirkungsmodus von Digitalis. *Klin. Wochenschr.* 42:157–162.

11. Reuter, H., and Seitz, N. 1968. The dependence of calcium efflux from cardiac muscle on temperature and external ion composition. *J. Physiol.* 195:451–470.

12. Baker, P. F., Blaustein, M. P., Hodgkin, A. L., and Steinhardt, R. A. 1969. The influence of calcium on sodium efflux in squid axons. *J. Physiol.* 200:431–458.

13. Glitsch, H. G., Reuter, H., and Scholz, H. 1970. The effect of the internal sodium concentration on calcium fluxes in isolated guinea-pig auricles. *J. Physiol.* 209:25–43.

14. Blaustein, M. P., and Hodgkin, A. L. 1969. The effect of cyanide on the efflux of calcium from squid axons. *J. Physiol.* 200:497–527.

15. Reuter, H. 1970. Calcium transport in cardiac muscle. In: L. Bolis, A. Katchalsky, R. D. Keynes, and W. R. Lowenstein (eds.), *Permeability and Function of Biological Membranes*. pp. 342–347. North-Holland, Amsterdam.

16. Blaustein, M. P. 1974. The interrelationship between sodium and calcium fluxes across cell membranes. *Rev. Physiol. Biochem. Pharmacol.* 70:33–82.

17. Mullins, L. J. 1979. The generation of electric currents in cardiac fibres by Na/Ca exchange. *Am. J. Physiol.* 236:C103–110.

18. Caroni, P., and Carafoli, E. 1980. An ATP-dependent Ca^{2+} pumping system in dog heart sarcolemma. *Nature (London)* 283:765–767.

19. Caroni, P., Reinlib, L., and Carafoli, E. 1980. Charge movement during the Na^+–Ca^{2+} exchange in heart sarcolemmal vesicles. *Proc. Natl. Acad. Sci. U.S.A.* 77:6354–6358.

20. Sommer, J. R., and Johnson, E. A. 1969. Cardiac muscle: A comparative study with special reference to frog and chicken hearts. *Z. Zellforsch.* 98:437–468.

21. Page, S. G., and Niedergerke, R. 1972. Structures of physiological interest in frog heart ventricle. *J. Cell Sci.* 11:179–203.

22. Chapman, R. A. 1974. A study of the contractures induced in frog atrial trabeculae by a reduction of the bathing sodium concentration. *J. Physiol.* 237:295–313.

23. Chapman, R. A., and Tunstall, J. 1980. The interaction of sodium and calcium ions at the cell membrane and the control of contractile strength in frog atrial muscle. *J. Physiol.* 305:109–124.

24. Chapman, R. A., and Ochi, R. 1971. The effects of manganese ions on the contractile responses of isolated frog atrial trabeculae. *J. Physiol.* 222:56–58P.

25. Chapman, R. A., and Ellis, D. 1977. The effects of manganese ions on the contraction of the frog's heart. *J. Physiol.* 272:331–354.

26. Ellis, D. 1977. The effects of external cations and ouabain on the sodium activity in sheep heart Purkinje fibres. *J. Physiol.* 273:211–240.

27. Ellis, D., and Deitmer, J. W. 1978. The relationship between the intra- and extracellular sodium activity of sheep heart Purkinje fibres during inhibition of the Na–K pump. *Pfluegers Arch.* 377:209–215.

28. Horakova, M., and Vassort, G. 1979. Sodium–calcium exchange in regulation of cardiac contractility: Evidence for an electrogenic, voltage-dependent mechanism. *J. Gen. Physiol.* 73:403–424.

29. Bers, D. M., and Ellis, D. 1982. Intracellular calcium and sodium activity in sheep heart Purkinje fibres: Effect of changes of external sodium and intracellular pH. *Pfluegers Arch.* 393:171–178.

30. Vaughan-Jones, R. D., Lederer, W. J., and Eisner, D. A. 1983. Ca^{2+} ions can affect intracellular pH in mammalian cardiac muscle. *Nature (London)* 301:522–524.
31. Fabiato, A., and Fabiato, F. 1978. Effects of pH on the myofilaments and the sarcoplasmic reticulum of skinned cells from cardiac and skeletal muscles. *J. Physiol.* 276:233–255.
32. Philipson, K. D., Bers, D. M., Nishimoto, A. Y., and Langer, G. A. 1980. Binding of Ca^{2+} and Na^+ to sarcolemmal membranes: Relation to control of myocardial contractility. *Am. J. Physiol.* 238:H373–378.
33. Bers, D. M., Philipson, K. D., and Langer, G. A. 1981. Cardiac contractility and sarcolemmal calcium binding in several cardiac muscle preparations. *Am. J. Physiol.* 240:H576–H583.
34. Tillisch, J. H., Fung, L. K., Horn, P. M., and Langer, G. A. 1979. Transient and steady-state effects of sodium and calcium on myocardial contractile response. *J. Mol. Cell. Cardiol.* 11:137–148.
35. Langer, G. A., Nudd, L. M., and Ricchiuti, N. V. 1976. The effect of sodium deficient perfusion on calcium exchange in cardiac tissue culture. *J. Mol. Cell. Cardiol.* 8:321–328.
36. Wendt, I. R., and Langer, G. A. 1977. The sodium–calcium relationship in mammalian myocardium: Effect of sodium deficient perfusion on calcium fluxes. *J. Mol. Cell. Cardiol.* 9:551–564.
37. Fosset, M. de Barry, J., Lenoir, M. C., and Lazdunski, M. 1977. Analysis of molecular aspects of Na^+ and Ca^{2+} uptake by embryonic cardiac cells in culture. *J. Biol. Chem.* 252:6112–6117.
38. Murphy, E., Wheeler, D. M., Anderson, L., Horres, C. R., and Lieberman, M. 1981. Sodium calcium exchange in cultured chick heart cells. *J. Gen. Physiol.* 78:4a.
39. Mas-Oliva, J., Williams, A. J., and Naylor, W. G. 1980. Two orientations of isolated cardiac sarcolemmal vesicles separated by affinity chromatography. *Anal. Biochem.* 103:222–226.
40. Reinlib, L., Caroni, P., and Carafoli, E. 1981. Studies on heart sarcolemma: Vesicles of opposite orientation and the effect of ATP on the Na^+/Ca^{2+} exchange. *FEBS Lett.* 126:74–76.
41. Reeves, J. P., and Sutko, J. L. 1980. Sodium–calcium exchange affinity generates a current in cardiac membrane vesicles. *Science* 208:1461–1464.
42. Pitts, B. J. R. 1979. Stoichiometry of sodium–calcium exchange in cardiac sarcolemmal vesicles: Coupling to the sodium pump. *J. Biol. Chem.* 254:6232–6235.
43. Bers, D. M., Philipson, K. D., and Nishimoto, A. Y. 1980. Sodium calcium exchange and sidedness of isolated cardiac sarcolemmal vesicles. *Biochem. Biophys. Acta* 601:358–371.
44. Philipson, K. D., and Nishimoto, A. Y. 1980. $Na^+–Ca^{2+}$ exchange is affected by membrane potential in cardiac sarcolemmal vesicles. *J. Biol. Chem.* 255:6880–6882.
45. Caroni, P., Reinlib, L., and Carafoli, E. 1980. Charge movements during the Na^+/Ca^{2+} exchange in heart sarcolemmal vesicles. *Proc. Natl. Acad. Sci. U.S.A.* 77:6354–6358.
46. Brown, A. M. 1979. Evidence for a magnesium- and ATP-dependent calcium extrusion pump in dog erythrocytes. *Biochim. Biophys. Acta* 554:195–203.
47. Parker, J. C. 1979. Active and passive Ca movements in dog red blood cells and resealed ghosts. *Am. J. Physiol.* 237:C10–C16.
48. Philipson, K. D., Bersohn, M. M., and Nishimoto, A. Y. 1982. Effects of pH on Na^+ and Ca^{2+} exchange in canine cardiac sarcolemmal vesicles. *Circ. Res.* 50:287–293.
49. Lee, C. O., and Fozzard, H. A. 1975. Activities of potassium and sodium ions in rabbit heart muscle. *J. Gen. Physiol.* 65:695–708.
50. Deitmer, J. W., and Ellis, D. 1978. Changes in the intracellular sodium activity of sheep heart Purkinje fibres produced by calcium and other divalent cations. *J. Physiol.* 277:437–453.
51. Coray, A., Fry, C. H., Hess, P., McGuigan, J. A. S., and Weingart, R. 1980. Resting calcium in sheep cardiac tissues and in frog skeletal muscle measured with ion-selective microelectrodes. *J. Physiol.* 305:60–61P.
52. Marban, E., Rink, T. J., Tsien, R. W., and Tsien, R. Y. 1980. Free calcium in heart muscle at rest and during contraction measured with Ca^{2+}-sensitive microelectrodes. *Nature (London)* 286:845–850.

53. Sheu, S-S., and Fozzard, H. A. 1982. Transmembrane Na^+ and Ca^{2+} electrochemical gradients in cardiac muscle and their relationship to force development. *J. Gen. Physiol.* 80:325–351.

54. Macknight, A. D. C., and Leaf, A. 1977. Regulation of cellular volume. *Physiol. Rev.* 57:510–573.

55. Chapman, R. A., Coray, A., and McGuigan, J. A. S. 1983. Sodium/calcium exchange in mammalian heart: The maintenance of low intracellular calcium concentration. In: A. Drake and M. I. M. Noble (eds.), *Cardiac Metabolism.* pp. 117–149. John Wiley, New York.

56. Lee, C. O., Uhm, D. Y., and Dresdner, K. 1980. Sodium–calcium exchange in rabbit heart muscle cells: Direct measurement of sarcoplasmic Ca^{2+} activity. *Science* 209:699–701.

57. Deitmer, J. W., and Ellis, D. 1980. Interactions between the regulation of the intracellular pH and sodium activity of sheep cardiac Purkinje fibres. *J. Physiol.* 304:471–488.

58. Noble, D. 1980. Mechanism of action of therapeutic levels of cardiac glycosides. *Cardiovasc. Res.* 14:495–514.

59. Ponce-Hornos, J. E., and Langer, G. A. 1980. Sodium–calcium exchange in mammalian myocardium: The effects of lithium. *J. Mol. Cell. Cardiol.* 12:1367–1382.

60. Lee, C. O., and Dagostino, M. 1982. Effect of strophanthidin on intracellular Na ion activity and twitch tension of constantly driven canine cardiac Purkinje fibres. *Biophys. J.* 40:185–198.

61. Cohen, C. J., Fozzard, H. A., and Sheu, S-S. 1982. Increase in intracellular sodium ion activity during stimulation in mammalian cardiac muscle. *Circ. Res.* 50:651–662.

62. Lado, M. G., Sheu, S-S., and Fozzard, H. A. 1982. Changes in intracellular Ca^{2+} activity with stimulation in sheep cardiac Purkinje strands. *Am. J. Physiol.* 243:H133–H137.

63. Glitsch, H. G., Pusch, H., and Vassort, G. 1979. An estimation of the intracellular Na activity in guinea-pig atrial cells. *Pfluegers Arch. Suppl.* 379:R2.

64. Lee, C. O., Kang, D. H., Sokol, J. H., and Lee, K. S. 1980. Relation between intracellular Na ion activity and tension of sheep cardiac Purkinje fibres exposed to dihydro-ouabain. *Biophys. J.* 29:315–330.

65. Glitsch, H. G., and Pusch, H. 1980. Correlation between changes in membrane potential and intracellular Na activity during K activated response in sheep Purkinje fibres. *Pfluegers Arch.* 384:189–191.

66. Sheu, S-S., Korth, M., Lathrop, D. A., and Fozzard, H. A. 1980. Intra- and extracellular K^+ and Na^+ activities and resting membrane potential in sheep cardiac Purkinje strands. *Circ. Res.* 47:692–700.

67. Cohen, C. J., and Fozzard, H. A. 1979. Intracellular K and Na activities in papillary muscle during inotropic interventions. *Biophys. J.* 25:144.

68. Eisner, D. A., Lederer, W. J., and Vaughan-Jones, R. D. 1981. The dependence of sodium pumping and tension on intracellular sodium activity in voltage-clamped sheep Purkinje fibres. *J. Physiol.* 317:163–187.

69. Sokol, J. H., Lee, C. O., and Lupo, F. J. 1979. Measurement of the free calcium ion concentration in sheep cardiac Purkinje fibres with neutral carrier Ca^{++}-selective microelectrodes. *Biophys. J.* 25:143.

70. Dahl, G., and Isenberg, G. 1980. Decoupling of heart muscle cells: Correlation with increased cytoplasmic calcium activity and with changes of nexus ultrastructure. *J. Membr. Biol.* 53:63–75.

The Effects of Intracellular Na on Contraction and Intracellular pH in Mammalian Cardiac Muscle

R. D. Vaughan-Jones

University Laboratory of Physiology
Oxford OXl 3PT, England

D. A. Eisner

Department of Physiology
University College London
London WC1E 6BT, England

W. J. Lederer

Department of Physiology
University of Maryland Medical School
Baltimore, Maryland 21201

Abstract. Intracelluar Na and pH were measured with recessed-tip ion-selective microelectrodes in voltage-clamped sheep cardiac Purkinje fibers. Intracellular Na activity (a_{Na}^i) was elevated by inhibiting the Na/K pump. This produced an increase of twitch tension that had a steep dependence on the increase of a_{Na}^i. These effects of a_{Na}^i on twitch tension are probably mediated by an Na–Ca exchange. An increase of a_{Na}^i also produced a component of tonic tension that appears to be produced directly by the Na–Ca exchange. The dependence of tonic tension and a_{Na}^i on membrane potential suggests that this exchange process may be voltage-sensitive. The increase of a_{Na}^i is associated with an intracellular acidification that appears to be secondary to an increase of $[Ca^{2+}]_i$ produced by Na–Ca exchange. Therefore, as well as affecting $[Ca^{2+}]_i$, Na–Ca exchange can under some circumstances influence pH_i indirectly, and this complicates the interpretation of changes in tension, since protons and Ca ions have opposite effects on contractile force.

INTRODUCTION

Calcium ions are required for the heart to contract [1]. Following the more recent descriptions of sarcolemmal Na–Ca exchange in heart, it has become apparent that Na must also play an important role, albeit an indirect one, in regulating contraction. This is because a change in the transmembrane Na gradient will, via Na–Ca exchange, change the intracellular Ca^{2+} concentration ($[Ca^{2+}]_i$) [2,3], and this in turn will alter the force of contraction. One important way in which this chain of events may be triggered is via a

313

rise of intracellular Na^+ ($[Na^+]_i$). Because $[Na^+]_i$ is normally quite low (about 10 mM [4]), a rise of only a few millimolar units will result in a large change in the transmembrane Na gradient, and this will produce significant changes in $[Ca^{2+}]_i$. Therefore, mechanisms that influence intracellular Na will be important for controlling $[Ca^{2+}]_i$ and hence contraction in the heart.

With the development of ion-selective microelectrodes, it has become possible to measure directly the intracellular Na activity, a^i_{Na}, of cardiac cells [4]. More recently, it has proved possible to measure a^i_{Na} in beating preparations [5–8]. We can therefore examine the sensitivity of contraction in heart to changes in a^i_{Na}. In this chapter, we examine the effects on contraction of a rise of intracellular Na produced by inhibiting the Na/K pump. This is of interest not only because of the effects on contraction, but also because it probably reproduces the toxic and possibly the therapeutic effects of cardiac glycosides [9]. The experiments indicate that contraction is extremely sensitive to small changes in a^i_{Na}. We consider some of the reasons for this and, in particular, the possible role played by Na–Ca exchange. To do this, we look at the influence of intracellular Na on tonic as well as twitch tension. Finally, we examine the influence of intracellular Na on intracellular pH. Acid is known to depress concentration [10], and this effect seems to be independent of any change in $[Ca^{2+}]_i$ [11]. Therefore, because of the important influence of pH on contraction, we investigate one of the mechanisms responsible for linking Na and pH in heart.

METHODS

In the work discussed herein, a^i_{Na} and pH_i have been measured in isolated sheep cardiac Purkinje fibers. The measurements were made with recessed-tip, glass, ion-selective microelectrodes [12]. The Purkinje fiber was shortened to less than 2 mm so that it could also be voltage-clamped using a two-microelectrode technique. One end of the fiber was pinned to the bottom of the experimental chamber, while the other end was connected to a piezoresistive tension transducer so that tonic and twitch tension could be recorded (see Figure 1 and Eisner et al. [7] for details). All measurements of intracellular Na have been expressed in terms of activities (a^i_{Na}) rather than concentration ($[Na^+]_i$). The electrodes were calibrated in solutions of various $[Na^+]$, and an activity coefficient of 0.75 for Na^+ was assumed [7].

Purkinje fibers have been used in this work because (1) they can be voltage-clamped reasonably easily and (2) their contractions are fairly weak, so that they do not usually dislodge the intracellular microelectrodes. One can therefore measure contraction and one or more intracellular ion levels simultaneously under voltage-clamp conditions. One should bear in mind that similar experiments have not yet been achieved in other cardiac tissues, largely because of the immense technical problems involved. Therefore, we only tentatively extrapolate results obtained in Purkinje fibers to cardiac

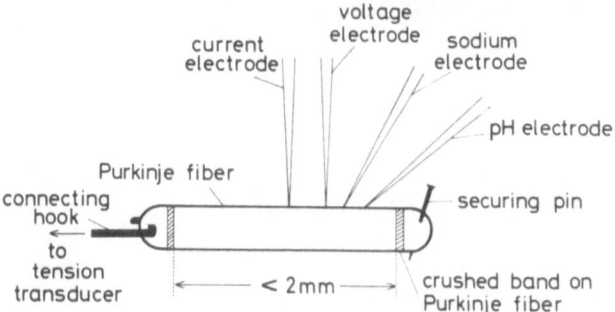

Figure 1.   Diagram illustrating placement of microelectrodes and position of tension transducer. The current-passing electrode was inserted in the center of the preparation; the other electrodes were inserted roughly in a line. The interelectrode spacing was 50–100 μm. An ion activity (pH$_i$ and a$^i_{Na}$ in this case) was measured as the signal of the relevant ion-selective microelectrode relative to that of the intracellular voltage electrode.

muscle in general. Nevertheless, there are already indications that much of the contractile behavior of Purkinje fibers is mimicked, at least qualitatively, by other mammalian cardiac tissues [13].

Solutions. The standard modified Tyrode's solution consisted of: 145 mM NaCl, 4 mM KCl, 2 mM CaCl$_2$, 1 mM MgCl$_2$, 10 mM Tris, and 10 mM glucose, pH 7.4, at 37°C. Modifications of this solution are described in the text. The solution was bubbled with 100% O$_2$ in some experiments and equilibrated with air in others; no differences were found between these two procedures.

RESULTS AND DISCUSSION

Relationship between Twitch Tension and Intracellular Na

Figure 2 shows the effects on contraction of raising the intracellular Na activity, a$^i_{Na}$. This was done by inhibiting the Na/K pump in a K-free, Rb-free solution (see the Figure 2 caption for details). The resulting rise of a$^i_{Na}$ was accompanied by an increase of twitch tension and the development of a tonic contracture. The Na pump was then reactivated by adding back 4 mM Rb to the bathing solution. An elevated a$^i_{Na}$ stimulates the Na/K pump [4,7] so that in Figure 2, the excess Na was rapidly expelled from the cell, resulting in a fall of a$^i_{Na}$. This fall was accompanied by a fall of both twitch and tonic tension. Of incidental interest in Figure 2 is the upper trace, which shows current at the holding potential of −68 mV. On stimulation of the Na/K pump, there was an overshoot of outward current that relaxed along with the fall of a$^i_{Na}$. This outward current is the electrogenic current generated by the Na/K pump [7,14,15].

The effects on tension of changing a$^i_{Na}$ are consistent with the idea that

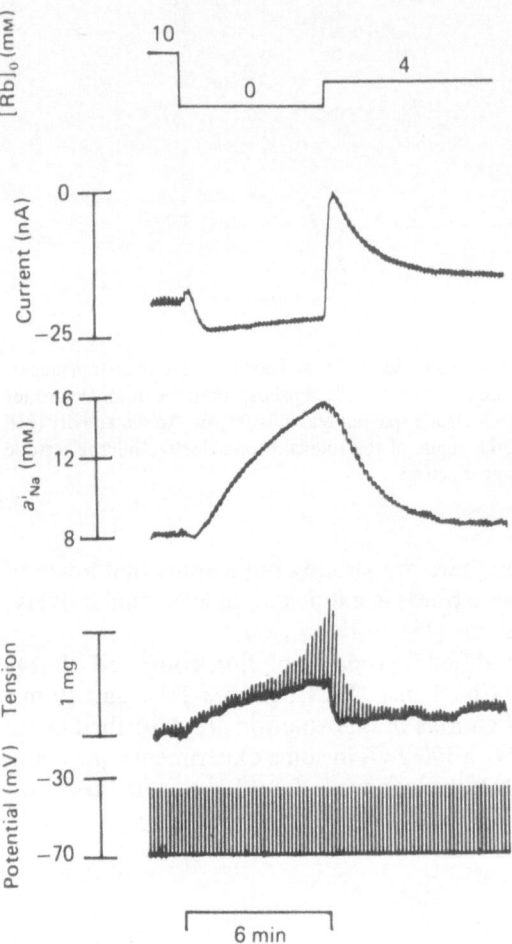

Figure 2.   The effects on tension of changing the intracellular Na activity (a_{Na}^i). Traces show (from top to bottom): membrane current, a_{Na}^i, tension, and voltage-clamped membrane potential. The bathing-solution protocol is shown at the top of the figure. A 500-msec depolarization to -34 mV was applied at 0.1 Hz from a holding potential of -68 mV. This evoked a twitch, seen here as a spike on the tension trace. All solutions were K-free and contained the concentration of Rb indicated. Removal of Rb_o inhibits the Na pump so that a_{Na}^i rises. Readmission of Rb_o reactivates the pump so that a_{Na}^i falls again. From Eisner et al. [7].

raising a_{Na}^i produces a rise of $[Ca^{2+}]_i$ via an Na–Ca exchange at the sarcolemma [2]. The elevated $[Ca^{2+}]_i$, if large enough, is then expressed as a tonic contracture and also as an increase in twitch tension, although in this latter case, the precise link between resting $[Ca^{2+}]_i$ and the magnitude of the twitch is not known.

It is of interest to determine the quantitative relationship between a_{Na}^i and twitch tension. Figure 3A shows an experiment in which a_{Na}^i was again raised by inhibiting the Na/K pump in a K-free, Rb-free solution. Sample records of tension and voltage obtained at a faster time scale and at different levels of a_{Na}^i are shown in Figure 3B. Evidently, raising a_{Na}^i has little effect on the time–course of the twitch, its main effect being to elevate peak tension. This is emphasized in Figure 3C, in which twitch tension is plotted vs. a_{Na}^i. It is clear that the relationship is highly nonlinear, and this is in contrast to a recent report [5] in which a linear relationship was found. We have never found a linear relationship unless measurements are made over a range of a_{Na}^i sufficiently small that the relationship may appear approximately linear. The striking feature of Figure 3C is that twitch tension is extremely sensitive to small rises of a_{Na}^i. At levels close to resting a_{Na}^i, tension can be described empirically as

$$\text{Tension} = K\,(a_{Na}^i)^n$$

where, at a given membrane potential, K is a constant and (in Figure 3C) $n = 7$. In other experiments, values of n closer to 3 or 4 are more commonly observed [16]. Such a relationship means that the sarcolemmal control of a_{Na}^i is extremely important in determining the contractile state of the tissue, since small changes in a_{Na}^i are amplified into large changes of twitch tension. Small changes in a_{Na}^i of approximately 1 mM can be produced by various physiological maneuvers such as an increase in the frequency of contraction [6,8]. While such changes in a_{Na}^i are small, the relationship displayed in Figure 3C indicates that they are likely to have significant effects on contraction.

As yet, we do not know the reason for the steep dependence of twitch tension on a_{Na}^i. Many processes that increase the phasic delivery of Ca^{2+} to the contractile proteins may be involved. In addition, tension may be a steep function of $[Ca^{2+}]_i$. However, sarcolemmal Na–Ca exchange will most likely play an important role, if only to provide the link between intracellular Na^+ and Ca^{2+}. This exchange helps to set resting $[Ca^{2+}]_i$, and an elevated $[Ca^{2+}]_i$ may increase the loading of Ca^{2+} into releasable intracellular stores such as the sarcoplasmic reticulum. An elevated resting $[Ca^{2+}]_i$ also appears to promote the voltage-gated Ca^{2+} influx that forms much of the slow inward current (I_{si}) [17,18], and this could further amplify the effects of an elevated a_{Na}^i. Finally, if Na–Ca exchange involves the movement of 2 or more Na ions per Ca ion (see later), this will also contribute to the observed steep relationship between tension and a_{Na}^i.

An additional property of Na–Ca exchange that may also influence tension is that it may be sensitive to membrane potential. Mullins and Requena [19] have presented evidence that Na–Ca exchange in the squid giant axon can produce a net Ca influx on depolarization. One explanation of such behavior is that the Na–Ca exchange is electrogenic. If the exchange moves 3–4 Na ions per Ca ion, net positive charge will accompany the movement of Na ion through the system. Furthermore, if the exchange is at equilibrium somewhere between systolic and diastolic potentials, then a sufficiently large depolarization will favor the outward movement of the exchanger's net positive charge and hence will promote a net influx of Ca^{2+} in exchange for the efflux of Na^+. Conversely, a hyperpolarization will favor ion movements in the opposite direction. Consequently, the exchange may provide another source of Ca^{2+} entry during the course of an action potential, and this Ca^{2+} may contribute directly to twitch contraction. Such an idea is still contro-

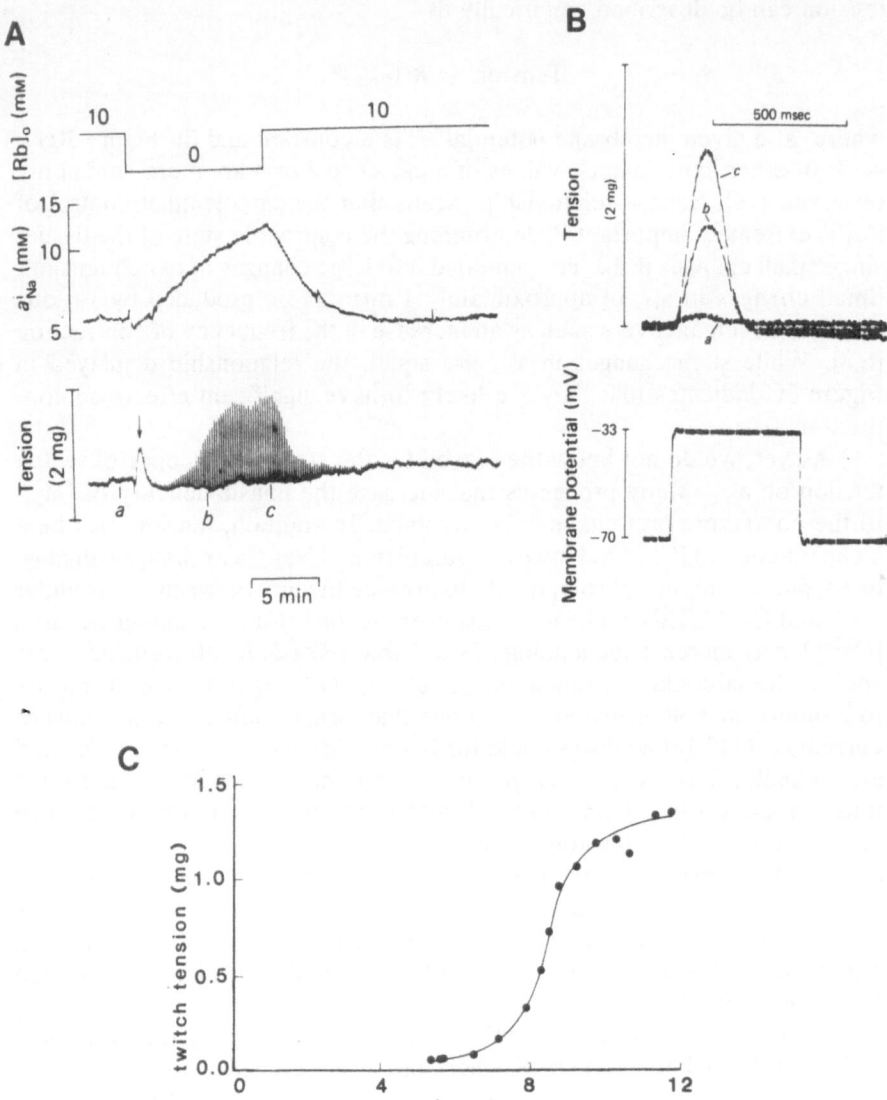

Figure 3.   Relationship between tension and a^i_{Na}. (A) Time–course of the effects of inhibiting and then reactivating the Na/K pump. Traces show a^i_{Na} (*top*) and tension (*bottom*). All solutions were K-free and contained the concentration of Rb indicated at the top of the figure. A 500-msec depolarization was applied to -33 mV from a holding potential of -70 mV at 0.1 Hz.

versial, and as we shall see, it is a moot point whether the kinetics of Na–Ca exchange are fast enough to permit the translocation of sufficient amounts of Ca^{2+} to influence twitch tension significantly. Nevertheless, as described in the next section, there is evidence that tonic tension is influenced by a^i_{Na} and membrane potential in a manner consistent with a voltage-sensitive Na–Ca exchange. Therefore, the system may exist, although its possible direct contribution to twitch tension remains to be established.

Dependence of Tonic Tension on a^i_{Na} and Membrane Potential

Evidence for the voltage sensitivity of Na–Ca exchange in intact cardiac muscle has come from studies of tonic tension [20–22]. Tonic tension is of interest, since it can give information about the control of the resting level of $[Ca^{2+}]_i$, although the effects of other factors, such as changes in pH_i, must also be considered. We have seen already that tonic tension and presumably $[Ca^{2+}]_i$ can be elevated by a rise of a^i_{Na} (Figure 2). This is consistent with the rise of a^i_{Na} producing a rise of $[Ca^{2+}]_i$ via Na–Ca exchange. However, the ability of a^i_{Na} to produce a tonic contracture also depends on the membrane potential. This is illustrated in Figure 4. In this experiment, a rise of a^i_{Na} is produced by inhibiting the Na/K pump by exposure to a K-free, Rb-free solution (Figure 4A). Figure 4B demonstrates that depolarization in 10-mV steps produces initially no increment of tonic tension (i). However, as a^i_{Na} rises (ii–iv), similar depolarizations result in increasingly larger tonic contractures, an effect that can be reversed readily on reactivation of the Na/K pump, producing a fall in a^i_{Na}. This effect can be expressed another way by noting that a rise of a^i_{Na} produces only a small tonic contracture at −60 mV, whereas at more positive potentials, the contracture and presumably the elevation of $[Ca^{2+}]_i$ are much more pronounced. Thus, the ability to raise tonic tension and hence resting $[Ca^{2+}]_i$ appears to depend on (1) a sufficiently high level of a^i_{Na} and (2) a large enough depolarization. Indeed, at sufficiently negative potentials, raising a^i_{Na} produces *no* contracture [22].

The tonic contracture produced by depolarization is decreased by reducing the extracellular Ca^{2+} concentration, suggesting that it is caused by an influx of Ca [23]. Further evidence that the tonic contracture is produced by a Ca influx rather than, for example, a release of Ca from intracellular stores comes from the observation that it is not reduced in the presence of 10 mM caffeine [24], a drug that interferes with Ca metabolism of the sarcoplasmic reticulum. However, the experiment of Figure 5 suggests that this Ca influx must occur by some mechanism other than the conventional slow

---

The arrow indicates a transient disturbance of the tension transducer following the first solution change. (B) Superimposed records of twitch tension and membrane potential obtained from the experiment shown in (A), at various levels of a^i_{Na}. (a–c) Points indicated in (A). (C) Graph illustrating the dependence of twitch tension on a^i_{Na}. Data from (A) obtained as a^i_{Na} was increasing in K-free, Rb-free solution. From Eisner et al. [7].

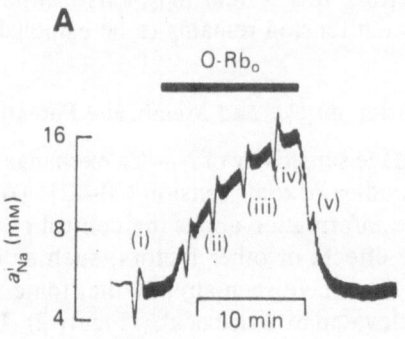

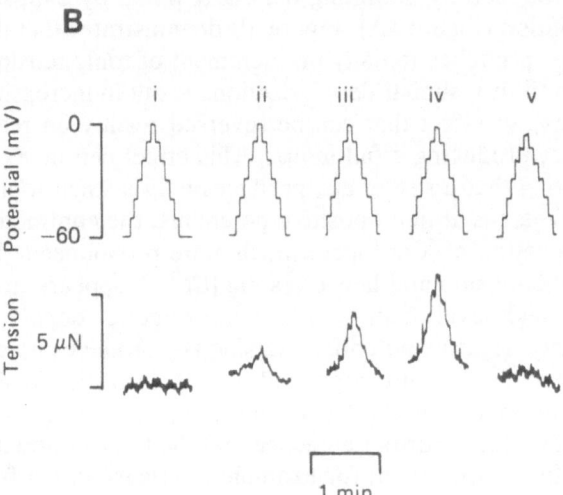

Figure 4.   Effects of membrane potential on the increase of tonic tension produced by an increase of a_{Na}^i. (A) Time–course of change of a_{Na}^i. [Rb]$_o$ was reduced from 4 to 0 mM for the period shown. The artifacts [(i)–(v)] indicate where the membrane potential was stepped to investigate tonic tension. (B) Specimen tension records. Traces show membrane potential (*top*) and tension (*bottom*). From Eisner et al. [22].

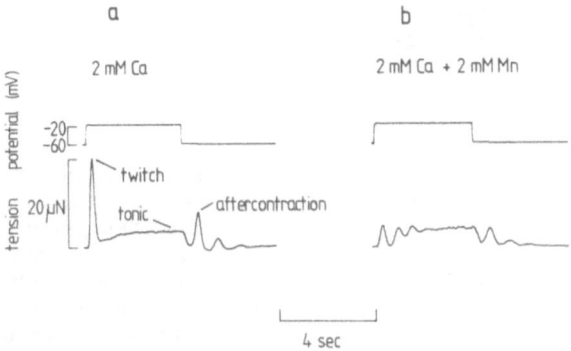

Figure 5.   Effects on twitch and tonic tension of inhibiting the slow inward calcium channel. Traces show membrane potential (*top*) and tension (*bottom*). In both panels, a 4-sec voltage-clamp pulse was applied from a holding potential of -60 to -20 mV at 0.1 Hz. The Na pump had been inhibited by exposure to a K-free, Rb-free solution. The records were obtained in the following solutions: (a) 2mM Ca; (b) 2mM Ca + 2 mM Mn.

inward Ca current (I_{si}). This experiment shows that Mn, which inhibits I_{si}, does not abolish tonic tension, although (as expected [25]) it does decrease the size of the twitch, which does presumably depend on I_{si}. Similar results were obtained with D600 (20 μM). Hence, we appear to have a voltage-sensitive, [a_{Na}^i]-sensitive Ca influx that does not occur through conventional, voltage-gated Ca channels. A possible explanation, therefore, is that it is mediated via a voltage-sensitive Na–Ca exchange. Consistent with this is the observation that tonic contractures cannot be evoked by depolarization in Na-free solutions even when external Ca is raised to 20 mM (Eisner, Lederer, and Vaughan-Jones, unpublished observations).

We can look more quantitatively at the effects of a_{Na}^i and membrane potential on tonic tension by referring to Figure 6A. This graph was obtained from an experiment in which the Na/K pump was inhibited with the cardiac glycoside strophanthidin (10^{-5} M) to increase a_{Na}^i. As a_{Na}^i was rising, the membrane potential was depolarized from a holding potential of -64 mV to any one of five different potentials. When tonic tension had stabilized at the new potential (usually within 2 sec), the change in tonic tension was measured and the level of a_{Na}^i noted. This process was repeated so that measurements could be made at increasingly higher levels of a_{Na}^i. The procedure allowed plotting of the series of curves in Figure 6A, relating tonic tension to a_{Na}^i at five different membrane potentials. At all potentials, there is an equally steep dependence of tension on a_{Na}^i, which resembles the situation for twitch tension already described.

We can now compare the relative effectiveness on tonic tension of changes in a_{Na}^i and membrane potential. The method is outlined in the inset of Figure 6B. Briefly, if one refers to the -13-mV curve in Figure 6A, then at a given level of a_{Na}^i (y), a hyperpolarization to -34 mV (for example) will

A

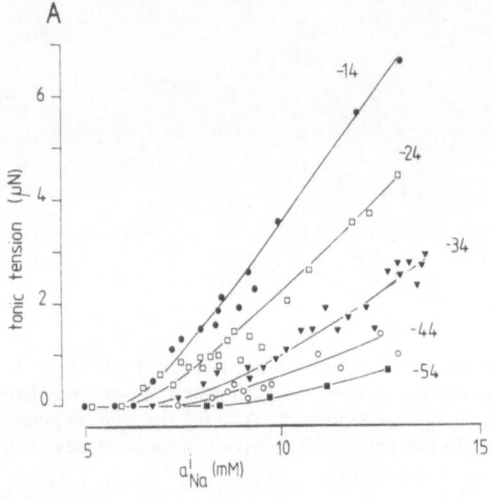

B

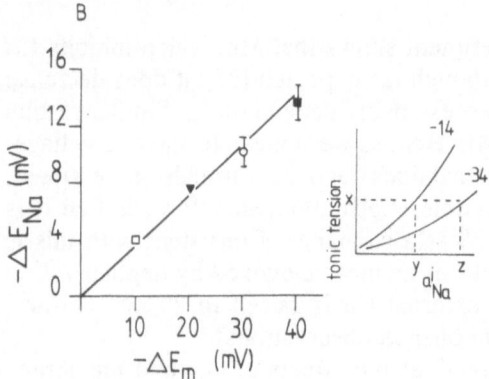

Figure 6. Relative effects of membrane potential and a^i_{Na} on tonic tension. (A) Dependence of tonic tension on a^i_{Na} at various membrane potentials. Tonic tension is plotted as a function of a^i_{Na} at the following membrane potentials: (●) −14 mV; (□) −24 mV; (▼) −34 mV; (○) −44 mV; (■) −54 mV. Tonic tension measurements were obtained at the end of a 2-sec depolarizing voltage-clamp pulse from a holding potential of −64 mV to the potential indicated. (B) Comparison of the effects of E_m and E_{Na} on tonic tension. Data taken from (A). The method used to obtain the graph is shown in the inset. All data are referred to the points measured at −14 mV. A hyperpolarization (ΔE_m) to another membrane potential would decrease tension. This can be compensated for by increasing a^i_{Na}, and the change of E_{Na} required (ΔE_{Na}) has been plotted as a function of ΔE_m. Several such comparisons have been made between the points measured for each pair of membrane potentials in (A), and these are shown in the main figure. Further details are given in the text. From Eisner et al. [22].

produce a relaxation of tonic tension. One can now move up the −34-mV curve and determine the level of a^i_{Na} (z) required to bring tonic tension back to its original control value. The change of a^i_{Na} can then be expressed as a change in E_{Na}, the Na equilibrium potential:

$$\Delta E_{Na} = RT/F \ln(y/z)$$

This, therefore, is the change in E_{Na} required to offset the effects on tension and presumably on $[Ca^{2+}]_i$ of a 20-mV hyperpolarization. The calculation has been repeated for different levels of a^i_{Na} and for different hyperpolarizations, and the results are plotted in Figure 6B. We see that to keep tonic tension constant, a change of membrane potential must always be compensated for by a much smaller change in E_{Na}.

It is interesting to note that such behavior can be accounted for quite easily in terms of an Na–Ca exchange model that is at equilibrium. If n Na ions are transported per Ca ion, then one can obtain the equilibrium condition [26]:

$$2(E_m - E_{Ca}) = n(E_m - E_{Na})$$

where all the symbols have their usual meaning. Rearranging, we obtain

$$2E_{Ca} = nE_{Na} - (n - 2)E_m$$

Hence, we see that to maintain a constant E_{Ca} and hence a constant tonic tension, a change of membrane potential, E_m, must be offset by a change of E_{Na} equal to $[(n - 2)/n]E_m$. The slope of the line in Figure 6B relating ΔE_{Na} and ΔE_m is 0.37, which gives a value of 3.2 for n. Hence, the behavior of tonic tension in the Purkinje fiber is consistent with an Na–Ca exchange at equilibrium with a stoichiometry of about 3 Na : 1 Ca. This agrees with the conclusions of other work on Na–Ca exchange in heart using a variety of techniques [27–30]. However, it should be stressed that the exchange may not be at equilibrium under the conditions of our experiments [22]. In addition, the possible changes of pH$_i$ described in the next section may distort the relationship between tension and a_{Na}^i, especially at high levels of $[Ca^{2+}]_i$. Finally, it has been shown recently that resting $[Ca^{2+}]_i$ is not always stable; it can oscillate, most notably at high $[Ca^{2+}]_i$ [31,32]. This phenomenon may be caused by the presence of intracellular stores that, at a high $[Ca^{2+}]_i$, sequester and release Ca^{2+} phasically. As a result, $[Ca^{2+}]_i$ can never be strictly at equilibrium with a given a_{Na}^i and membrane potential. All these problems could lead to an erroneous estimate of the coupling ratio for Na–Ca exchange when determined by the aforediscussed method. Nevertheless, it is worth reemphasizing that the Na and voltage dependence of tonic tension observed in this work cannot easily be accounted for in other ways, unless the Na dependence of tension resides in an electroneutral Na–Ca exchange and the voltage-dependence in an, as yet undiscovered, D600- and Mn-insensitive, voltage-gated Ca channel.

If Na–Ca exchange is indeed influenced by membrane potential, then one must now ask: (1) Does it reverse during the course of an action potential? (2) Is the Ca influx sufficient to influence the twitch? Unfortunately, both questions must remain unanswered. The first question is perhaps less important, since if Na–Ca exchange always mediates a net Ca efflux, then a depolarization will reduce this efflux, so that even if there is no net reversal, the reduction of Ca efflux will allow other mechanisms to raise $[Ca^{2+}]_i$. The second question is more of a problem. Reference to Figure 5A may provide a clue. We see here that the tonic contracture produced by depolarization is rising long after the spontaneous relaxation of the twitch. If the time-course of development of tonic tension represents the rate of delivery of

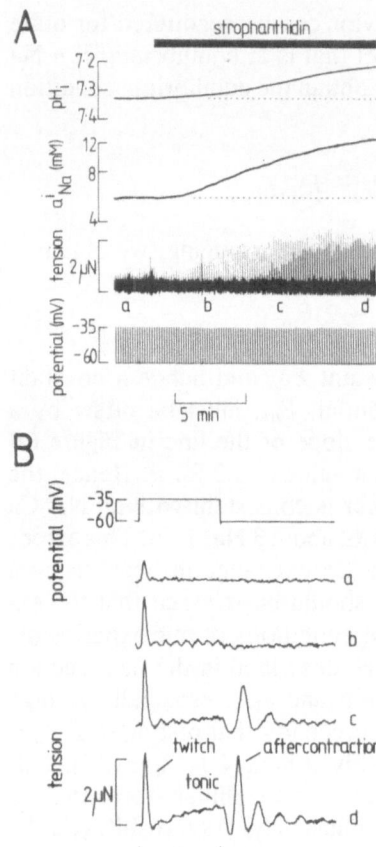

Figure 7. Effects of Na pump inhibition on pH_i, a^i_{Na}, and tension. (A) Time–course of the onset of effects. Traces show (top to bottom): pH_i, a^i_{Na}, tension, and membrane potential. Strophanthidin (10 μM) was applied for the period shown. Throughout the experiment, the membrane potential was held at -60 mV and depolarizing steps of 2-sec duration were applied to -35 mV at 0.1 Hz to elicit contractions. The tension trace has been high-pass-filtered (time constant 10 sec) to remove D.C. changes of tension and therefore only allows accurate resolution of the twitch. (B) Specimen tension records of contraction produced by the voltage-clamp pulse shown at the top of the record. These records have not been filtered. The records were obtained at the points [(a)–(d)] shown on (A). From Vaughan-Jones, et al. [38].

Ca^{2+} by a voltage-sensitive Na–Ca exchange, it would appear that the system is simply too slow to contribute directly to twitch tension. On the other hand, it will clearly contribute to the resting $[Ca^{2+}]_i$, which is established at the end of the plateau phase of an action potential. Consequently, the exchange might be expected to influence the degree of loading of releasable intracellular Ca stores if these rely for their Ca on cytoplasmic $[Ca^{2+}]_i$. The indirect influence of such a mechanism on contraction would then depend partly on the level of a^i_{Na} and partly on the electrical behavior of the tissue.

Influence of Intracellular Na on Intracellular pH

Raising a^i_{Na} alters not only $[Ca^{2+}]_i$ but also pH_i. This is shown in Figure 7A, in which pH_i was measured in addition to a^i_{Na} and tension while the Na/K pump was inhibited by adding 10^{-5} M strophanthidin. The rise in a^i_{Na} and the positive inotropy (Figure 7B) were accompanied by an intracellular acidification of about 0.15 pH unit. Two explanations have been proposed for this acidification [33]: (1) It is produced by the increase of a^i_{Na} acting on a

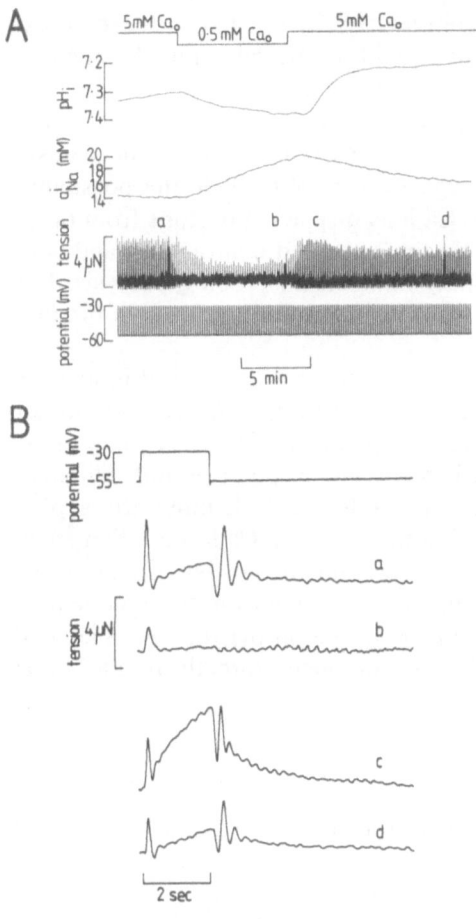

Figure 8.   Effects of changing the external Ca concentration ($[Ca^{2+}]_o$) on pH_i, a^i_{Na}, and tension. (A) Time-course of effects. Traces show (top to bottom): pH_i, a^i_{Na}, tension, and membrane potential. The fiber had been exposed to a K-free, Rb-free solution for 20 min to inhibit the Na pump before this record was obtained. As shown above the record, $[Ca^{2+}]_o$ was changed from 5 to 0.5 and then back to 5 mM. Throughout the experiment, the membrane potential was held at -55 mV and 2-sec voltage-clamp pulses were applied at 0.1 Hz. The tension trace was filtered as in Figure 7A. (B) Specimen records of contraction produced by the depolarizing voltage-clamp pulse shown at the top. From Vaughan-Jones, et al. [38].

sarcolemmal Na–H exchange. (2) It results from the rise of $[Ca^{2+}]_i$ displacing protons from common intracellular sites [cf. 34]. These possibilities were distinguished by the experiment of Figure 8. In this experiment, the Na–K pump was again inhibited so that a^i_{Na} had risen and pH_i was decreasing. A reduction of external Ca from 5 to 0.5 mM decreased all components of tension (cf. Figures 8A and B), indicating a fall in $[Ca^{2+}]_i$. This was accompanied by an intracellular alkalinization. Raising external Ca reversed these effects; i.e., $[Ca^{2+}]_i$ increased, as evidenced by the increase in tension, and pH_i became acid. It is now accepted that the main influence of external Ca on $[Ca^{2+}]_i$ under these conditions (i.e., at a high intracellular Na) is mediated via Na–Ca exchange [35,36]. Hence, raising external Ca leads to a Ca influx in exchange for the efflux of Na, which therefore reduces a^i_{Na}. The fact that this fall of a^i_{Na} is accompanied by an acidification rules out a major role for Na–H exchange, since a fall of a^i_{Na} would act on Na–H exchange to produce an alkalinization. On the other hand, the acidification is still consistent with a Ca–H interaction. Such Ca–H interaction in the control of pH_i in heart has been suggested previously [33,37], but in these cases, the possible effects of Na–H exchange could not be ruled out. Meech and Thomas [34] have also demonstrated that Ca injection into snail neurons produces an acidification. In their experiments, the site of Ca–H interaction appeared to be mostly at the mitochondrial membrane. A similar mechanism may be operating in the heart, although we cannot exclude the possibility that the acidification is produced by Ca ions displacing protons from other intracellular buffer sites. Alternatively the increased contractility and consequent increase of ATP hydrolysis may stimulate anaerobic glycolysis. The acidosis would then result from the consequent increase of lactate production.

These results therefore show that Na–Ca exchange in heart influences not only $[Ca^{2+}]_i$ but also (via changes of $[Ca^{2+}]_i$) pH_i. As yet, we do not know the extent to which the exchange helps to set pH_i under more physiological conditions, in particular when the Na–K pump is not inhibited. Under these conditions, we find that external Ca has little influence on pH_i, although this may simply reflect the fact that external Ca has a rather small effect on $[Ca^{2+}]_i$ when a^i_{Na} is low [38]. The influence of Na–Ca exchange on pH_i means that pH_i becomes indirectly dependent on Na. One should therefore be careful not to confuse effects of Na on pH that are mediated indirectly by Na–Ca exchange with those produced directly by an Na–H exchange mechanism.

Effects of Intracellular pH on Tension

The Na-dependent changes of pH described above may have significant effects on contraction. It has been known since the work of Gaskell [10] that acid depresses contraction. Much, if not all, of this influence seems to be mediated via changes of intracellular rather than extracellular pH [39]. The experiment shown in Figure 9 investigates the sensitivity of contraction in the Purkinje fiber to changes in pH_i induced at a constant external pH (pH_o). This was achieved by using external NH_4Cl. This raises pH_i because the molecular NH_3 that exists at a pH_o of 7.4 crosses the sarcolemma very rapidly. Once inside the cell, it takes up H^+ ions to form NH_4^+, so that pH_i becomes rapidly alkaline. Removal of external NH_4Cl reverses this situation, and if exposure to NH_4Cl has been sufficiently prolonged, there will also be a transient intracellular acidification as all the intracellular NH_4^+ leaves the cell as NH_3. We can now look at the effects of this maneuver on contraction. The changes of pH_i are mirrored by changes of contraction: alkalinization increases tension. Figure 10 shows the results of an experiment similar to that shown in Figure 9. Here, the exposure to NH_4Cl was more prolonged, so that the acidification following NH_4Cl removal was more pronounced. Hence, a wider excursion in pH_i could be examined. An acidification of 0.2 pH unit from a resting pH_i of about 7.0 approximately halved contraction, whereas a similar alkalinization doubled contraction. These effects of pH

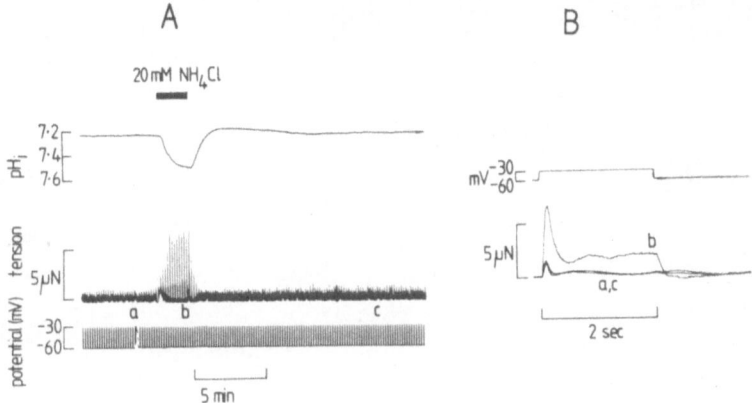

Figure 9.   Effects of changes of pH_i on contraction. (A) Time–course of the effects of adding 20 mM NH_4Cl for the period shown. Traces show (top to bottom): pH_i, tension, and membrane potential. The membrane potential was held at -60 mV and 2-sec voltage-clamp pulses were applied to -30 mV at 0.1 Hz. The tension trace has been filtered (cf. Figure 7). (B) Specimen tension records produced by the depolarizing voltage-clamp pulse shown above at the points indicated on (A). From Eisner et al. [41].

are similar in magnitude to the effects found by Fabiato and Fabiato [40] for skinned cardiac fibers. Nevertheless, it is clear that pH_i exerts a large influence on contraction. This has been interpreted as an inhibitory effect of protons on the contractile apparatus [40]. Consistent with this is the finding that brief changes of pH_i do not alter the phasic changes of $[Ca^{2+}]_i$ associated with the twitch in papillary muscle, even though contraction itself is modified [11].

Since a change of a_{Na}^i can lead to a change of *both* $[Ca^{2+}]_i$ *and* pH_i, both of these will affect contraction. We can write the sequence of ionic changes as

$$\downarrow \text{Na–K pumping} \rightarrow \uparrow [Na^+]_i \xrightarrow{\text{Na–Ca exchange}} \uparrow [Ca^{2+}]_i \xrightarrow{\text{Ca–H interaction}} \downarrow pH_i$$

$$\qquad\qquad\qquad\qquad\qquad\qquad\quad \downarrow \qquad\qquad\qquad\qquad\quad \downarrow$$

$$\qquad\qquad\qquad\qquad\qquad\qquad +\text{ve inotropy} \qquad -\text{ve inotropy}$$

An important consequence of this is that the positive inotropic effect of a rise in a_{Na}^i will be attenuated if pH_i also becomes more acid. In other words, the observed steep dependence of both twitch and tonic tension on a_{Na}^i (see Figures 3C and 6A) would be even steeper if pH_i did not decrease as a_{Na}^i increased. This emphasizes further the powerful influence of a_{Na}^i on contraction. The effects of a change of a_{Na}^i on contraction are therefore the sum of the relative effects on $[Ca^{2+}]_i$ and pH_i, and it is this sum that de-

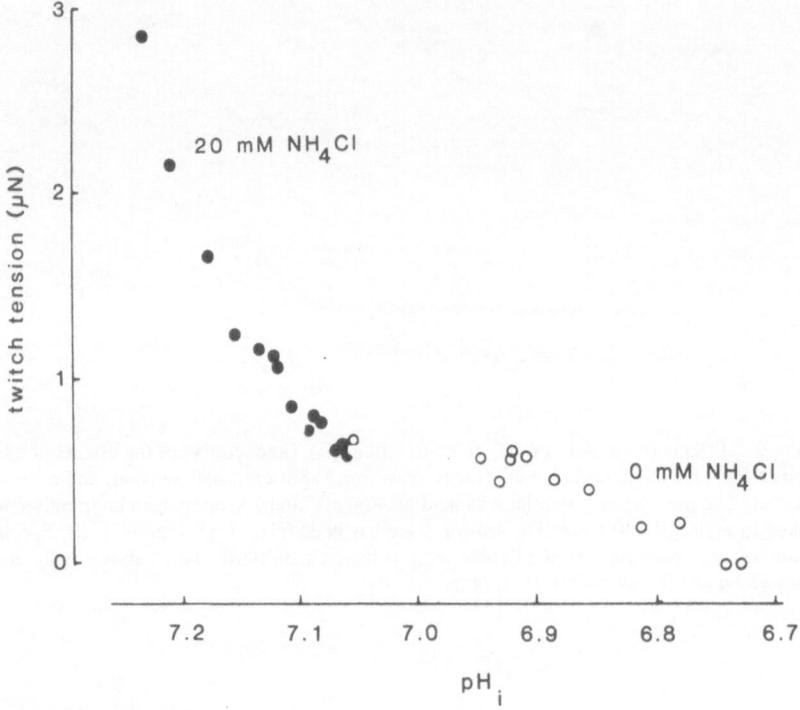

Figure 10.   Dependence of twitch tension on pH_i. The pH_i was changed by first adding (to alkalinize) and then removing (to acidify) 20 mM NH_4Cl. Tension was produced by a 2-sec voltage-clamp pulse to -30 mV from a holding potential of -60 mV. Symbols show points obtained in 20 mM NH_4Cl (●) or during the removal of NH_4Cl (O).

termines whether one observes finally either a positive or a negative inotropy.

ACKNOWLEDGMENTS

The work described in this chapter was supported by the British Heart Foundation, the MRC, and the Wellcome Trust (D.A.E.); the March of Dimes Birth Defects Foundation, the NIH (HL-25675), and the American Heart Association and its Maryland Affiliate (W.J.L.); and the MRC (R.D.V.-J.).

REFERENCES

1. Ringer, S. 1883. A further contribution regarding the influence of the different constituents of the blood on the contraction of the heart. *J. Physiol.* 4:29–42.
2. Baker, P. F., Blaustein, M. P., Hodgkin, A. L., and Steinhardt, R. A. 1969. The influence of calcium on sodium efflux in squid axons. *J. Physiol.* 200:431–458.

3. Glitsch, H. G., Reuter, H., and Scholz, H. 1970. The effect of the internal sodium concentration on calcium fluxes in isolated guinea-pig auricles. *J. Physiol.* 204:25–43.

4. Ellis, D. 1977. The effects of external cations and ouabain on the intracellular sodium activity of sheep heart Purkinje fibres. *J. Physiol.* 273:211–240.

5. Lee, C. O., Kang, D. H., Sokol, J. H., and Lee, K. S. 1980. Relation between intracellular Na ion activity and tension of sheep cardiac Purkinje fibers exposed to dihydro-ouabain. *Biophys. J.* 29:315–330.

6. Cohen, C. J., Fozzard, H. A., and Sheu, S.-S. 1982. Increase in intracellular sodium ion activity during stimulation in mammalian cardiac muscle. *Circ. Res.* 50:651–662.

7. Eisner, D. A., Lederer, W. J., and Vaughan-Jones, R. D. 1981. The dependence of sodium pumping and tension on intracellular sodium activity in voltage-clamped sheep cardiac Purkinje fibres. *J. Physiol.* 317:163–187.

8. Lederer, W. J., and Sheu, S.-S. 1983. Heart-rate dependent changes in intracellular sodium activity and twitch tension in sheep cardiac Purkinje fibres. *J. Physiol.* 345:44P.

9. Noble, D. 1980. Mechanism of action of therapeutic levels of cardiac glycosides. *Cardiovasc. Res.* 14:495–514.

10. Gaskell, W. H. 1880. On the tonicity of the heart and blood vessels. *J. Physiol.* 3:48–75.

11. Allen, D. G., and Orchard, C. H. 1983. The effect of changes of pH on intracellular calcium transients in mammalian cardiac muscle. *J. Physiol.* 335:555–567.

12. Thomas, R. C. 1978. *Ion-sensitive Micro-electrodes.* Academic Press, New York and London.

13. Karagueuzian, H. S., and Katzung, B. G. 1982. Voltage-clamp studies of transient inward current and mechanical oscillations induced by ouabain in ferret papillary muscle. *J. Physiol.* 327:255–271.

14. Eisner, D. A., and Lederer, W. J. 1980. Characterization of the electrogenic sodium pump in cardiac Purkinje fibres. *J. Physiol.* 303:441–474.

15. Gadsby, D. C., and Cranefield, P. F. 1979. Direct measurement of changes in sodium pump current in canine cardiac Purkinje fibres. *Proc. Natl. Acad. Sci. U.S.A.* 76:1783–1787.

16. Eisner, D. A., Lederer, W. J., and Vaughan-Jones, R. D. 1983. The relationship between twitch tension and intracellular Na activity in sheep cardiac Purkinje fibres. *J. Physiol.* 341:28–29P.

17. Marban, E., and Tsien, R. W. 1982. Enhancement of cardiac calcium current during digitalis inotropy: Positive feedback regulation by intracellular calcium? *J. Physiol.* 329:589–614.

18. Lederer, W. J., and Eisner, D. A. 1982. The effects of sodium pump activity on the slow inward current in sheep cardiac Purkinje fibres. *Proc. R. Soc. Lond.* 214:249–262.

19. Mullins, L. J., and Requena, J. 1981. The "late" Ca channel in squid axons. *J. Gen. Physiol.* 78:683–700.

20. Horackova, M., and Vassort, G. 1979. Sodium–calcium exchange in regulation of cardiac contractility: Evidence for an electrogenic, voltage-dependent mechanism. *J. Gen. Phsyiol.* 73:403–424.

21. Chapman, R. A., and Tunstall, J. 1980. The interaction of sodium and calcium ions at the cell membrane and the control of contractile strength in frog atrial muscle. *J. Physiol.* 305:109–123.

22. Eisner, D. A., Lederer, W. J., and Vaughan-Jones, R. D. 1983. The control of tonic tension by membrane potential and intracellular Na activity in the sheep cardiac Purkinje fibre. *J. Physiol.* 335:723–743.

23. Eisner, D. A., and Lederer, W. J. 1979. Inotropic and arrhythmogenic effects of potassium depleted solutions on mammalian cardiac muscle. *J. Physiol.* 294:255–277.

24. Eisner, D. A., and Lederer, W. J. 1982. Effects of caffeine on the transient inward current in cardiac Purkinje fibres. *J. Physiol.* 322:48–49P.

25. Leoty, C., and Raymond, G. 1972. Mechanical activity and ionic currents in frog atrial trabeculae. *Pfluegers Arch.* 334:114–128.

26. Blaustein, M. P., and Hodgkin, A. L. 1969. The effect of cyanide on the efflux of calcium from squid axons. *J. Physiol.* 200:497–528.

27. Sheu, S-S., and Fozzard, H. A. 1982. Transmembrane Na^+ and Ca^{2+} electrochemical gradients in cardiac muscle and their relationship to force development. *J. Gen. Physiol.* 80:325–351.
28. Pitts, B. J. R. 1979. Stoichiometry of sodium-calcium exchange in cardiac sarcolemmal vesicles. *J. Biol. Chem.* 254:6232–6235.
29. Reeves, J. P., and Sutko, J. L. 1979. Sodium-calcium ion exchange in cardiac sarcolemmal vesicles. *Proc. Natl. Acad. Sci. U.S.A.* 76:590–594.
30. Philipson, K. D., and Nishimoto, A. Y. 1980. Na^+-Ca^{2+} exchange is affected by membrane potential in cardiac sarcolemmal vesicles. *J. Biol. Chem.* 255:6880–6882.
31. Orchard, C. H., Eisner, D. A., and Allen, D. G. 1983. Oscillations of intracellular Ca^{2+} in mammalian cardiac muscle. *Nature* 304:735–738.
32. Wier, W. G., Kort, A. A., Stern, M. D., Lakatta, E. G., and Marban E. 1983. Cellular calcium fluctuations in mammalian heart: Direct evidence from noise analysis of aequorin signals in Purkinje fibers. *Proc. Natl. Acad. Sci. U.S.A.* 80:7361–7371.
33. Deitmer, J. W., and Ellis, D. 1980. Interactions between the regulation of the intracellular pH and sodium activity of sheep cardiac Purkinje fibres. *J. Physiol.* 304:471–488.
34. Meech, R. W., and Thomas, R. C. 1980. Effect of measured calcium chloride injections on the membrane potential and internal pH of snail neurones. *J. Physiol.* 298:111–129.
35. Deitmer, J. W., and Ellis, D. 1978. Changes in the intracellular sodium activity of sheep heart Purkinje fibres produced by calcium and other divalent cations. *J. Physiol.* 277:437–453.
36. Eisner, D. A., Orchard, C. H., and Allen, D. G. 1984. Control of intracellular ionized calcium concentration by sarcolemmal and intracellular mechanisms. *J. Mol. Cell. Cardiol.* 16:137–146.
37. Bers, D. M., and Ellis, D. 1982. Intracellular calcium and sodium activity in sheep heart Purkinje fibres: Effects of changes of external sodium and intracellular pH. *Pfluegers Arch.* 393:171–178.
38. Vaughan-Jones, R. D., Lederer, W. J., and Eisner, D. A. 1983. Ca^{2+} ions can affect intracellular pH in mammalian cardiac muscle. *Nature* 301:522–524.
39. Poole-Wilson, P. A. 1978. Measurement of myocardial intracellular pH in pathological states. *J. Mol. Cell. Cardiol.* 10:511–526.
40. Fabiato, A., and Fabiato, F. 1978. Effects of pH on the myofilaments and the sarcoplasmic reticulum of skinned cells from cardiac and skeletal muscles. *J. Physiol.* 276:233–255.
41. Eisner, D. A., Lederer, W. J., and Vaughan-Jones, R. D. 1983. The relationship between intracellular pH and contraction in sheep cardiac Purkinje fibres. *J. Physiol.* 334:106–107P.

INFLUENCE OF LIPIDS ON MEMBRANES

Interaction of Amphiphilic Molecules with Biological Membranes

A Model for Nonspecific and Specific Drug Effects with Membranes

L. Herbette

Departments of Medicine and Biochemistry
University of Connecticut Health Center
Farmington, Connecticut 06032

C. A. Napolitano, F. C. Messineo, and A. M. Katz

Department of Medicine
University of Connecticut Health Center
Farmington, Connecticut 06032

Abstract. The nonspecific interactions of propranolol, timolol, and ethanol with model and sarcoplasmic reticulum membranes were determined utilizing radioisotopic association, differential scanning calorimetry, and neutron diffraction. Differential scanning calorimetry performed on mixtures of these amphiphilic compounds and model membrane bilayers composed of dimyristoyllecithin showed that propranolol was approximately 25 times more lipid-soluble than timolol and at least 100 times more lipid-soluble than ethanol. Neutron diffraction showed that the solvation of propranolol was within the fatty acyl chain region of the lipid bilayer. This solvation correlated with the effect of propranolol to inhibit ATP-dependent calcium transport in isolated rabbit skeletal muscle sarcoplasmic reticulum, a membrane that lacks β-adrenergic receptors. In contrast, the major site of interaction of ethanol was within the aqueous compartment hydrating the sarcoplasmic reticulum membrane. A model for nonspecific drug interaction with the sarcoplasmic reticulum membrane based on the site of interaction of these amphiphiles and their relative potencies to inhibit calcium transport by these membranes is proposed. In principle, this model could be extended to specific drug interactions with membranes.

INTRODUCTION

Amphiphilic molecules can interact with either or both protein and lipid components of biological membranes [1–3]. The interactions of these amphiphiles with membrane lipids are complex and may be only partially dependent on the lipid solubility of the amphiphile [4,5]. To investigate the molecular basis for these interactions, we compared the lipid solubility of several amphiphiles with their ability to alter membrane structure in both model membranes (dimyristoyllecithin) and rabbit skeletal sarcoplasmic reticulum. This latter membrane was examined because it is devoid of specific

333

receptors for the compounds investigated. The effects of these amphiphiles to alter membrane structure were then correlated with their ability to inhibit calcium transport by the sarcoplasmic reticulum.

Ethanol and two β-adrenergic receptor blocking drugs, propranolol and timolol, were chosen for study because their partition coefficients for pure lipid–aqueous systems cover a broad range. Radioisotopic association, differential scanning calorimetry, and neutron diffraction were used to determine the sites of interaction of these compounds with model membranes and the sarcoplasmic reticulum. A model for the nonspecific membrane effects of these amphiphiles, based on their sites of interaction with the membrane systems, could be conceptually extended to include a possible mechanism for specific drug–membrane interaction.

METHODS

A "light" fraction of sarcoplasmic reticulum vesicles prepared from rabbit white skeletal muscle as previously described [6] was used in all experiments. Model membrane liposomes were prepared as previously described [7], amphiphilic drugs being comixed with dimyristoyllecithin prior to lipid-bilayer formation and used for radioisotope and calorimetric measurements.

Calcium Uptake Measurements

Calcium uptake velocity was measured either by dual-wavelength spectrophotometry (Johnson Research Foundation Multichannel Spectrophotometer) using the calcium indicator antipyralazo III (720, 790 nm) [8,9] or by a radioisotopic procedure [10]. Unless otherwise specified, reaction media contained 120 mM KCl, 40 mM histidine (pH 6.8, 25°C), 50 mM KH_2PO_4, 1 mM $MgCl_2$, 60 μM $CaCl_2$, 1 mM MgATP, 100 μM antipyralazo III, and 6 μg/ml sarcoplasmic reticulum. Recordings were calibrated by three serial additions of $CaCl_2$, and reactions were initiated by MgATP. The small baseline shift caused by MgATP addition was subtracted from all recordings.

Calorimetric Measurements

The thermotropic behavior of multilamellar dimyristoyllecithin (DML) in the presence and absence of drugs was observed in a high-sensitivity differential scanning calorimeter [11]. A scan rate of 0.5 K min^{-1} was used throughout, and scanning was from temperatures below the gel-to-liquid-crystalline-phase transition to temperatures above the transition. The temperature, T_m, of maximal excess heat capacity was taken as a measure of the transition temperature. The baseline for most of the calorimetric scans was readily established, because there was no permanent change in heat

capacity accompanying the transition. The transition enthalpy could therefore be evaluated by planimeter integration of the scan. Cooling and res-
canning of several of the samples showed that the transitions were fully
reversible.

Neutron Diffraction Methods

DML and propranolol in a ratio of 1.25:1 (mg/mg) was prepared in
chloroform as described [7] (20 mM Tris, pH 7.5) with propranolol deuterated
in the naphthalene moiety. Alternatively, DML was sonicated in a buffer
solution (20 mM, pH 7.5) of deuterated propranolol at 23°C and used to make
multilayers for diffraction. Control samples using fully protonated propranolol were prepared in an identical manner. These dispersions were centrifuged onto aluminum foil and glued to a glass slide [9]. The glass slide was
suspended over a saturated salt solution (66% relative humidity) and hydrated at different H_2O/D_2O ratios [12]. Sarcoplasmic reticulum membrane
multilayers prepared as previously described [9] were equilibrated with deuterated or protonated ethanol in the vapor phase for several hours following
partial dehydration at 88% relative humidity overnight.

Lamellar neutron diffraction data were collected at the high-flux beam
reactor using the Brookhaven low-angle diffractometer operating at 2.36 Å
[13]. The equipment design and detection system have been described previously [12]. For these experiments, the two-dimensional position-sensitive
counter had a spatial resolution of either 0.7 or 1.5 mm in the meridional
(horizontal) and 1.5 mm in the equatorial (vertical) direction. The specimen
geometry was similar to that previously described [12]. Lamellar diffraction
data ($0.019 \, A^{-1} < s < 0.057 \, A^{-1}$, where s is the reciprocal space coordinate)
were collected at or above the phase-transition temperature of DML at a
specimen-to-detector distance of 80–85 cm via ω-scans ($0° \leq \omega \leq 4.5°$; $\Delta\omega$
= 0.1°). For sarcoplasmic reticulum membranes, lamellar diffraction data
($0.004 < s < 0.028 \, A^{-1}$) were collected at 10°C at a specimen-to-detector
distance of 300 cm ($0° \leq \omega \leq 2.5°$; $\Delta\omega$ = 0.1°). Data reduction and analysis
were as described in a previous study [12,14].

Radioisotope Measurements of the Association of Amphiphilic Molecules with Membranes

The association of propranolol and timolol with DML and isolated sarcoplasmic reticulum membranes was quantified using ^{3}H-labeled propranolol
or timolol. The term "association" is used for radioisotope measurements,
since these studies provided no information regarding the localization of the
drug molecules in the membrane. Various concentrations of each drug were
added to model and sarcoplasmic reticulum membrane preparations, and the
samples were allowed to equilibrate at various temperatures between 0 and
45°C. Samples were centrifuged at 100,000 g in microcentrifuge tubes (400

μl) for 1 hr in a Beckman SW27 swinging-bucket rotor at the equilibration temperature. Aliquots (50 μl) of the supernatant were sampled before and after centrifugation and added to a Biofluor scintillation mixture, and ^{3}H radioactivity was determined. The pellets were cut from the centrifuge tubes and carefully blotted dry, added to Biofluor, and counted for radioactivity. The mixing of the drug and lipid prior to the formation of multilamellar lipid structures by vortexing was essential because the addition of drugs to preformed lipid dispersions consistently yielded lower drug–lipid association values that were a function of incubation time. The aforedescribed procedure in which drug and lipid were covortexed yielded association values that were independent of equilibration time.

Association of ethanol with the sarcoplasmic reticulum membrane was carried out using ^{14}C-labeled ethanol and hydrated oriented sarcoplasmic reticulum membrane multilayers, similar to those used for diffraction studies [9]. [^{14}C]Ethanol was allowed to equilibrate with the multilayer in the vapor phase, and the ^{14}C radioactivity present in these multilayers was then determined by scintillation counting.

Protein concentration was determined by the method of Lowry et al. [15]. Determination of inorganic phosphate by the method of Chen et al. [16] was used to estimate total phospholipid content. Drug association is expressed as moles drug per mole phospholipid throughout this chapter.

Materials

All reagents used were reagent-grade, and deionized water was glass-distilled prior to use. Unlabeled propranolol was purchased from Sigma Chemical Company (St. Louis, Missouri) and was used without further purification. [^{3}H]Propranolol (19.0 Ci/mmole) was obtained from New England Nuclear Corporation (Boston, Massachuetts), and ^{3}H$_2$O (0.1 Ci/mmol) was obtained from ICN (Irvine, California). Unlabeled timolol and [^{3}H]timolol (34.7 Ci/mmol) were gifts from Merck, Sharpe & Dohme (Rahway, New Jersey). DML was purchased from Calbiochem-Behring Company (San Diego, California). Deuterated propranolol and deuterated ethanol were obtained from Merck, Sharpe & Dohme (Canada). Protonated ethanol was distilled prior to use (95% ethanol).

RESULTS

Interaction of Propranolol with the Sarcoplasmic Reticulum Membrane

The interaction of propranolol with membranes was initially investigated by differential scanning calorimetry using the DML model lipid bilayer system. The decrease in phase-transition temperature of the lipid bilayer, T_m, was linearly related to the concentration of propranolol, C_p, and could be described by the equation

$$T_m = (23.96 \pm 0.10) - (1.64 \pm 0.08)C_p$$

This decrease in T_m was interpreted to reflect partitioning of drug into the fatty acyl chain structure of the lipid bilayer.

Inspection of the shapes of the differential scanning calorimetry curves suggests that ideal solutions are not formed in either the liquid crystal or the gel phase. Although this nonideality prohibits absolute quantification of the partitioning of the drugs between the aqueous and lipid phases, application of a simple Hill-type analysis [17] indicated that for propranolol in the DML system, the partition coefficient, defined as the ratio of the amount of drug solvated in the membrane lipids to the amount of drug in the aqueous medium, was approximately 90. Although this value is an approximation, it can be assumed that the true partition coefficient remains constant over the concentration ranges where the transition temperature varies linearly with drug concentration [7]. Therefore, the partition coefficient can be compared on a relative basis with values obtained for other drugs.

Neutron diffraction with propranolol deuterated in the naphthalene moiety was employed to define the location of this drug molecule in the DML lipid bilayer. The unit cell dimensions for DML bilayers with and without propranolol differed by less than 1 Å, suggesting that propranolol did not cause significant perturbation of the lipid-bilayer structure. Significant differences in the lamellar intensities were observed for DML lipid bilayers with protonated as compared to deuterated propranolol. This study was done at 23°C and repeated with similar results at 30°C, temperatures at which the DML bilayer was in the liquid crystalline state. A low-resolution study was sufficient to determine the average position of both the phospholipid headgroups and the naphthalene moiety of propranolol within the unit-cell profile structures. The fine-structure details of the hydrocarbon core of the DML lipid bilayer are not evident at this resolution (Figure 1). The neutron scattering difference profile function for deuterated (naphthalene moiety) vs. protonated propranolol calculated from the differences in lamellar intensities demonstrated average peak densities at ±9 Å about the center of the hydrocarbon core of the DML lipid bilayer (Figure 1). This value corresponds to the separation of the central maxima within the difference profile for deuterated vs. protonated propranolol given in Figure 1 (real-space approach). It has been shown that a reciprocal space approach in which the difference structure factors are model-refined can provide a more accurate determination of these peak locations [18]. This procedure showed that the peak densities attributable to the deuterated naphthalene moiety of propranolol were located 11 ± 1 Å from the center of the hydrocarbon core of the DML lipid bilayer. In separate experiments carried out on the same samples, H_2O–D_2O exchange was used to obtain the water-profile structure. This water-profile structure was used to define the hydrocarbon core of the DML lipid bilayer from which water was excluded. When the average peak densities for the naphthalene moiety of propranolol were

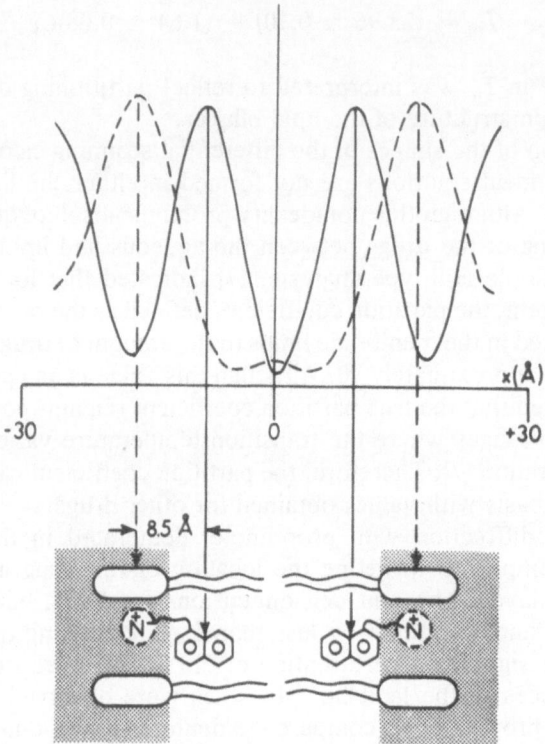

Figure 1.   Neutron scattering profiles for the propranolol–DML system at 23°C. (– – –) Scattering profile of DML with protonated propranolol in 100% H_2O, which provides the positions of the headgroups of the DML lipid bilayer; (——) neutron scattering difference profile for DML lipid bilayers with propranolol deuterated vs. protonated in the naphthalene moiety. The drawing shows the average location of the naphthalene moiety of propranolol (peak densities 11 ± 1 Å about the center of the DML hydrocarbon core) mapped directly along the profile axis of the DML lipid bilayer. The increase in density at the edges of the unit cell (±D/2) within this difference profile can be attributed to Fourier truncation artifacts, since the lamellar intensity function for deuterated propranolol contained a very weak third-order reflection relative to the corresponding lamellar intensity function for protonated propranolol.

mapped along the profile axis of the DML lipid bilayer, the naphthalene moiety of the propranolol molecule was found to be within the hydrocarbon core region of the DML lipid bilayer (Figure 2). This location of the naphthalene moiety would position the charged amine moiety of propranolol within the water layer that hydrates the phospholipid headgroups of the DML lipid bilayer (Figure 2). This result, which is consistent with the calorimetric and radioisotope measurements [7], supports the view that the lowering of the phase-transition temperature of DML was due to direct solvation of propranolol into the DML lipid bilayer.

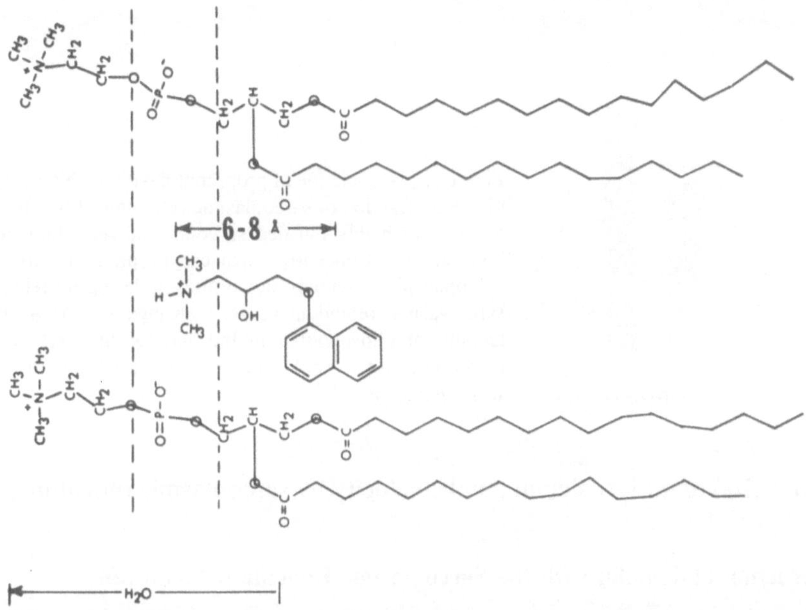

Figure 2. Location of the propranolol molecule within the DML lipid bilayer as determined by neutron diffraction. The distance between the center of the naphthalene moiety and the charged amine group is 6–8 Å.

These studies were extended to the sarcoplasmic reticulum membrane by measuring the association of propranolol with the sarcoplasmic reticulum membrane using ^{3}H-labeled propranolol. The molar association ratio, expressed as moles propranolol/mole total sarcoplasmic reticulum phospholipids, was compared in intact sarcoplasmic reticulum vesicles and extracted lipids from the sarcoplasmic reticulum membrane. Experiments with deproteinated highly purified sarcoplasmic reticulum lipids indicated that removal of protein significantly ($p < 0.001$) enhanced the association of the drug, raising the molar association ratio to a value similar to that observed with DML above its phase-transition temperature (Figure 3). This is not surprising, since X-ray diffraction data indicate that the purified sarcoplasmic reticulum lipids remain in the liquid crystalline state at temperatures as low as $-5°C$ [9,19].

The concentration dependence of the molar association ratio of propranolol for light sarcoplasmic reticulum membranes correlates with the concentration dependence of the inhibitory effects of this drug on calcium uptake [7]. Double-reciprocal plots of the association data provided estimates of the concentrations at which half-maximal association with the sarcoplasmic reticulum membrane occurred. The value of 0.88 mM for propranolol was similar to the propranolol concentration of 0.79 mM that caused 50% inhi-

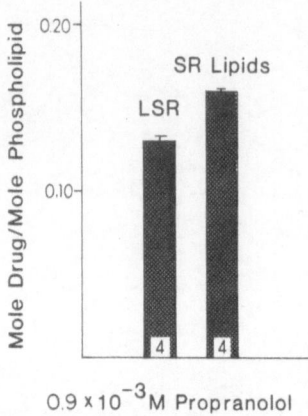

Figure 3.   Association of propranolol with the highly purified light fraction of sarcoplasmic reticulum (LSR) membranes and highly purified sarcoplasmic reticulum (SR) lipids at 10°C. Concentrations were: propranolol, 1.0 mm; sarcoplasmic reticulum membranes, 1.25 mg protein/ml; sarcoplasmic reticulum lipids, 0.88 mg/ml, n = 4. The amount of phospholipid in the sarcoplasmic reticulum membrane and sarcoplasmic reticulum lipid experiments was equivalent.

bition* (I_{50}) of initial calcium uptake velocity by sarcoplasmic reticulum [9].

Interaction of Timolol with the Sarcoplasmic Reticulum Membrane

Calorimetric measurements of the effects of timolol, another β-adrenergic blocking drug, on the DML model membrane system demonstrated that timolol was less potent than propranolol in lowering the phase-transition temperature. The concentration dependence of the ability of timolol to lower the phase-transition temperature is given by the equation

$$T_m = (23.40 \pm 0.11) - (0.07 \pm 0.01)C_T$$

Neglecting nonideality (as for propranolol), simple Hill analysis of these data yielded a partition coefficient of approximately 3–4 for timolol. Although the absolute value is subject to error, the relative ratio of these coefficients indicates that timolol is approximately 25 times less lipid-soluble than propranolol. Because of the present excessive cost to deuterate timolol, neutron diffraction experiments were not possible, so that a more precise location of this molecule in membranes could not be determined.

Studies with timolol were extended to the sarcoplasmic reticulum membrane using ^{3}H-labeled drug. The molar association ratio for extracted sarcoplasmic reticulum lipids was significantly ($p < 0.001$) higher than that of intact LSR, as shown in Figure 4. In accord with the data of the calorimetric studies, less timolol than propranolol is associated with the sarcoplasmic

---

* The I_{50} value is defined as the amphiphile concentration that results in 50% inhibition of calcium uptake velocity by the sarcoplasmic reticulum membrane relative to the total inhibition at saturating concentrations of these amphiphiles. Radioisotope methods for measuring calcium uptake velocity by sarcoplasmic reticulum are described by Messineo and Katz [3]. The spectrophotometric approach using calcium-sensitive metallochromic indicators is described in the Methods section, and these data are given in Table 1.

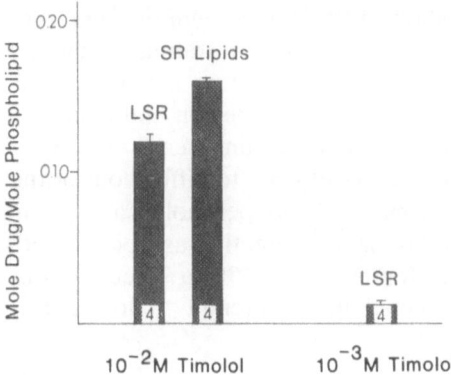

Figure 4. Association of timolol with the highly purified light fraction of sarcoplasmic reticulum (LSR) membranes and highly purified sarcoplasmic reticulum (SR) lipids at 10°C. Concentrations were: timolol, 10 mM; sarcoplasmic reticulum membrane, 1.25 mg protein/ml; sarcoplasmic reticulum lipids, 0.88 mg/ml, n = 4. The far-right-hand bar shows the molar association ratio for 1.0 mM timolol with sarcoplasmic reticulum to compare to the data in Figure 3.

reticulum membrane at equal drug concentrations (compare Figures 3 and 4). The concentration at which half-maximal association of timolol (36 mM) with the sarcoplasmic reticulum membrane occurs is significantly greater than the concentration required for half-maximal inhibition (see footnote, p. 340) of calcium transport (11 mM), suggesting that timolol has more than one site of interaction with the sarcoplasmic reticulum membrane.

Interactions of Ethanol with the Sarcoplasmic Reticulum Membrane

Previous calorimetric studies [20–22] have shown that the partitioning of ethanol between an aqueous buffer–lipid system favors the aqueous domain; i.e., partition coefficients are less than 1, unlike those of propranolol and timolol, which are significantly greater than 1. However, ethanol inhibited calcium transport by sarcoplasmic reticulum in a concentration-dependent manner. Over a concentration range of 0–0.85 M, ethanol-induced inhibition of calcium uptake by sarcoplasmic reticulum was correlated with increasing concentrations. The concentration of ethanol at which inhibition of calcium transport was half-maximal (see footnote, p. 340) is 80.5 mM, consistent with its low partition coefficient. At ethanol concentrations above 0.85 M, both stimulation and inhibition can occur and the dose–response curve is complex. To correlate the effects of ethanol on calcium transport with the possible site of ethanol interaction with the sarcoplasmic reticulum membrane, ^{14}C-labeled ethanol was allowed to equilibrate with hydrated oriented sarcoplasmic reticulum membrane multilayers under conditions similar to those used in neutron diffraction studies. Approximately 11 moles ethanol per mole Ca^{2+}-pump ATPase (1 mole ethanol/10 moles lipid) were found to be "loosely" associated with the sarcoplasmic reticulum membrane at saturating ethanol concentrations. (A "saturated condition" is defined as that which results when a reservoir of ethanol is maintained throughout the experiment following ethanol equilibration with the multilayer in the vapor phase.)

Neutron diffraction experiments showed that the ethanol-profile structure for the sarcoplasmic reticulum membrane under saturating conditions was similar to the water-profile structure, thus indicating that ethanol is distributed primarily throughout the membrane water region and excluded from the hydrocarbon core of the sarcoplasmic reticulum membrane. After removal of the ethanol reservoir, which allows ethanol to diffuse out of the membrane water layer, approximately 1 mole ethanol per mole Ca^{2+}-pump ATPase (1 mole ethanol/110 moles lipid) remained "tightly" associated with the sarcoplasmic reticulum membrane for more than 30 hr. Neutron diffraction data are currently being collected in an attempt to locate this "tightly" bound ethanol component.

DISCUSSION

Model for Nonspecific Drug–Membrane Interaction

Rabbit fast skeletal muscle sarcoplasmic reticulum is particularly suitable for studying nonspecific effects of β-adrenergic receptor blocking drugs for several reasons: (1) These membranes do not contain *specific* β-adrenergic receptors; (2) calcium transport by these membranes can be used to study the functional consequences of nonspecific interactions with the membrane; (3) detailed structural analysis of the sarcoplasmic reticulum membrane allows sites of drug action to be determined; and (4) the simple composition of the purified sarcoplasmic reticulum membrane, which contains a single essential protein, the Ca^{2+}/Mg^{2+}-sensitive ATPase, embedded in a lipid bilayer allows only a minimal number of potential drug interaction sites.

The relative partitioning of propranolol, timolol, and ethanol into model membrane systems is schematically depicted in Figure 5, and their ability to inhibit calcium transport in the sarcoplasmic reticulum membrane is quantitatively given in Table 1. Although the absolute values of the partition coefficients as determined by differential scanning calorimetry are subject to error, as evidenced by recent studies that discredit simple Hill analysis of the data [7,17], the relative ratio of these values is probably correct. The relative ratios of the partition coefficients of these amphiphilic molecules in the sarcoplasmic reticulum correlate well with the relative ratios of the I_{50} values for inhibition of calcium transport in sarcoplasmic reticulum. These data suggest that propranolol, timolol, and ethanol share a common site of interaction with the sarcoplasmic reticulum membrane and that their potency to inhibit calcium transport may be related to their ability to incorporate into the sarcoplasmic reticulum membrane bilayer. Thus, higher exogenous concentrations of an amphiphile with a lower partition coefficient are needed in order to attain higher concentrations of the amphiphile in the sarcoplasmic reticulum membrane bilayer resulting in calcium-transport inhibition.

The interpretations derived from a comparison of the partition coefficients and the I_{50} values could be confirmed in the case of propranolol and

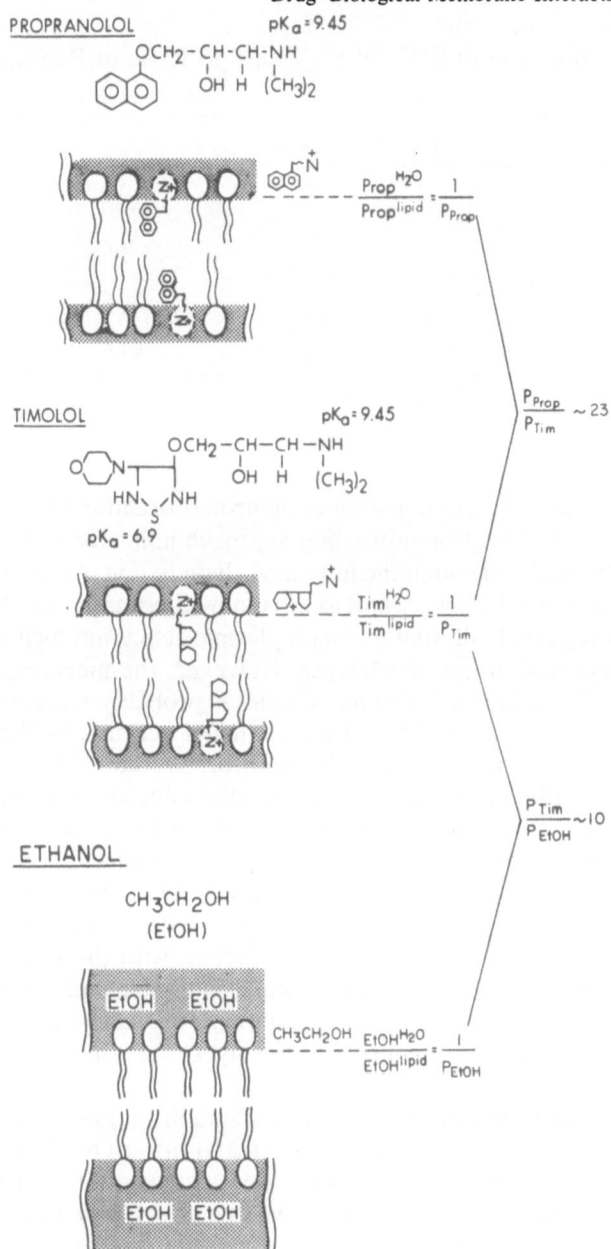

Figure 5.   Schematic representation of the location of propranolol, timolol, and ethanol in the model membrane system depicted as a partitioning between the lipid and aqueous phases of this system. The naphthalene ring of propranolol anchors the charged amine side chain as shown. The partially charged morphine ring of timolol in contrast to the aromatic naphthalene ring of propranolol may explain the dramatic partitioning (aqueous–hydrocarbon core) difference for these two β-receptor blocking drugs, which is approximately a factor of 23. Timolol, however, would appear to have another site of interaction in addition to the less complex partitioning of propranolol. Ethanol is seen to associate primarily with the aqueous layers hydrating the lipid bilayer structure.

Table 1.   Comparison of Ratio of I_{50} Values to Ratio of Partition Coefficients

Amphiphile	Estimated partition coefficient		I_{50} (mM)	
		Ratio[a]		Inverse ratio[a]
Propranolol	90		0.79	
		23		14
Timolol	4		11	
		8		7
Ethanol	<1[b]		80.5	

[a] I_{50} values are inversely related to partition coefficient values.
[b] Values of 0.4–0.6 were obtained from the literature [20–22].

ethanol by the use of a combination of neutron diffraction and radioisotope measurements. The neutron diffraction approach indicated that propranolol was primarily localized within the fatty acyl chain region of the sarcoplasmic reticulum membrane bilayer, whereas ethanol was primarily localized within the aqueous regions hydrating the sarcoplasmic reticulum membrane, with minimal incorporation into the bilayer. However, the mechanism of interaction of these amphiphiles with membranes is probably more complicated. For example, we have found that 1 mole ethanol per mole ATPase remains tightly bound when membrane multilayers pretreated with ethanol vapor were subsequently equilibrated with an ethanol-free environment. This "tightly bound" component may increase the ATPase turnover rate (A. Scarpa, personal communication). Thus, ethanol may have different sites of interaction with the sarcoplasmic reticulum membrane that can account for its complex dose–response curve on sarcoplasmic reticulum function. In addition to ethanol's multiple sites of interaction with the sarcoplasmic reticulum membrane, timolol both incorporates into the membrane bilayer and appears to have another site of interaction with the sarcoplasmic reticulum membrane different from the membrane bilayer that is not involved in calcium transport inhibition [7].

The data discussed in the previous paragraphs suggest that the *net* inhibitory effect of these amphiphiles on calcium transport by the sarcoplasmic reticulum membrane may be caused by direct effects on the permeability of the membrane bilayer and/or by perturbations to the bulk lipid matrix that may indirectly alter the molecular function of the intramembraneous calcium pump ATPase. This latter effect may be stimulation, an additional and variable inhibition, or no change in the ATPase or calcium pump turnover rate. These effects could also be mediated by a direct drug–protein interaction. In a study of fatty acid effects, for example, we have found complex phenomena that depend on the ratio of amphiphile and membrane concentrations such that not only a *net* inhibition but also a stimulation of calcium transport by sarcoplasmic reticulum could be observed [23]. In conclusion, this model for nonspecific drug–membrane interaction may have relevance to specific drug–membrane action [24].

ACKNOWLEDGMENTS

Calorimetric results were taken from Herbette et al. [7] and carried out by Dr. J. M. Sturtevant at Yale University. Mr. K. Segalman carried out the sarcoplasmic reticulum calcium uptake velocity experiments in the presence of drugs using the spectrophotometric approach. This work was supported by NIH Grants HL-27630, HL-18708, HL-21812, HL-22135, HL-26903, and HL-00911, and by a grant from the American Heart Association. Dr. Napolitano is a postdoctoral fellow supported by NIH Training Grant HL-07420. Dr. Messineo is a clinical investigator of the NIH.

REFERENCES

1. Seeman, P. 1972. The membrane actions of anesthetics and tranquilizers. *Pharmacol. Rev.* 24:583–655.
2. Katz, A. M., and Messineo, F. C. 1981. Lipid–membrane interactions and the pathogenesis of ischemic damage in the myocardium. *Circ. Res.* 48:1–16.
3. Herbette, L., Messineo, F. C., and Katz, A. M. 1981. The interaction of drugs with the sarcoplasmic reticulum. *Annu. Rev. Pharmacol. Toxicol.* 22:413–434.
4. Moules, I. K., Rooney, E. K., and Lee, A. G. 1982. Binding of amphipathic drugs and probes to biological membranes. *FEBS Lett.* 138:95–100.
5. Conrad, M. J., and Singer, S. J. 1981. The solubility of amphipathic molecules in biological membranes and lipid bilayers and its implications for membrane structure. *Biochemistry* 20:807–818.
6. Katz, A. M., Repke, D. I., and Hassalback, W. 1977. Dependence of ionophore and caffeine-induced calcium release from sarcoplasmic reticulum vesicles on external and internal calcium ion concentrations. *J. Biol. Chem.* 252:1938–1949.
7. Herbette, L., Katz, A. M., and Sturtevant, J. M. 1983. Comparisons of the interaction of propranolol and timolol with model and biological membrane systems. *Mol. Pharmacol.* 24:259–269.
8. Scarpa, A. 1979. Measurement of calcium ion concentrations with metallochromic indicators. In: *Detection and Measurement of Free Calcium in Cells.* C. Ashley and A. Campbell (eds.), pp. 85–115, Elsevier, Amsterdam.
9. Herbette, L., Marquardt, J., Scarpa, A., and Blasie, J. K. 1977. A direct analysis of lamellar x-ray diffraction from hydrated oriented multilayers of fully functional sarcoplasmic reticulum. *Biophys. J.* 20:245–272.
10. Messineo, F. C., and Katz, A. M. 1979. Effects of propranolol and timolol on calcium uptake by sarcoplasmic reticulum vesicles. *J. Cardiovasc. Pharmacol.* 1:449–459.
11. Privalov, P. L., Plotniko, V. V., and Filimono, V. V. 1975. Precision scanning microcalorimeter for study of liquids. *J. Chem. Thermodynam.* 7:41–47.
12. Herbette, L., Wang, C. T., Saito, A., Fleischer, S., Scarpa, A., and Blasie, J. K. 1981. A comparison of the profile structures of isolated and reconstituted sarcoplasmic reticulum membranes. *Biophys. J.* 36:47–72.
13. Schoenborn, B. P., and Nunes, A. C. 1972. Neutron scattering. *Annu. Rev. Biophys. Bioeng.* 1:529–552.
14. Herbette, L., Scarpa, A., Blasie, J. K., Wang, C. T., Hymel, L., Seelig, J., and Fleischer, S. 1983. The determination of the separate Ca^{2+} pump protein and phospholipid profile structures within reconstituted sarcoplasmic reticulum membranes via x-ray and neutron diffraction. *Biochim. Biophys. Acta* 730:369–378.

15. Lowry, O. H., Rosenbrough, N. J., Farr, A. L., and Randall, R. J. 1951. Protein measurement with Folin reagent. *J. Biol. Chem.* 193:265–275.
16. Chen, P. S., Toribara, T. B., and Warner, H. 1956. Microdetermination of phosphorus. *Anal. Chem.* 28:1756–1758.
17. Hill, M. W. 1974 The effect of anesthetic-like molecules on the phase transition in smectic mesophases of dipalmitoyllecithin. I. The normal alcohol up to C = 9 and three inhalation anesthetics. *Biochim. Biophys. Acta* 356:117–124.
18. Buldt, G., Gally, H. U., Seelig, J., and Zaccai, G. 1979. Neutron diffraction studies on phosphatidylcholine model membranes. I. Head group conformation. *J. Mol. Biol.* 134:673–691.
19. Davis, D. G., Inesi, G., and Gulik-Krzywicki, T. 1976. Lipid molecular motion and enzyme activity in sarcoplasmic reticulum membrane. *Biochemistry* 15:1271–1276.
20. Vanderkooi, J. M., Landesberg, R., Selick, H., and McDonald, G. G. 1977. Interaction of general anesthetics with phospholipid vesicles and biological membranes. *Biochim. Biophys. Acta* 464:1–16.
21. Pringle, M. J., Brown, K. B., and Miller, K. W. 1981. Can the lipid theories of anesthesia account for the cutoff in anesthetic potency in homologous series of alcohols? *Mol. Pharmacol.* 19:49–55.
22. Katz, Y., and Diamond, J. M. 1974. Thermodynamic constants for nonelectrolyte partition between dimyristoyl lecithin and water. *J. Membrane Biol.* 17:101–120.
23. Katz, A. M., Nash-Adler, P., Watras, J., Messineo, F. C., Takenaka, H., and Louis, C. F. 1982. Fatty acid effects on calcium influx and efflux in sarcoplasmic reticulum vesicles from rabbit skeletal muscle. *Biochim. Biophys. Acta* 687:17–26.
24. Herbette, L. G., Sarmiento, J. G., and Rhodes, D. G. 1984. Mechanism for cardiovascular drug binding to membrane associated receptors: Approach to the binding site through the lipid bilayer. *Biophys. J.* 45:312a.

Phospholipid Alterations and Membrane Injury during Myocardial Ischemia

Kenneth R. Chien and James T. Willerson

Department of Internal Medicine (Cardiology Division)
University of Texas Health Science Center
Dallas, Texas 75238

L. Maximilian Buja

Department of Pathology
University of Texas Health Science Center
Dallas, Texas 75238

Abstract. Several independent studies have demonstrated that there is a degradation of membrane phospholipids during myocardial ischemia. At present, most of the data support the initial activation of a phospholipase A pathway of phospholipid degradation. The extent of total phospholipid degradation is in the nanomole per gram wet weight quantity, as opposed to ischemic liver, in which the extent of phospholipid depletion approaches the micromole per gram wet weight level. However, in vitro studies suggest that calcium permeability properties and other myocardial cell membrane functions are sensitive to nanomole levels of phospholipid degradation. Clearly, further work is necessary in intact cell and heart preparations to correlate the degradation of phospholipid with the development of irreversible membrane injury during ATP depletion and hypoxia.

INTRODUCTION

The biochemical mechanisms responsible for membrane injury during myocardial ischemia are currently unknown. However, several recent studies have suggested that alterations in myocardial phospholipid metabolism may contribute to membrane damage during ischemia. In an ischemic-liver model, the degradation of membrane phospholipids was related temporally to the development of membrane calcium permeability defect, a severalfold increase in tissue calcium content, and the development of irreversible damage in ischemically injured cells [1–3]. Pharmacological inhibition of the phospholipid degradation resulted in protection against the alterations in calcium homeostasis and the development of irreversible cell injury [4].

Recently, these initial studies have been confirmed by other investigators [5,6]. There are now several reports of phospholipid degradation during ischemia of the kidney [7,8], brain [9], and myocardium [10–15]. The purpose of this chapter is to review our current understanding of the metabolism of phospholipids during myocardial ischemia and to explore the possible relationship of these alterations to the development of membrane dysfunction during ischemia.

PHOSPHOLIPID METABOLISM DURING MYOCARDIAL ISCHEMIA

Myocardial cells contain at least two distinct phospholipases [16,17]. The phospholipase C cleaves the water-soluble headgroup from phosphatidylcholine, yielding phosphorylcholine and diacylglycerol. The diaclyglycerol lipase can subsequently release free arachidonate and other fatty acids from the Sn-1 and Sn-2 positions of the phospholipid molecule [18]. Since the phospholipase C pathway has not been extensively characterized in myocardial cells, the contribution of this enzyme to phospholipid depletion during myocardial ischemia is currently unknown.

Myocardial cells also contain phospholipase A_2 activities that remove a fatty acyl group from the Sn-2 position, resulting in the formation of lysophosphatidylcholine and free fatty acids. The newly generated lysophosphatidylcholine can then enter one of two major pathways. First, it can be further degraded by a lysophospholipase, resulting in glycerophosphorylcholine and in other free fatty acids [19]. The action of the lysophospholipase would result in the loss of the phosphatidylcholine molecule. Alternatively, the lysophosphatidylcholine can be reacylated by the lysophosphatidylcholine acyl transferase to regenerate the intact phosphatidylcholine molecule [19]. It is obvious that the net loss of phosphatidylcholine from the membrane will be dependent on the relative rates of deacylation and reacylation. In addition, this deacylation–reacylation cycle strictly controls the fatty acyl composition of membrane phospholipids.

Recent evidence from several laboratories now suggests that the phospholipase A pathway is responsible for most of the degradation of membrane phospholipid during myocardial ischemia. In initial reports, lysophosphatidylcholine was found to accumulate in ischemic rabbit myocardium to levels approaching 13% of the total phospholipid content [20]. However, it was subsequently demonstrated that the markedly elevated lysophosphatidylcholine content in this study was secondary to lipid extraction with acidified solvents. Myocardial phospholipids contain large amounts of ether-linked lipids (plasmologens) that can be artifactually converted to lysolipids [14,21]. However, in recent studies utilizing neutral solvents, there is evidence of a transient increase in lysophosphatidylcholine in some models of myocardial ischemia, but it does not exceed 1% of the total phospholipid content [11,14]. It should be noted that these increases may not be proportional to the extent of total phospholipid degradation, since lysophosphatidylcholine can be subsequently reacylated, further deacylated, or released into the venous effluent during ischemia. Shaikh and Downar [22] have provided evidence of a deacylation–reacylation cycle during myocardial ischemia involving the Sn-2 position of phosphatidylcholine. Additional support for the activation of a phospholipase A_2 during myocardial ischemia is provided by the demonstration of the accumulation of unesterified arachidonate in ischemic canine myocardium [23]. Under normoxic conditions, arachidonic acid is found almost entirely esterified in membrane phospholipids. Since arachidonic acid is poorly oxidized by myocardial cells and cannot be converted to prostaglandins in isolated myocardial cells during ATP depletion [24], the accumulation of arachidonate may be an effective marker of phospholipid degradation. Several groups have now demonstrated that the time–course of accumulation of unesterified arachidonate correlates with the development of irreversible injury in ischemic canine myocardium [23,25]. It should be noted that the rate and extent of phospholipid degradation during myocardial ischemia appear to be markedly decreased compared to previous studies in ischemic liver [1]. After 1 hr of liver ischemia, there was a greater than 20% decrease in the phospholipid content of microsomal membranes. However, there is no detectable decrease in total phospholipid content after 1 hr of fixed coronary occlusion in ischemic canine myocardium [15]. This result may be secondary to the lower amount of phospholipase activity present in myocardium. Therefore, examining phospholipid degradation simply by measuring total phospholipid content will not provide the necessary sensitivity to measure phospholipid depletion and degradation during early myocardial ischemia.

PHOSPHOLIPID ALTERATIONS AND MEMBRANE FUNCTION

For several years, it was thought that the total membrane lipid content and composition were not directly involved in the regulation of membrane protein function. In the original Singer model of membrane structure, the lipid bilayer merely provided a matrix for the insertion of the membrane proteins. However, recent work by several investigators has demonstrated that changes in the "fluidity" of the membrane lipid bilayer can have a marked influence on membrane function. The fluidity of the membrane is determined not only by the total phospholipid/cholesterol ratio, but also by the degree of saturation of the fatty acyl chains. Accordingly, these parameters are strictly controlled in the cell membrane under normal conditions. Any acute change in the fatty acyl composition or total phospholipid/cholesterol ratio of the membrane during ischemia might have a marked effect on membrane fluidity and a secondary effect on membrane-bound enzymes and permeability properties of the membranes. In cultured liver cells, increasing the lateral mobility of β-adrenergic receptors by enrichment with exogenous phospholipid resulted in a marked decrease in receptor–adenylate cyclase coupling [26]. In a cultured-myocardial-cell model, Hasin et al. [27] have shown that the enrichment in linoleic acid of membrane lipids caused a rise in the flux of Cl^- and K^+ through their respective channels.

The loss of arachidonate and other unsaturated fatty acids, as well as a net loss of phospholipid during myocardial ischemia, would be expected to decrease membrane fluidity. Clearly, further work is necessary to correlate the alterations in phospholipid content and fatty acyl composition with changes in the membrane lipid fluidity and membrane protein function.

In addition to changes in the fatty acyl composition, several studies have now suggested that the net loss of nanomole or lesser amounts of phospholipid from myocardial membranes can have deleterious effects on membrane function. Exposure of sarcolemmal vesicles to an exogenous phospholipase C resulted in a markedly increased rate of passive calcium permeability [15]. Similarly, it has now been shown that phospholipase C treatment can produce a cation permeability defect in cultured myocardial cells [28], as well as a release of creatine phosphokinase activity into the medium [29]. Treatment of isolated Purkinje fibers with phospholipase C can produce marked derangements in the cellular action potentials [30]. These changes can be measured at levels of phospholipid degradation similar to those found during in vivo myocardial ischemia. Since the phospholipase C activity does not generate lysophospholipids, this effect cannot be ascribed to the accumulation of lysolipids, but rather must be due to the net loss of phospholipid from the membrane. Thus, the myocardial-cell membrane appears to be quite sensitive to small levels of phospholipid depletion.

The accumulation of the hydrolysis products of phospholipase A degradation represents an alternative mechanism of membrane injury during ischemia. Lysophospholipids are potent amphiphilic detergents and have been demonstrated to have deleterious effects on the in vitro electrophysiological properties of myocardial cells. In addition, exogenous administration of lysophosphatidylcholine can result in a marked increase in the rate of intracellular calcium accumulation [31]. The basis of these effects of lysophosphatides most likely is due to the nonspecific disruption of the sarcolemmal membrane. It should be noted that the detergent effects of amphiphiles are dependent more on the amphiphile/membrane lipid ratio than on the absolute concentrations of the amphiphile and the myocardium [32]. Since lysophosphatidylcholine levels do not account for more than 1% of the total phospholipid content, the role of lysophosphatides in membrane injury during in vivo ischemia is not yet clear [32].

As a result of the phospholipase A activities, there is also an increase in the unesterified fatty acid content of ischemic myocardium [10,23]. The work of Messineo and Katz has demonstrated that incubation of sarcoplasmic reticulum vesicles with unsaturated fatty acids can result in an increased rate of passive calcium efflux [33]. The basis of this effect is unknown, but it may be the ability of the fatty acids to intercalate into the membrane lipid bilayer. The increase in unesterified arachidonate may have particular importance in the development of membrane injury during ischemia. As opposed to the other fatty acids released during ischemia, arachidonate can be converted to prostaglandins and other oxygenated metabolites that may have direct biological effects on the intact heart and vasculature. The release of arachidonate from membrane phospholipids is considered to be the rate-limiting step of prostaglandin synthesis. The metabolic fate of the unesterified arachidonate in ischemic myocardium is unknown and clearly is an area for future research. In an ischemic canine model, the time–course of the accumulation of unesterified arachidonate closely correlated with the development of irreversible myocardial cell injury [23].

SUMMARY

In conclusion, several independent studies have demonstrated that there is a degradation of membrane phospholipids during myocardial ischemia. At present, most of the data support the initial activation of a phospholipase A pathway of phospholipid degradation. The extent of total phospholipid degradation is in the nanomole per gram wet weight quantity, as opposed to ischemic liver, in which the extent of phospholipid depletion approaches the micromole per gram wet weight level. However, in vitro studies suggest that the calcium permeability properties and other myocardial-cell-membrane functions are sensitive to nanomole levels of phospholipid degradation. Clearly, further work is necessary in intact cell and heart preparations to correlate the degradation of phospholipid with the development of irreversible membrane injury during ATP depletion and hypoxia.

ACKNOWLEDGMENTS

This work was supported by NIH Ischemic SCOR Grant HL 17669 and the Harry S. Moss Heart Fund.

REFERENCES

1. Chien, K. R., Abrams, J., Serroni, A., Martin, J. T., and Farber, J. L. 1978. Accelerated phospholipid degradation and associated membrane dysfunction in irreversible ischemic liver cell injury. *J. Biol. Chem.* 253:4809–4817.
2. Chien, K. R., Abrams, J., Pfau, R. G., and Farber, J. L. 1977. Prevention by chlorpromazine of ischemic liver cell death. *Am. J. Pathol.* 88:539–558.
3. Chien, K. R., Sherman, C., Mittnacht, S., and Farber, J. L. 1980. Microsomal membrane structure and function consequent to calcium activation of an endogenous phospholipase. *Arch. Biochem. Biophys.* 205:614–622.
4. Farber, J. L., Chien, K. R., and Mittnacht, S. 1982. The pathogenesis of irreversible cell injury in ischemia. *Am. J. Pathol.* 102:271–278.
5. Wattiaux, R., and Wattiaux-DeConinck, S. 1980. Reversible and irreversible alterations of lysosomes in ischemic rat liver: Effects of chlorpromazine. *Biochem. Pharmacol.* 29:963–966.

6. Matsumoto, J., Tanaka, T., Gamo, M., Saito, K., and Honjo, I. 1981. Phospholipid metabolism of dog liver under hypoxic conditions induced by ligation of the hepatic artery. *Biochim. Biophys. Acta* 664:527–537.

7. Patel, Y. Stewart, J., Matthys, E., and Venkatacham, M. A. 1982. Renal cortical free fatty acid and 1,2 diglyceride in renal ischemic injury. *Clin. Res.* 30:541A.

8. Smith, M. W., Collan, Y., Kaling, M., and Trump, B. F. 1980. Changes in mitochondrial lipids of rat kidney during ischemia. *Biochim. Biophys. Acta.* 618:192–201.

9. Bazan, N. G. 1970. Effects of ischemia and electroconvulsive shock on free fatty acid pool in the brain. *Biochim. Biophys. Acta* 218:1–14.

10. Van der Vusse, G. I., Roeman, T. H. M., Prinzen, F. W., Coumans, W. A., and Reneman, R. S. 1982. Uptake and tissue content of fatty acids in dog myocardium under normoxic and ischemic conditions. *Circ. Res.* 50:538–546.

11. Corr, P. D., Snyder, D. W., Lee, B. I., Gross, R. W., Keim, C. R., and Sobel, B. E. 1982. Pathophysiological concentrations of lysophosphatides and the slow response. *Am. J. Physiol.* 243:H187–H195.

12. Hsueh, W., Isaksan, P. C., and Needleman, P. 1977. Hormone selective lipase activation in the isolated rabbit heart. *Prostaglandins* 13:1073–1090.

13. Vasdev, S. C., Kako, K. J., and Biro, G. P. 1979. Phospholipid composition of cardiac mitochondria and lysosomes in experimental myocardial ischemia in the dog. *J. Mol. Cell. Cardiol.* 11:1195–1200.

14. Shaikh, N. A., and Downar, E. 1981. Time course of changes in porcine myocardial phospholipid levels during ischemia: A reassessment of the lysolipid hypothesis. *Circ. Res.* 49:316–325.

15. Chien, K. R., Reeves, J. P., Buja, L. M., Bonte, F., Parkey, R. W., and Willerson, J. T. 1981. Phospholipid alterations in canine ischemic myocardium: Temporal and topographical correlations with Tc-99m-PPi accumulation and an in vitro sarcolemmal Ca^{+2} permeability defect. *Circ. Res.* 48:711–719.

16. Hostetler, K. Y., and Hall, L. B. 1980. Phospholipase C activity of rat tissues. *Biochem. Biophys. Res. Commun.* 96:388–393.

17. Weglicki, W. B. 1980. Degradation of phospholipids of myocardial membranes. In: Wildenthal, K. (ed.), *Degradative Processes in Heart and Skeletal Muscle.* pp. 377–388. Elsevier/North-Holland, Amsterdam.

18. Prescott, S. M., and Majerus, P. W. 1981. The fatty acid composition of phosphatidylinositol from thrombin-stimulated human platelets. *J. Biol. Chem.* 256:579–582.

19. Gross, R. E., and Sobel, B. E. 1982. Lysophosphatidylcholine metabolism in the rabbit heart. *J. Biol. Chem.* 257:6702–6708.

20. Sobel, B. E., Corr, P. B., Robison, A. K., Goldstein, R. A., Witkowski, F. X., and Klein, M. S. 1978. Accumulation of lysophosphoglycerides with arrhythmogenic properties in ischemic myocardium. *J. Clin. Invest.* 62:546–553.

21. Mogelson, S., Wilson, G. E., and Sobel, B. E. 1980. Characterization of rabbit myocardial phospholipids with ^{31}P nuclear magnetic resonance. *Biochim. Biophys. Acta* 619:688.

22. Shaikh, N. A., and Downar, E. 1983. Ischemic induced phospholipase(s) activation in isolated perfused cat hearts. *J. Mol. Cell. Cardiol.* 15:171.

23. Chien, H. R., Han, A., Bush, L. R., Buja, L. M., and Willerson, J. T. 1984. Accumulation of unesterified arachidonate in ischemic canine myocardium: Relationship to a phosphatioylcholine deacylation–reacylation cycle and the depletion of membrane phospholipids. *Circ. Res.* 54:313–322.

24. Gunn, M. D., Sen, H., Kim, Y. M., Revtyak, G., Buja, L. M., Campbell, W. B., and Chien, K. R. Arachidonate metabolism of cultured myocardial cells during ATP depletion: Deacylation of arachidonate without conversion to prostaglandins. Submitted.

25. Prinzen, F. W., van der Vusse, G. J., Coumans, W. A., Roemen, T. H. M., and Reneman, R. S. 1983. Accumulation of non-esterified fatty acids in ischemic myocardium in relation to residual blood flow and ATP content. *J. Mol. Cell. Cardiol.* 15:370.

26. Bakardjieva, A., Galla, H. J., and Helmreich, E. J. M. 1979. Modulation of the β-receptor adenylate cyclase interactions in cultured Chang liver cells by phospholipid enrichment. *Biochem.* 18:3016–3023.
27. Hasin, Y., Sapoznikov, D., Stein, O., and Stein, Y. 1982. Effect of fatty acid composition of rat heart myocytes on their electrical activity. *J. Mol. Cell. Cardiol.* 14:163–171.
28. Langer, G. A., Frank, J. S., and Philipson, K. D. 1981. Correlation of alterations in cation exchange and sarcolemmal ultrastructure produced by neuraminidase and phospholipases in cardiac cell tissue culture. *Circ Res.* 49:1289–1299.
29. Higgins, T. J. C., Bailey, P. J., and Allsopp, D. 1982. Interrelationship between cellular metabolic status and susceptibility of heart cells to attack by phospholipase. *J. Mol. Cell. Cardiol.* 14:645–654.
30. Shaikh, N. A., and Downar, E. 1983. Effects of exogenous and endogenous lysophospholipids on the excitability of cardiac muscle and Purkinje fibres of sheep heart. *J. Mol. Cell. Cardiol* . 15:170.
31. Sedlis, S. P., Corr, P. B., Sobel, B. E., and Ahumada, G. G. 1983. Lysophosphatidylcholine potentiates Ca^{++} accumulation in rat cardiac myocytes. *Am. J. Physiol.* 13:H32–H38.
32. Katz, A. M. 1982. Membrane derived lipids and the pathogenesis of ischemic myocardial damage. *J. Mol. Cell. Cardiol.* 14:627–632.
33. Ashavaid, T. F., Colvin, R. A., MacAlister, T., Messineo, F. C., and Katz, A. M. 1983. Fatty acid effects on Na/Ca exchange in sarcolemmal vesicles. *J. Mol. Cell. Cardiol.* 15:362.

Contributors

DAVID G. ALLEN, Department of Physiology, University College London, London WC1E 6BT, England

L. MAXIMILIAN BUJA, Department of Pathology, University of Texas Health Science Center, Dallas, Texas 75238

CLAUDIO M. CALDARERA, Istituto di Chimica Biologica, Centro Studi e Ricerche del Metabolismo del Miocardio, Università di Bologna, 40216 Bologna, Italy

JOSEPH M. CAPASSO, Cardiovascular Center, Department of Medicine, Albert Einstein College of Medicine, Bronx, New York 10461

MARTIN CAPLAN, Department of Medicine (Cardiology), Medical College of Virgina, Richmond, Virgina 23298

ERNESTO CARAFOLI, Laboratory of Biochemistry, Swiss Federal Institute of Technology (ETH), 8092 Zurich, Switzerland

JAMES B. CAULFIELD, Department of Pathology, School of Medicine, University of South Carolina, Columbia, South Carolina 29208

MICHAIL A. CHERNOUSOV, USSR Cardiology Research Center, Academy of Medical Sciences, Moscow 121552, USSR

KENNETH R. CHIEN, Department of Internal Medicine (Cardiology Division), University of Texas Health Science Center, Dallas, Texas 75238

LEONA COHEN-GOULD, Cardiovascular Center, Department of Medicine, Albert Einstein College of Medicine, Bronx, New York 10461

J. S. CRIE, Pauline and Adolph Weinberger Laboratory for Cardiopulmonary Research, Departments of Physiology and Internal Medicine, The University of Texas Health Science Center at Dallas, Dallas, Texas 75235

D. A. EISNER, Department of Physiology, University College London, London WC1E 6BT, England

D. ELLIS, Department of Physiology, University Medical School, Edinburgh EH8 9AG, Scotland

CAROLE D. EVANS, Department of Nuclear Medicine, Veterans Administration Medical Center, and Department of Medicine, New York University School of Medicine, New York, New York 10016

M. E. EVSEVIEVA, Institute of General Pathology and Pathological Physiology of the USSR AMS, Laboratory of Heart Pathophysiology, Moscow 121552, USSR

STEPHEN M. FACTOR, Department of Pathology, Albert Einstein College of Medicine, Bronx, New York 10461

D. R. FERRY, Rudolf Buchheim-Institut für Pharmakologie, Justus Liebig Universität, Giessen, D-63 Giessen, Federal Republic of Germany

DAVID C. GADSBY, Laboratory of Cardiac Physiology, The Rockefeller University, New York, New York 10021

PAMELA B. GARLICK, Department of Pharmacology, Columbia University College of Physicians and Surgeons, New York, New York 10032; present address: Heart Research Unit, The Rayne Institute, St. Thomas' Hospital, London S. E. 1

H. GLOSSMANN, Rudolf Buchheim-Institut für Pharmakologie, Justus Liebig Universität, Giessen, D-63 Giessen, Federal Republic of Germany

GENNADY N. GNEUSHEV, USSR Cardiology Research Center, Academy of Medical Sciences, Moscow 121552, USSR

A. GOLL, Rudolf Buchheim-Institut für Pharmakologie, Justus Liebig Universität, Giessen, D-63 Giessen, Federal Republic of Germany

ELLEN E. GORDON, Department of Physiology, The Milton S. Hershey Medical Center, The Pennsylvania State University, Hershey, Pennsylvania 17033

CARLO GUARNIERI, Istituto di Chimica Biologica, Centro Studi e Ricerche del Metabolismo del Miocardio, Università di Bologna, 40216 Bologna, Italy

PETER HARRIS, Cardiothoracic Institute, London W1N 2DX, England

L. HERBETTE, Departments of Medicine and Biochemistry, University of Connecticut Health Center, Farmington, Connecticut 06032

MICHAEL L. HESS, Department of Medicine (Cardiology), Medical College of Virginia, Richmond, Virginia 23298

FRANZ HOFMANN, Pharmakologisches Institut der Universität Heidelberg, D-6900 Heidelberg, Federal Republic of Germany

A. M. KATZ, Department of Medicine, University of Connecticut Health Center, Farmington, Connecticut 06032

YUJI KIRA, Department of Physiology, The Milton S. Hershey Medical Center, The Pennsylvania State University, Hershey, Pennsylvania 17033

VICTOR E. KOTELIANSKY, USSR Cardiology Research Center, Academy of Medical Sciences, Moscow 121552, USSR

W. J. LEDERER, Department of Physiology, University of Maryland Medical School, Baltimore, Maryland 21201

T. LINN, Rudolf Buchheim-Institut für Pharmakologie, Justus Liebig Universität, Giessen, D-63 Giessen, Federal Republic of Germany

BENEDICT LUCCHESI, Department of Pharmacology, University of Michigan School of Medicine, Ann Arbor, Michigan 48109

NANCY H. MANSON, Department of Medicine (Cardiology), Medical College of Virginia, Richmond, Virgina 23298

JOE M. McCORD, Department of Biochemistry, College of Medicine, University of South Alabama, Mobile, Alabama 36688

F. Z. MEERSON, Institute of General Pathology and Pathological Physiology of the USSR AMS, Laboratory of Heart Pathophysiology, Moscow 121552, USSR

F. C. MESSINEO, Department of Medicine, University of Connecticut Health Center, Farmington, Connecticut 06032

HOWARD E. MORGAN, Department of Physiology, The Milton S. Hershey Medical Center, The Pennsylvania State University, Hershey, Pennsylvania 17033

PETER GORDON MORRIS, MRC Biomedical NMR Centre, National Institute for Medical Research, London NW7 1AA, England

CLAUDIO MUSCARI, Istituto di Chimica Biologica, Centro Studi e Ricerche del Metabolismo del Miocardio, Università di Bologna, 40216 Bologna, Italy

MAURICE NACHTIGAL, Department of Pathology, School of Medicine, University of South Carolina, Columbia, South Carolina 29208

C. A. NAPOLITANO, Department of Medicine, University of Connecticut Health Center, Farmington, Connecticut 06032

MURRAY ORATZ, Department of Nuclear Medicine, Veterans Administration Medical Center, and Department of Medicine, New York University School of Medicine, New York, New York 10016

CLIVE H. ORCHARD, Department of Physiology, University College London, London WC1E 6BT, England

J. M. ORD, Pauline and Adolph Weinberger Laboratory for Cardiopulmonary Research, Departments of Physiology and Internal Medicine, The University of Texas Health Science Center at Dallas, Dallas, Texas 75235

TREVOR POWELL, University Laboratory of Physiology, Oxford OX1 3PT, England

RENEE M. REMILY, Cardiovascular Center, Department of Medicine, Albert Einstein College of Medicine, Bronx, New York 10461

THOMAS F. ROBINSON, Cardiovascular Center, Department of Medicine, and Department of Physiology and Biophysics, Albert Einstein College of Medicine, Bronx, New York 10461

JOSEPH L. ROMSON, Department of Pharmacology, University of Michigan School of Medicine, Ann Arbor, Michigan 48109

MARCUS A. ROTHSCHILD, Department of Nuclear Medicine, Veterans Administration Medical Center, and Department of Medicine, New York University School of Medicine, New York, New York 10016

G. THOMAS ROWE, Department of Medicine (Cardiology), Medical College of Virginia, Richmond, Virginia 23298

RANJAN S. ROY, Department of Biochemistry, College of Medicine, University of South Alabama, Mobile, Alabama 36688

STEPHEN W. SCHAFFER, Department of Pharmacology, College of Medicine, University of South Alabama, Mobile, Alabama 36688

SIDNEY S. SCHREIBER, Department of Nuclear Medicine, Veterans Administration Medical Center, and Department of Medicine, New York University School of Medicine, New York, New York 10016

N. J. SEVERS, Department of Cardiac Medicine, Cardiothoracic Institute (University of London), London W1N 2DX, England

VLADIMIR P. SHIRINSKY, USSR Cardiology Research Center, Academy of Medical Sciences, Moscow 121552, USSR

PETER H. SUGDEN, Department of Cardiac Medicine, Cardiothoracic Institute, London W1N 2DX, England

SUN BEN TAO, Department of Pathology, School of Medicine, University of South Carolina, Columbia, South Carolina 29208

CHRISTOPHER J. TURNER, Department of Chemistry, Columbia University, New York, New York 10027

R. D. VAUGHAN-JONES, University Laboratory of Physiology, Oxford OX1 3PT, England

J. R. WAKELAND, Pauline and Adolph Weinberger Laboratory for Cardiopulmonary Research, Departments of Physiology and Internal Medicine, The University of Texas Health Science Center at Dallas, Dallas, Texas 75235

K. WILDENTHAL, Pauline and Adolph Weinberger Laboratory for Cardiopulmonary Research, Departments of Physiology and Internal Medicine, The University of Texas Health Science Center at Dallas, Dallas, Texas 75235

JAMES T. WILLERSON, Department of Internal Medicine (Cardiology Division), University of Texas Health Science Center, Dallas, Texas 75238

A. J. WILLIAMS, Department of Cardiac Medicine, Cardiothoracic Institute, University of London, London W1N 2DX, England

MANFRED ZIMMER, Pharmakologisches Institut der Universität Heidelberg, D-6900 Heidelberg, Federal Republic of Germany

Index